WOMEN
AND
PAIN

WOMEN
AND
PAIN

Why It Hurts and What You Can Do

Including Complementary and Holistic Remedies,
as Well as Traditional Medicine

MARK ALLEN YOUNG, M.D., F.A.C.P.
with KAREN BAAR, M.P.H.

HYPERION

New York

All names and identifying characteristics of patients have been changed.

The ideas, suggestions and procedures in this book do not replace the medical advice of a trained medical professional. You should consult with your physician before adopting the suggestions and procedures in this book, especially if you have any preexisting medical or psychological conditions, or if you are currently taking medicine. Any changes in your dosage should be made only in cooperation with your prescribing physician.

Before using any remedies mentioned in this book, be sure to consult with the appropriate medical authorities and check the product's label for any warnings or cautions. Keep in mind that herbal remedies are not as strictly regulated as drugs. Pregnant women are advised that special precautions may pertain regarding the use of any healing agent. If you are pregnant, talk to your doctor before taking any medicine, herbal remedy or nutritional supplement.

The names of patients mentioned in the case reports and studies in this book have been changed to protect confidentiality. Where relevant, signed consent was obtained from persons whose case reports are cited in this book.

Any application of the recommendations set forth in the following pages is at the reader's discretion and sole risk. Trade names of specific products appear throughout this book only as examples. The inclusion of a particular trade name in no way represents an endorsement by the publisher, nor does the exclusion of a trade name represent a negative judgment of any kind.

Library of Congress Cataloging-in-Publication Data

Young, Mark A.
women and pain : why it hurts and what you can do including
complementary and holistic remedies, as well as traditional
medicine / Mark Young with Karen Baar.
p. cm.
Includes bibliographical references and index.
ISBN 0-7868-8679-X
1. Pain—Popular works. 2. Women—Diseases—Popular works.
I. Baar, Karen. II. Title.

RB127.Y68 2002
616'.0472'082—dc21
2001039248

FIRST TRADE PAPERBACK EDITION

10 9 8 7 6 5 4 3 2

Book design by JoAnne Metsch

ACKNOWLEDGMENTS

I wish to lovingly acknowledge the help and ever-present support of my wife, Marlene Malka Young, whose supreme culinary skills contributed greatly to this work. Her devotion and stalwart dedication to her physician-author husband and to our children, Michelle, Michael, and Jennifer, have helped to make this book a success.

Kindest gratitude is due my agent, Janis Vallely, who brought the idea for this book to life and helped me navigate the uncharted waters of book publishing; to Karen Baar whose literary skill and editorial expertise were invaluable to the process; and to my editor, Leslie Wells, who truly helped to make this book a reality.

Acknowledgments also are due to my many colleagues in academic medicine and to the many scientists and researchers around the world who have helped us fathom the mystery of pain, its effects on women, and its treatment using the best of traditional and complementary medicine.

Special thanks to Debra Walters, Nicole Royer, Jennifer Ryan, Stanley Kornhauser, Joseph Powers, Howard Hoffberg, Michael Lesser, and Evan Young for technical assistance.

—*Mark Young, M.D.*

Thanks to Mark Young, for his innovative approach to pain, to our editor, Leslie Wells, whose enthusiasm for this project was so exciting, and to Janis Vallely, who got this book off the ground and helped keep it afloat. I also appreciate Carrie Covert's flexibility in the face of an impossibly tight schedule.

Love and gratitude to the people who have sustained me during a very difficult time—Sally Connolly, Katherine Grady, Pamela Hort, Jean Larson,

David Paskin, Semeon Tsalbins, and Carol Ripple—I couldn't have done this without your love, encouragement, and support. And to my agent, Angela Miller, who is always a staunch ally and trusted friend and adviser.

Finally, to my treasures, Kate and Emma: I cherish you more each day.

—*Karen Baar*

CONTENTS

Tell Me Where It Hurts

Do you suffer from constant, agonizing pain? Have you been to doctor after doctor, only to receive nothing that helps or be told "it's all in your head," "it's stress," or "you're just getting old"? If so, you're not alone.

Women have said it—and men have denied it—for years. Now we know that it's true: Women feel more pain, seek help more aggressively, and make more active attempts to cope with pain than men.

Unfortunately, we also know that too frequently women aren't taken seriously. Although we think of medicine as a professional discipline, rooted in science and free of bias, this isn't always the case. Frankly, our health care system often disregards women in pain. At best, it's ignorance of gender differences. But some physicians stereotype women as complainers who are less self-controlled and more likely to overreport symptoms than men. They dismiss female patients with antidepressants, antianxiety drugs, and platitudes. This adds insult to injury. When you're in pain, it's the last thing you need.

Given how much we know about pain, it's scandalous that women suffer needlessly. As a physiatrist, a physician board certified in physical medicine and rehabilitation, I specialize in treating disabling painful conditions with gentle, simple conservative modalities. Using my skills in acupuncture and complementary medicine, I have helped thousands of people find relief from pain. My background as a member of the teaching faculty of Johns Hopkins University has instilled in me a strong commitment to patient education and empowerment. Since my specialty places so much emphasis on properly balancing the emotional and physical needs of patients, often people with painful chronic disabilities, I am keenly aware of the frustration, anger, and depression that many women patients face when they are in pain and don't know where to turn for help.

IRENE'S STORY

Irene is a sixty-four-year-old woman who works as a stadium vendor, selling pretzels at the local ballpark. She spends most of her workday on her feet.

She came in to see me complaining of a dull ache in her right heel, along with pain, swelling, and decreased movement in her knee. She'd had discomfort for a while, but the pain was becoming considerably more disabling. Although she had developed a mild limp, that wasn't the worst of it: "Doc, at the end of the day, my foot feels like it's about to fall off and my knee hurts like the dickens."

Irene was feeling desperate. She had been to a couple of other doctors and had gotten little relief. But something else was also eating away at her: "They keep telling me that it's just because I'm getting old, and they say I have to quit my job. But I love my work; it's so much fun to be out there, especially when the Orioles win! Besides, I need the money," she confided.

When I examined Irene, I discovered that she had a large heel spur and an osteoarthritic knee. I knew right away that we could come up with a plan that would relieve her pain and let her keep working.

Irene usually wore the same shoes day in and day out, a pair of worn-out espadrilles she picked up at Payless. I told her she needed to invest in comfortable, cushioned sneakers to wear at work. I also recommended that she buy a viscoelastic horseshoe-shaped heel cushion (which allows the spur to "float" without direct contact) and to think about getting fitted for custom-made orthotics. It was essential that she provide some padding for that heel. Also, what goes on in your foot affects the rest of your leg, so good footwear would also have a positive impact on her arthritic knee.

In addition, I suggested that she soak her feet in an herbal bath after work each day. She laughed when I suggested that her husband learn the arts of foot massage and acupressure, but she took the handouts and put them in her purse.

For her knee, I suggested glucosamine and chondroitin supplements, two nutritional remedies that effectively relieve osteoarthritis. I also showed her how to do quadriceps strengthening exercises to bolster the stability of her knee joint, and urged her to add some light aerobic exercise to her daily routine.

I ran into Irene the next time I went to a game. She was in the next section of the stadium, but when she spotted me, she flashed a big smile and gave me a thumbs-up. After the game, she caught up with me. "The pain is so much better, Doc, and my limp is gone." Then, she winked and said: "And those foot massages are great!"

GENDER MATTERS

Happily, times are changing. Gender has become a "hot button" issue on the national research agenda, so important that a conference on gender and pain was held at the National Institutes of Health (NIH) in 1998. Eye-opening biomedical research presented there concluded that:

- Women experience more pain than men.
- Women discuss pain more than men.
- Women cope better with pain than men.
- Society's attitudes toward men and women in pain may influence physicians' treatment.
- The open expression of pain sometimes helps people obtain better pain control, but being seen as "too emotional" may work against a woman and lead to inadequate care.
- Pain treatment that works for one sex may not work as well, or at all, for the other.

Some of the most galvanizing research concerns the medications we use to treat pain. This work calls into question the age-old pain management practice of "one size (or one drug) fits all." For example, a series of landmark studies has shown that morphine-like drugs, called kappa-opioids, produce significantly greater pain relief in women than in men. (These drugs work through receptors in the central nervous system. There are multiple types of opioid receptors—kappa, mu, delta, and sigma. The mu and kappa categories are the two major classes thought to be responsible for analgesia.) Kappa-opioids are not as commonly used as other narcotic pain medications. Drugs that work on the mu-receptors are the standard of care and are much more frequently prescribed. Yet they cause more nausea, itching, cardiac effects, constipation, and depression of the respiratory system. Treating women with kappa-opioids, then, may provide better pain relief with fewer side effects.

Other studies show that common pain relievers do less for women than for men. For example, in a recent study of experimentally induced pain, ibuprofen—the key ingredient in Advil, Motrin, and other over-the-counter analgesics known as NSAIDS (for nonsteroidal anti-inflammatory drugs) — was less effective at providing pain relief for women than men. Perhaps dosages for NSAIDS need to take gender into account.

In addition, many painful diseases and injuries disproportionately affect women. Even when men and women suffer from the same illness, the symptoms may be different:

- Osteoarthritis (OA), or degenerative joint disease, is far more common among women over the age of fifty-five, and women may suffer from a more severe form of this disease. In one recent study, women experienced 40 percent more pain, as well as worse pain. In addition, women are more likely to develop inflammatory types of OA that lead to knobby deformities of the DIP and PIP joints (the two sets of joints below the knuckles).
- Rheumatoid arthritis (RA) occurs two and a half times more often among women, and it may also affect them more severely. Women have reported more painful joints, more swollen joints, and worse function. And the majority of studies show that RA is slightly more disabling for women than it is for men.
- Migraine headaches are more severe, longer lasting, and more frequent in women than in men. In addition, women have more nausea, vomiting, numbness, and tingling with their headaches, while men are more likely to have a visual aura.
- Tension headaches occur two to three times more frequently among women, who also experience much higher levels of tenderness in all the muscles surrounding the skull.
- Women athletes experience knee injuries two to eight times more frequently than their male counterparts. This is particularly true for tears of the anterior cruciate ligament (ACL).
- Osteoporosis affects both sexes, but women develop it at a much younger age and in far greater numbers because of hormonal differences.

Gender differences play out on the operating table, too. In a study recently published in the *British Medical Journal*, women emerged from general anesthesia faster than men. However, they returned to their presurgery health status significantly more slowly and they experienced more postoperative complications.

WOMEN AREN'T JUST SMALL MEN

We don't know why these differences exist, but a wide range of scientific studies shows that the sexes differ on nearly every level. From the molecular to the psychological, from the basic genetic codes to the hormones, biology, physiology, and the overall functioning of the immune response systems — men and women are different.

We aren't doing enough to understand and close this gender gap. The prestigious Institute of Medicine (IOM) of the National Academy of Sciences recently issued a call for biomedical researchers to "study sex differences from womb to tomb." The IOM's report recommended that researchers take sex differences into account in clinical trials, including studies of new drugs.

Even when women participate in clinical trials — and more women do now than five years ago — there is little gender-specific information coming out of the studies. Scientists at drug companies and research institutions have largely ignored sex-based differences in their data analysis.

We also know precious little about how drugs behave during pregnancy or breast-feeding. Most women who participate in research are postmenopausal. Admittedly, there are serious ethical concerns about allowing women of childbearing age to enter studies. But there may be other, less worthy issues at stake: Perhaps pharmaceutical companies are worried about the marketing consequences of defining a drug as more effective in one sex than another.

Sticking our heads in the sand is not the answer. We must develop guidelines that allow all women to fully participate in research. Failure to do this has serious ramifications; it could, in fact, be a matter of life and death. For example, of the ten prescription drugs withdrawn by the FDA from the market since 1997 because of adverse reactions, eight posed greater risks for women than for men. (In some cases, the drugs were more widely prescribed to women; however, even with medications prescribed equally to males and females, they were more dangerous for women.) And when you are pregnant, physiological changes may affect your response to a drug; you may be more vulnerable to its toxicity or its effectiveness. When you take a drug, you need to know that it is safe and effective for you.

TAKE CHARGE OF YOUR PAIN NOW

It's going to take a while until these changes come about. Meanwhile, you're in pain, and pain can leave you feeling powerless. My message is that you can regain control of your life with gentle yet potent pain relief strategies geared to your needs as a woman.

JENNY'S STORY

Jenny is a twenty-two-year-old college student. While driving on campus during a late-spring rainstorm, she had to stop short suddenly and was rear-ended by the car in back of her. "My neck snapped back and forth, but it didn't hurt," she said. "Later on, though, this dull, aching pain started up, and it just kept getting worse. I guess it's what you call whiplash."

By that evening, Jenny's pain was so terrible she couldn't sleep. She couldn't move her neck freely because every move provoked a new onslaught of excruciating spasms. The next day, a nurse-practitioner in the Department of Student Health referred her to me for an evaluation.

Jenny had a considerable amount of pain, spasm, and range of motion restriction in her neck. I ordered X rays, which were negative, although they did show a flattening in the cervical neck, a common finding in whiplash victims. Her neurological exam was normal and she had no motor deficits or weakness, no sensory loss, and no reflex changes.

Jenny is a rarity—one of the few patients I've had who refuses to take any conventional medications—so I had to be creative. For starters, I recommended white willow bark, an herb that has the same analgesic and anti-inflammatory effects as conventional painkillers. For her spasms, I suggested valerian root tea and long, relaxing aromatherapy baths with lavender. I also told her to take advantage of this opportunity and get her boyfriend to give her a gentle neck massage. In addition, I showed her how to apply a moist heat pack, and I referred her for a couple of sessions of physical therapy.

What really did the trick, though, were my acupuncture treatments. She looked more and more relaxed after every session. To prolong those effects, I sent her home with acupressure exercises to do on her own.

It took about two full weeks, but Jenny made a full recovery.

I have always been deeply motivated by modern medicine's quest to alleviate pain, especially for individuals suffering the indignities of disabling disease. During my early days as a medical student at the Finch University

Health Sciences/Chicago Medical School, I was inspired by the examples of my professors, who conducted research in the pharmacology and physiology of pain. As an intern at the University of Chicago/Louis A. Weiss Memorial Hospital, working at the bedsides of people in pain strengthened my commitment to the art and science of pain management and impelled me to pursue a physiatry residency training at the Albert Einstein College of Medicine/Montefiore Medical Center in New York. And because I enjoy research and teaching in addition to caring for patients, I joined the faculty of the Johns Hopkins University School of Medicine in 1991.

Throughout my career, I've observed the strengths that conventional pharmaceuticals and therapeutic procedures bring to the battle against pain. But I also know their limitations. I am a practitioner of integrative medicine, which combines the best of conventional and so-called alternative — I prefer the term *complementary* — care. Of course, I prescribe drugs and use other conventional pain relief techniques when necessary. But the emphasis in my practice, and what you'll find in this book, is a multifaceted program of complementary alternatives, including dietary, herbal and homeopathic remedies, exercise, recipes, and mind-body techniques.

The therapies in this book are all safe and supported by scientific research, as well as my own experience. They are the treatments most frequently chosen by, and most effective for, women. These remedies, easily incorporated into your lifestyle, will let you finally take charge of your pain and, in many instances, free yourself from it entirely.

At its most fundamental level, medicine is about the relief of pain and suffering. As a rehabilitation doctor, I pay special attention to pain, recognizing that not every patient reports pain or responds to it in the same way. I know how important it is to tailor treatments to each individual's need. Gender affects how we perceive, report, and cope with pain. As scientists continue to untangle the threads — hormonal cycles, genetics, brain structure, anatomical, physiological and biological differences — that weave the intricate web of gender-based pain perception, it's imperative that you receive selective, customized care. I hope *Women and Pain* enables you to take the first step forward into the pain-free future you deserve.

NOTES ON DOSING

Herbal remedies: Doses have been standardized according to the German Commission E Monograph (CEM) and/or the *Physicians' Desk Reference for Herbals* (*PDR-H*). The German Commission E is the rough equivalent of our FDA. Their monographs about specific herbs, which document the herbs' health risks, benefits, and side effects, are based on decades of clinical trials. Dosages from the *PDR-H* and Commission E are confirmed by the American Botanical Council. Please consult your physician before taking any herbal medicines.

Dietary supplements: Quantities are in accordance with the U.S. Dietary Reference Intake (DRI). The DRI are quantitative estimates of nutrient intakes that are useful for assessing and planning diets in healthy people. The DRI standards were established by a consensus of the Food and Nutrition Board of the Institute of Medicine and the National Academy of Science. For vitamins, minerals, or supplements listed, a dose range composed of two values has been included: a lower limit and an upper limit. The lower limit is the recommended dietary allowance (RDA). The upper limit is the tolerable upper intake level (UL). Please note that the UL is not the recommended dose, but is the maximum amount that has been determined scientifically to be tolerated without adverse effects. Both the RDA and UL may vary according to age, pregnancy, nutrition, and lactation status. Please consult a physician.

WOMEN

AND

PAIN

1

—

The Gender Gap

Beth is a forty-one-year-old woman who works as an inventory clerk at a local bookstore. She'd been my patient for years, ever since her orthopedist referred her to me for "conservative management." I saw her periodically for mild scoliosis (a sidewise spine curvature), which causes fleeting aches and pains. Otherwise, she had been essentially healthy and strong.

Beth was usually pretty cheerful. But on this day, I knew something was wrong as soon as she walked in the door. She was worried because she had recently noticed the gradual onset of a dull, aching pain in her neck and upper shoulders, as well as increasing fatigue. "These days, it often hurts in the small of my back, too, and I tire easily," she told me. But it wasn't just her physical pain that had her keyed up; there was more going on. She'd been to an Urgent Care Center (she could not get in to see her primary care doctor, since he was too busy), where she was told that there was nothing wrong with her, that it was "just stress," and sent off with a prescription for Xanax, an antianxiety drug.

"I just don't believe it," Beth said. "There's nothing particularly worrisome going on in my life right now. They just didn't take me seriously; besides, they seemed awfully rushed."

Still, she was puzzled and disturbed; what was causing her pain? "It's too soon to be falling apart, isn't it?" she joked. "Seriously, though, I know I'm getting older, but I still feel like I'm in good shape. And I'm not doing anything different at work. So what's up?"

After a thorough review of her most recent spine films, laboratory workup, bone mineral density, and pulmonary function test results (breathing can go bad when the spine is deformed), which were all normal, I performed a thorough physical, including a spine examination. Although her posture appeared to be the same as in prior office visits, she did indeed have more tenderness and spasm in her neck and back. Fortunately, her scoliosis and degree of spine angle were unchanged. Her height, leg lengths, and angle of back inclination, reflecting the degree of spine rotation, had not worsened. Because she hadn't exercised in some time, she did exhibit some weakness in her back extensor and abdominal muscle strength, and her overall hip and back flexibility were not quite up to snuff.

As I explained to Beth, these changes had a major biomechanical impact on her spine, and were probably contributing to her neck, shoulder, and back pain. Making matters worse, Beth spends a lot of time at her job sitting at a desk, punching numbers into a computer to keep track of merchandise. And her neglect of exercise wasn't helping either. She used to work out regularly, but she'd grown increasingly sedentary, especially during the winter months.

Unfortunately, Beth has an ailment for which there is no "cure"; her condition is chronic. Based on her X rays, the degree of curvature in her spine was less than 20 degrees—too small to recommend any specific surgery or bracing measure. And there is no way to reverse or improve her long-standing scoliosis.

My job, then, was to help her cope with her current level of pain and make sure it didn't get worse. I was optimistic, since I knew there was a lot of room for improvement. Beth used to be an avid runner. I suggested that at this time she take up swimming instead, which exerts less wear and tear on the body. Not only would swimming help quell the pain, but it would improve her general level of flexibility, muscle strength, and conditioning. I explained, however, that it would not reverse the scoliosis.

To further increase her flexibility, I recommended that she take up yoga or tai chi. And if she had the time, I suggested she take a light aerobic exercise class to enhance her endurance and lessen her fatigue. High-quality, supportive shoes would provide more stability and dampen the impact of her spine pain. And warm herbal baths at the end of her workday would also give her significant relief.

Finally, I advised Beth to tackle some ergonomic improvements at work. She needed a better chair, and it was important that she not sit scrunched up at her desk for long periods of time. Frequent rest breaks were also critical. Whether she stretched—and I suggested a few simple exercises she could do—or just walked around, she absolutely had to get away from her desk for a few minutes every hour. "My boss is a young guy who's a fitness fanatic. I hope he'll understand," she said.

A couple of months later, Beth returned for a follow-up visit. She had started swimming again and had noticed improvements already. But she waited until the end of her visit to tell me the big news: "I finally got up the courage to ask my boss for a new chair. When he told me he wasn't sure it was necessary, I got nervous. But then he told me why—in my new job, I'd be up and around a lot more. No more crunching numbers. He promoted me to office manager!"

This is an exciting time in medical science. We're unlocking so many mysteries, and learning an enormous amount about what makes us all tick. As they unravel nature's code, the scientists working on the Human Genome Project may ultimately reveal that our individual susceptibilities to disease depend on microscopic genetic differences. Why, then, should it be surprising that gender, a major genetic variation, profoundly affects the way we experience pain?

Yet women's pain has been largely ignored by the medical and scientific community, and women have been systematically excluded from biomedical research. As recently as 1984, the National Institute on Aging published a report called "Normal Human Aging" using data only from men! Except for studies centered on breasts and reproductive organs (sometimes derided as "bikini medicine"), most research on medications, pain, and other disorders was for men only, the misguided rationale being that women's pesky hormonal cycles would just confuse the results. Besides, researchers mistakenly assumed that many conditions don't affect women as frequently, or that when they do, the symptoms are the same. Even when studies included women, the results were not separately analyzed by gender.

Change has come, although it's too little and too slow. In 1990 the National Institutes of Health established the Office of Research on Women's Health. And in 1993, Congress passed a law mandating that sufficient numbers of women and minorities be included in research to allow a valid analysis of any differences. Also that year, the Food and Drug Administration (FDA) rescinded its restriction on permitting women in their childbearing years to participate in medical research. In 1998, the agency began requiring manufacturers of pharmaceuticals and medical devices to report the age, race, and gender of individuals participating in their research trials. Today, some legislators are hoping to pass a law that would mandate an office of women's health in every agency in the Department of Health and Human Services.

Even so, some scientists *still* fail to take women into account. An April 2000 article, "Studies Find Research on Women Lacking," in the *New York Times* reported that three new studies, including an investigation by the Government Accounting Office, found that medical researchers who receive federal money often ignore the requirement to analyze their data to see if women and men respond differently to a given treatment. I think this kind of behavior is reprehensible; and it certainly doesn't serve your needs as a health care consumer (and a taxpayer).

Despite these obstacles, the field of gender-based biology is producing some astounding results, although they are not yet widely accepted or even generally known. Some of the most important research shows that women experience more severe, longer lasting, and more frequent pain.

MEN AND WOMEN HAVE DIFFERENT "PAIN THERMOSTATS"

Here's the bottom line: Women feel more pain than men. In both experimental and clinical research, women consistently have both lower pain thresholds—the minimum amount of stimulation that reliably evokes pain in an individual—and less pain tolerance—the maximum time or intensity of a painful stimulus that a person can endure. Studies also suggest that women report greater pain than men even when they have the same degree of tissue injury.

The reason for this disparity is not just that women are more emotional or more willing to talk about their pain than men, although some doctors still fall back on that tired old excuse. No, the truth is, men and women are physiologically different. For example, in an experiment published in 1991, not only did the women rate pain from heat stimuli as more intense than the men, they were also better able to discriminate among various intensities of pain. We now know that there are profound, gender-based differences in how women and men perceive pain.

PAIN MEDICATIONS: ONCE SIZE DOES NOT FIT ALL

Besides differing in their perceptions of pain, men and women also respond differently to analgesics, or pain relievers. For instance, certain commonly used pain medications provide effective relief for men who suffer chronic pain in their reproductive organs, but rarely for women with chronic pelvic pain. Researchers at Johns Hopkins compared thirty-nine women with chronic pelvic pain and twenty-five men with chronic testicular pain. (None of the cases involved cancer.) Each person received one of several types of medications—antidepressants, anticonvulsants, and opioids—known to relieve other pain syndromes. A larger percentage of men than women improved in each case. For example, with antidepressants, the most frequently used medication, nine of eleven men (82 percent) improved, while only four of twenty-eight women (14 percent) did so.

We are also discovering that there are gender differences in how people respond to some of the most widely used pain relievers. In a recent study of experimentally induced pain, ibuprofen—the key ingredient in Advil, Motrin, and other over-the-counter analgesics—was less effective at providing pain relief for women than men. And a Dutch study of the effects of intravenous morphine, which is used for severe pain, revealed clear sex-related differences, even when men and women had similar levels of the drug in their blood. The morphine eased men's pain during the first hour, while women had no pain relief during that time. On the other hand, the effects dissipated fairly quickly among the men but lasted longer for the women. Wouldn't you want your doctors to know about research like this if you were suffering from terrible pain?

Recently, research in the United States on another class of painkillers, known as kappa-opioids, has also produced striking results. The drugs were given to twenty-eight young men and twenty young women who had their wisdom teeth removed. If you've ever been through this procedure, you know that it can produce moderate or severe pain. Women experienced long-lasting, high-quality pain relief from kappa-opioids, with few side effects. But the men received little benefit.

We haven't yet figured out the mechanisms behind these puzzling differences. It could have to do with hormones, the number of receptors on nerve cells, or the ways the brain regulates pain relief. Regardless of the reason, though, these findings matter when it comes to treating your pain. Kappa-opioids have been ignored, for the most part, even though they have fewer side effects than more commonly used painkillers such as codeine, Percodan, and morphine. Why? It's likely that when these drugs were tested by the pharmaceutical companies, their effects on women—if women even participated in the studies—were not analyzed separately. This kind of gender-blindness is outmoded and disgraceful. How much are we missing by ignoring potentially crucial gender differences in biomedical research?

LAUREN'S STORY

Lauren is a twenty-seven-year-old French-Canadian woman, who came to town to do an apprenticeship in architecture in a local firm. A talented pianist and rock climber, Lauren placed a lot of strain on her wrists. She came to my office complaining of pain in her right wrist, accompanied by numbness in her thumb and second finger. "I wake up in the dead of night with horrible pain and tingling. It's so weird; I have to shake out my hand to get it to ease up." She was also having a tough time opening jars. "I almost lost it the other night. I was preparing a Passover seder for fifteen people and I couldn't open the jar of horseradish!"

Lauren told me that her doctor back home attributed her pain to a "tight nerve" and offered few suggestions. "He minimized the importance of my symptoms and told me to 'just keep on trucking,'" she said. In a telephone conversation, her dad, a retired general practitioner, had urged her to see a specialist, and so she'd found her way to my office.

A careful history and physical revealed that Lauren's symptoms were probably caused by carpal tunnel syndrome, a condition that is particularly frequent among women. She had many of the classical features, including a positive Tinel's sign (tapping above her wrist crease caused numbness and tingling), and some weakness in her grip, as well as a tendency to drop things. Following my suggestion, she underwent a nerve conduction study, which confirmed my diagnosis.

Lauren was concerned about the impact this ailment might have on her life. "I play the piano all the time; besides, I use a keyboard all day at work," she said. At the same time, as a big fan of natural, noninvasive complementary treatments, she didn't want to do anything drastic; no steroid injections for her! I was happy to oblige, and assured her that she'd be back at her piano very soon.

First, we addressed her pain. Although she was only willing to use nonsteroidal anti-inflammatory drugs (NSAIDS) if it got really bad, she was thrilled when I gave her a sample of a natural topical treatment she could apply directly to her wrist. Because it works wonders for carpal tunnel syndrome, we got started with acupuncture right away. I also suggested that she try a TENS (transcutaneous electrical nerve stimulator) unit, which uses electrical impulses to stop the transmission of pain signals.

I taught Lauren some hand and wrist exercises and gave her a "cock-up splint," also known as a dorsiflexion or extension splint, which mechanically repositioned her wrist and took pressure off the carpal tunnel. In addition, to prevent her condition from worsening (or from recurring once she was better) I recommended some ergonomic strategies, including a wrist support to use while working on the keyboard, and taking frequent breaks. Finally, to speed healing, I suggested vitamin B6 and a number of other supplements.

Several months later, Lauren was symptom-free.

THE UNEQUAL BURDEN OF PAIN

A staggering array of painful illnesses and disorders disproportionately affect women. Of course, you are vulnerable to pain during many stages of your reproductive life cycle, including menstruation, pregnancy, childbirth, and menopause. But you are also far more likely to develop painful ailments that have nothing to do with reproductive health, simply because you're female. To name just a few, these include migraine and tension headaches, backaches, fibromyalgia, rheumatoid arthritis, facial pain, and carpal tunnel syndrome. In addition, women are at greater risk than men for developing chronic pain syndrome after they've suffered the same type of physical trauma.

What really muddies the waters, leading to missed diagnoses and ineffective treatments, is that men and women sometimes report different symptoms for the same disease. You've probably heard about the classic example, which is heart disease. Women less frequently suffer chest pain and more often report pain in the back, neck, and jaw. They experience more nausea, vomiting, abdominal complaints, fatigue, and shortness of breath. What's not as well known is that gender differences also play out in the symptoms of other diseases, such as irritable bowel syndrome, appendicitis, and migraine headaches.

I see this all the time in my own practice. Far more women than men come to see me because of chronic headache disorders. When it comes to migraines, it's probably three to one. My female patients have more nausea, vomiting, and aversion to light. Their headaches last longer, and more often disrupt their sleep. In addition, they have to miss work more often. Yet I know this isn't just psychosomatic, because many of the differences vanish after my patients go through menopause.

EXPLAINING THE GENDER GAP

We don't yet know why the gender disparities in pain perception, responses to medications, and prevalence of symptoms and diseases exist, but we're pursuing some hot leads. Some researchers believe it has to do with the varying expectations and roles society has for men and women. (Certainly, boys raised on a steady diet of Rambo and watching professional athletes "play through their pain" may grow up to feel that real men "grin and bear it.") Others put it down to psychological differences, such as anxiety or an individual's beliefs about his or her ability to tolerate pain. And biology, such as body size or differences in resting blood pressure, probably also comes into play. I think we're going to find that hormonal, genetic, anatomical, and psychological differences all play a role in explaining the gender gap. And men and women may also have different brain circuitry that partly accounts for this phenomenon.

This is a complex subject to unravel because pain is a complicated biochemical "fact." And it is very subjective. The way you perceive, interpret, and express pain is influenced by your philosophical or religious beliefs. Also, the threshold at which your pain becomes unbearable can vary, depending upon the culture you come from, or the situation you are in. There's a classic example in a book called *People in Pain*, published in 1969. The author, Mark Zborowski, a social anthropologist, studied Irish, Jewish, Italian, and "Old American" (i.e., WASP) World War II veterans and found that the way they reacted to pain—how uninhibited and expressive they were—was strongly associated with their ethnic group and social class.

What's more, your doctor brings his or her own biases into play when assessing your pain. For example, in an Israeli study, Jewish doctors and midwives evaluated the pain of 225 Jewish and 192 Bedouin women during labor; the women also assessed their own pain. Although the women evaluated their pain equivalently, the doctors and midwives reported less pain among the Bedouin women. So a caregiver's ethnic background or beliefs may influence how he evaluates someone's suffering.

What I find especially compelling is cutting-edge research showing that sex-linked genetic characteristics may be involved. In experiments with mice, whose genetic structure is similar to humans, scientists applied a technique called gene mapping to identify specific genes associated with pain and pain relief. They found that gender-linked genetic differences accounted for as much as 50 percent of the variability in pain responses. On female mice only, they found a gene on one chromosome linked to analgesic, or pain-relieving, activity; it appeared to be irrelevant to males. And conversely, a gene on another chromosome affected pain sensitivity, but only on male mice. The conclusion? Males and females have an entirely different genetic basis for pain. In other words, your tolerance for pain, your response to pain relievers, and even possibly your susceptibility to certain painful ailments may have nothing to do with your emotional makeup or with your being "a wimp." Instead, it may be hardwired into your genes. This is exciting news because once we learn more about the genes involved in sensitivity to pain, we may be able to develop innovative, individualized pain therapies.

Given the enormous influence they have in many aspects of your life, you might think that sex-related hormones also affect sensitivity and response to pain. You're right; the hormonal connection to pain is one of the most exciting areas of scientific research, with an impressive array of animal studies as well as experimental and clinical research on humans.

Men and women have different levels of the sex hormones, sometimes called steroid hormones: estrogen, progesterone, and testosterone. Hormones affect nerve conduction, so they may influence how your nerves send their pain messages. Sex steroids can also alter levels of neurotransmitters and other chemical messengers involved in transmitting pain through your central nervous system, as well as your body's own responses to pain. In addition, estrogen and other hormones affect how nerves respond to local anesthetics, and they may affect your body's response to other pain medications.

Besides the obvious hormonal differences between men and women, we also have to take into account the female hormonal cycle. Your estrogen, progesterone, and testosterone levels fluctuate over the course of a month, leading you to respond differently to pain during different phases of your menstrual cycle. You're probably more sensitive to pain during the days between ovulation and the start of menstruation. Known medically as the "luteal phase," it's more commonly called—you guessed it—the premenstrual period. Greater sensitivity to pain during this time may be due to the direct effects of hormones on pain processing. Or it may be indirect. For example, if you're one of the many women who suffer from sleep disturbances when you are premenstrual, it may affect how you react to pain.

What's more, in some conditions, painful symptoms worsen during the premenstrual phase. You may already know this if you have irritable bowel syndrome, headaches, rheumatoid arthritis, or fibromyalgia. And hormonal fluctuations also seem to play a role in the pain of temporomandibular disease. My belief is that as we continue to unravel the mystery of pain, innate hormonal differences, accentuated by the menstrual cycle, pregnancy, and oral contraceptives and other hormonal medications, will play a starring role.

Finally, new, controversial research has emerged on how anatomical features may at least partially explain men's and women's distinct responses to pain. It may be that the existence of the vaginal canal and of sensitive neural mechanisms known as "C-fibers" within the vagina play a key role in women's heightened sensitivity to pain. Here's one possible scenario: Because the vagina and cervix provide ready access to the body, they serve as an entrance for viral and other infectious agents, which may trigger a sequence of reactions through the C-fibers in the vagina, up through the spinal cord and brain. This could cause pain in parts of the body that are far from the original site, accounting for the fact that women more often have multiple areas of what is known as "referred pain," or pain that you feel at some distance from its source.

ARE WOMEN "BETTER SPORTS" ABOUT PAIN?

Before you go off in despair, let me assure you that the news isn't all bad. Although you may suffer more pain, you are also more adept at coping. The patients I see certainly belie the old notion that women are the "weaker sex." And research confirms my day-to-day observations.

For example, women appear to tolerate pain better than men. A recent study followed twenty-seven women and twenty-one men after they'd had surgery to implant a replacement tooth. In the ten days after the operation, the women handled low levels of pain better than the men, who were more disturbed by the persisting discomfort.

Nature tends to be an equalizer, and most body systems are inclined toward balance. So it's likely that because women experience more pain, they also have more physiological mechanisms for reducing it. Much research needs to be done, but we already know of one example. With the phenomenon known as pregnancy-induced analgesia, a woman's body produces higher levels of endorphins during the late stages of pregnancy to enhance her tolerance of pain. Maybe this is the biological underpinning for the old joke that if it were up to men to have babies, the human race would have been extinct long ago! Seriously, though, it wouldn't surprise me if we eventually discover that women tolerate pain better than men because of the sensitizing experience of childbirth.

Women also have an edge when we go beyond the physiological. You know that women are more likely than men to ask for directions when they are lost. Similarly, women tend to take more advantage of existing resources to deal with their pain. They use the health care system earlier, more aggressively, and more effectively than men. And they have a more open attitude toward innovative approaches to pain care, especially acupuncture, massage, meditation, yoga, and other complementary therapies.

Besides, women are better at taking care of themselves. You probably know how to lighten the emotional burden of pain by allowing yourself to vent your feelings, reaching out to friends and relatives, and listening to your body's warnings to slow down when you are in pain.

In one study, researchers compared men and women with arthritis. On "high pain" days, women were far more likely to use a variety of coping strategies, including relaxation, distraction, and seeking support from others. The day after a high pain day, men reported that their mood was poor, but women did not; suggesting that by taking charge of their pain, they were better able to limit its emotional consequences.

My patient Ramona is a perfect example of how well women cope with pain.

RAMONA'S STORY

Ramona is a twenty-eight-year-old mother of two, and a proud homemaker. At the tender age of seventeen, she was in a near-fatal car accident that resulted in a spine fracture and several bone fractures. She's experienced pain ever since.

Nevertheless, Ramona is a real trouper when it comes to contending with pain, and she comes to see me regularly. Although her pain can be troubling, she remains optimistic that she will ultimately conquer it. She has an open mind about complementary care, and over the years we have done acupuncture, relaxation and visualization, and biofeedback.

Ramona copes emotionally by relying on her own strength, as well as a solid support network of friends and family, with whom she talks regularly and extensively. Her husband, Rick, a manual laborer, has always been supportive. But he remains baffled by Ramona's ability to endure the pain as well as she does. "I'm a tough cookie, but if it were me, I would have thrown in the towel a long time ago," he told me.

•   •   •

Unfortunately, women like Ramona can't do it alone. Ignorance of gender differences has important practical ramifications. In the next chapter, I'll explain how misguided thinking about gender has affected women's medical care in the past, and may still have an impact on the care you receive today.

Why Gender Matters

When Professor Henry Higgins asked "Why can't a woman be more like a man?" in *My Fair Lady,* he might have been expressing the opinion of many pain doctors, who simply can't, don't, or won't take gender differences into account when they tailor pain-relief strategies.

But as bad as it is to deny the difference, it's inexcusable to dismiss women's pain as psychosomatic. Yet this has been part of the medical tradition since the time of ancient Greece. The word *hysteria* comes from the Greek word *hystera,* meaning womb. Plato and the other ancients compared the womb to an animal that roamed around a woman's body. The womb's wanderings were thought to be the source of many female maladies. Treatments often consisted of trying to lure that misbehaving womb back to its rightful place in the body.

Fast-forward to the nineteenth century. Any woman unfortunate enough to have pains incompatible with contemporary medical knowledge or symptoms that didn't respond to conventional treatment ran the risk of having her illness dismissed as imaginary. Maybe its source was now in her head, rather than her womb, but it was still hysteria. Hysteria was a shape-shifter, a unique ailment capable of imitating almost any known disease. And pain was one of its most common symptoms.

Unfortunately, this is not just ancient history. With distressing frequency, doctors *still* treat women as overly emotional or don't take their pain seriously. Even today, in the twenty-first century, outdated stereotypes often result in less-than-adequate care for women in pain.

NICOLE'S STORY

Nicole is a single, thirty-seven-year-old stockbroker who had intense pain in her right buttock. It had started as a dull ache nine months ago, appearing mostly when she sat for long periods of time, climbed stairs, or did squats in the gym. But it had escalated from a smoldering fire to a full-fledged conflagration after she participated in a charity bikeathon for breast cancer research.

A "fitness fiend" who took pride in being in excellent shape, Nicole simply couldn't fathom this angry pain that erupted after her marathon bike ride. "Doc, this burning pain is buried deep in my butt. It feels as though someone has taken a blowtorch to my derriere. Everything hurts; I can't even take pleasure in sitting on the floor with my nephew in my lap."

As we sat in my office and she described her condition, she appeared to be defensive and a bit wary. When I gently prodded, the rest of her all-too-familiar story emerged. Nicole had gone to her primary care doctor, who hadn't been sure what was happening. He ordered X rays of her hip, pelvis, and spine. When they were negative, he "went for the big guns" and ordered an MRI of her spine, which was also normal. Drawing a blank, he referred her to a chiropractor and, later, to a massage therapist.

Although she dutifully made the rounds to all the specialists, Nicole got nowhere. Still in agonizing pain, she'd returned in frustration to her internist. He now dismissed her condition as "psychological," implying that she was simply under too much stress because of the floundering stock market. She had left in tears. Finally, a friend at work, whom I had helped a number of years ago with acupuncture and exercise for a back problem, referred her to me.

After our interview and a thorough physical history, I reviewed her prior X rays and MRI. Indeed, they were negative. Still, I knew this was not a psychological problem; it was regrettable that she'd been treated so dismissively. I had a hunch she had an elusive malady called piriformis muscle syndrome. Because it's not an easy condition to pin down on diagnostic tests — in fact, a negative workup is a hallmark of this ailment — some doctors are skeptical about its existence.

Convinced that the "mystery" would most likely be solved by careful physical examination and muscle assessment, I tried several physical diagnostic maneuvers. We hit pay dirt when I asked Nicole to place all her weight on her left foot. At the same time, I asked her to move her right leg away from her body in a sideways fashion, while rotating it, so that her toes pointed up in the air. When she yelped, I had my diagnosis.

The piriformis muscle lies buried deep beneath the gluteal muscles in the buttocks. The piriformis has its origin at the sacral bone and attaches to the greater trochanter of the leg bone (femur), which is the "bump" on the outside top of the thigh. When this muscle contracts, it causes the leg to move out or away from the midline, and to rotate externally. The sciatic nerve is buried deep below the major muscles, including the piriformis, and in 15 percent of the population it runs right through the muscle. Any type of irritation or swelling of the piriformis sets the sciatic nerve, the largest nerve in the body, on fire.

Nicole was enormously relieved to know what the problem was. She was also highly motivated to get rid of it: "Just tell me what to do. I can't wait to feel better," she said. Because she was in such intense pain, I gave her a local injection of lidocaine and corticosteroid into her piriformis muscle to provide immediate relief. In addition, we started an acupuncture regimen. Once the pain had calmed down a bit, I explained that we had to "reeducate her muscles" with a program of stretching exercises. I also referred her to a physical therapist for ultrasound; by heating muscles, this modality promotes better stretch. Finally, because certain types of foot disorders such as overpronation can contribute to piriformis syndrome, I recommended that Nicole see a podiatrist for a foot orthotic.

Nicole left my office still in pain, but well on her way to relief. More gratifying, though, was that I had confirmed what she had known all along: This pain was not "all in her head."

BLAMING THE VICTIM

There is no way to measure pain objectively. Because it's an individual perception that we communicate through language and by crying or other nonverbal means, the interplay between doctor and patient is critical. When you see your doctor because you're in pain, how carefully he or she listens to you, and the preconceived notions he or she brings to the encounter, greatly influence the care you receive.

Women are more likely than men to seek medical attention for pain. They are better able—or more willing—to fully describe their pain sensations and to talk about their feelings. Besides, it's also more socially acceptable for women to express emotional distress. You would think that this ability to communicate the discomfort of pain would be an advantage. But I believe that women are, in effect, being punished for their strengths. Too often their reports are viewed with suspicion or their complaints are dismissed as "hysterical."

If you suffer from chronic pain, you're much more likely to be diagnosed with depression or histrionic and somatization disorders — ailments for which no physical cause can be found. In plain English, this means that many doctors will assume it's all in your head, or that you're just depressed.

Even worse, women are more often treated with psychotropic drugs than men. (These are medications that affect your mind; they are used for depression, anxiety, and other psychiatric ailments.) In 1989, researchers analyzed data from the National Ambulatory Medical Care Survey and found that even with the same complaint, diagnosis, and visit history, women were still 37 percent more likely than men to receive an antianxiety medication and a whopping 82 percent more likely to get an antidepressant! These results were confirmed in a later study published in 1998. Statistics like these are disgraceful. Despite enormous strides in improving our health care system's treatment of women, this kind of subtle sexism shows that we still have a long way to go.

Health care providers who doubt your experience of pain, blame you for the pain, or minimize your needs for pain relief add insult to injury. "Blaming the victim" can adversely affect your self-esteem, which escalates your distress and sense of isolation. It may also diminish the likelihood that any care you do receive will be effective. If you're suffering from chronic pain, the most important element in your doctor-patient relationship is whether you feel your doctor believes you. If your experience of pain is validated, you are more likely to be compliant and successful with pain relief strategies.

STEREOTYPES AFFECT YOUR CARE

Even when doctors or other caregivers know your pain isn't psychosomatic, their beliefs about pain and gender influence their attitudes, and they may treat you less aggressively. Several experiments have revealed that nurses make decisions based on gender stereotypes. For example, when nurses were asked to read and react to identical vignettes of men and women in pain, their care plans included more narcotic pain medication and emotional support for the men. In an actual clinical setting, these nursing care decisions would lead to inadequate treatment for female patients.

Sadly, we also have evidence that women do, in fact, get less pain medication. For instance, among 180 adults who'd had appendectomies, men received significantly more narcotic pain relievers than women for the initial postoperative dose, although the total dose during the recovery period was about the same. Gender bias must have come into play because the difference occurred while patients were still too groggy from surgery to express their needs!

When women do say what they need, however, nurses or doctors may take them less seriously or dismiss them as "whiny." In a study of people who'd undergone coronary artery bypass graft surgery, men received morphine significantly more often than women. Interestingly, women received more sedative drugs for anxiety or agitation. Perhaps this reflected the nurses' belief that women are more emotional and more likely to exaggerate complaints of pain than men. Regrettably, other research has shown that even among patients with metastatic cancer, being female is a significant predictor of inadequate pain management.

Even more chilling is this: Women may undergo surgery more frequently than men for similar pain syndromes. In a series of studies, a researcher compared men with chronic, nonmalignant testicular pain and women with chronic pelvic pain. Both of these ailments last at least three to six months and often have no obvious cause. One of fifteen men (7 percent) had undergone epididymectomy (the epididymis is a long, coiled tube that carries sperm from the testicles to the tip of the penis), while seventeen of thirty-nine women (44 percent) had had hysterectomies, without any resolution of their problems! The researcher concluded that male urologists may have greater reluctance to remove reproductive organs in male patients than male gynecologists have in female patients, a conclusion I find deeply disturbing.

PUTTING GENDER INTO THE EQUATION

We're at the beginning of a revolution. The science of gender-specific differences in health is relatively new, and some of the findings are speculative. Much more research needs to be done. Still, there are things that all of us—practitioners and patients—can do to increase awareness of gender issues and improve treatment for people in pain.

- Men and women may not experience the same symptoms or may express themselves differently when describing the pain associated with a specific problem. So "typical" descriptions of common pain problems and treatment protocols need to be changed, especially as we uncover more and more sex-related differences. For example, despite abundant information illustrating the importance of sex differences when it comes to heart disease, current recommendations for the evaluation of chest pain in women who have suspected coronary heart disease are *still* based on a male model of the disease.

- New models take a while to develop. In the meantime, I'd advise you to ask your doctor to search the scientific literature and be alert to any findings about potentially different diagnostic signs and symptoms in males and females. This will be especially important as more evidence emerges about the varying ways medications affect men and women. And bring this book with you to your doctor's office!
- Because your menstrual cycle may affect your pain, keep a pain diary to note any possible hormonal fluctuations in your symptoms. Whenever you notice regular variations, let your doctor know. If you have rheumatoid arthritis, for example, and you know it gets worse the week before your period, you might be able to adjust your medication or plan your schedule to avoid strenuous activities during that time.
- Other hormones, such as oral contraceptives or hormone replacement therapy, may also affect your painful symptoms. For instance, hormones can significantly increase the pain of temporomandibular disorder. If you notice a change after starting a prescription for hormones, let your doctor know right away.

Meanwhile, if you're reading this book, chances are you are in pain. In the next chapter, I'll explain how pain works, and how it may work differently for men and women.

3

The Mystery of Pain

Shakita is a forty-three-year-old woman who works as a nurse's aide for a home health and hospice agency. She has a heart of gold and her clients adore her. In fact, it was one of her geriatric patients who recommended that she see me.

Shakita is diabetic and overweight. When she came in, she told me she had ongoing, intermittent pain and numbness in the side of her left thigh. She had been to a string of doctors, including her family physician, a chiropractor, and several specialists. Although she'd been through an extensive and thorough workup, no one had found an identifiable cause for her pain. "They don't have a clue. I got so desperate, I even went to my neighborhood faith healer," she told me, a bit sheepishly.

Lately, her symptoms had gotten worse; the pain was so bad that she now reported a burning ache over the front and side of her thigh, along with some tingling. "It feels like water rippling down my side," she explained.

When I examined her, it soon became obvious that she fit the description of someone with meralgia paraesthetica, a nerve entrapment syndrome of the lateral femoral cutaneous nerve, which is located in the front, outer part of the thigh. This diagnosis would easily explain her pattern of alternating numbness and pain. Because this nerve is a purely sensory nerve, the ailment doesn't cause any motor loss or other deficits. (There are three types of nerves: sensory, motor, and mixed. Sensory nerves carry signals for sensation, such as numbness, tingling, light touch, or pain. Motor nerves provide power to your muscles and give them strength. Mixed nerves do both.)

Diabetes can be a risk factor for meralgia paraesthetica and can exacerbate its symptoms. So can a tight lumbar corset, or brace, which Shakita often wore because she needed to lift heavy patients. And she was obese, which further complicated her situation. When I advised her to lose some weight, she sighed and said: "Well, Doctor, I've been talking about going on a diet for years. If losing weight will ease this pain, maybe I'll finally have the motivation to do it."

In the meantime, I prescribed a capsaicin cream, made from hot peppers, or a lidoderm patch, a topical anesthetic, to dull her pain. I also started her on Neurontin, a medication used for seizures that also has powerful nerve stabilizing properties. She was intrigued by a chart of acupuncture points I had in my office, so I gave her a few acupressure exercises to try. I warned her to avoid corsets and other tight garments and urged her to start some kind of exercise. "There's a park across the street from my house. I'm up early anyway; maybe I'll take a walk before work," she said.

There's no motivator like pain. Over the next six months, Shakita exercised diligently and watched what she ate. Her symptoms gradually improved so much that she was able to stop the Neurontin and rely just on the topical analgesics.

WHAT IS PAIN?

When I care for patients, I find that illuminating how pain works demystifies it and makes it less frightening. Understanding the mechanics of pain can help you gain mastery over what may otherwise seem like a dark and powerful force that has taken over your life.

Human beings have tried to make sense of pain for millennia. Pain scares us, not only because it hurts, but because it is intimately connected to illness and hints at our mortality. Emily Dickinson understood this when she wrote: "Pain has but one Acquaintance / and that is Death."

Since the beginnings of time, our ancestors have tried to understand pain. In ancient days they thought it was a supernatural phenomenon—a form of spiritual possession or a punishment, gift, test, or means of redemption from the gods.

As we learned more about the natural world of biological processes, our conception of pain changed. In recent times, pain was reduced to a purely mechanistic model—electrical impulses speeding along nerves.

Today we know that pain is much more complicated. It involves a complex interaction between the mind *and* the body. To paraphrase Gertrude Stein, it is simply not true that a pain is a pain is a pain. Your experience of pain depends not only on cellular, molecular, genetic, and physiological factors, but it is also inextricably tied to your mental and emotional health, personal history, culture, and a host of other individual influences.

Still, gender may be the most crucial factor of all. It profoundly affects how we experience, communicate, and get care for pain. And there's experimental evidence that men and women may have different neuroanatomical and neurochemical pathways for processing, transmitting, and responding to pain.

HOW PAIN WORKS

What, then, is pain? The standard definition, developed by the International Association for the Study of Pain, is "an unpleasant sensory and emotional experience associated with actual or potential tissue damage or described in terms of such damage." But pain is much more than that. I consider pain the "fifth vital sign," along with blood pressure, temperature, respiratory rate, and pulse. It's a window into the body that shows whether something is awry, a sentinel that you should not ignore. Pain signals the possibility of lurking illness or pathology.

Acute and chronic pain are different. Simply put, acute pain flares up in response to a known cause and then it goes away, either in response to the body's own healing powers or with treatment. Not only is acute pain time-limited, but it also serves a purpose. Acute pain is how your body talks to you. Sometimes it's warning you that you're pushing yourself too hard— remember those sore legs the day after you first tried jogging? Or it may prod you to change your behavior. For example, mild back pain while sitting at your computer reminds you to shift your position or get up and take a break. And what compels you to snap your hand back from a hot stove? Searing pain. So important a messenger is acute pain that people born with a rare condition known as congenital insensitivity to pain suffer frequent injuries and tend to die early.

Chronic pain is another story. It's persistent, dragging on for weeks, months, or even years. And it's often a mystery. Chronic pain may be associated with a long-term incurable or intractable medical condition or disease, like cancer. Or a serious infection may be its initial trigger. Sometimes there's no identifiable cause at all. But for some reason the pain keeps going long after you've recovered from the original problem. And unlike acute pain, which is a biologically useful process, pain often loses its function when it becomes chronic. Worst of all, we can't treat the pain by removing or curing its cause.

RACHEL'S STORY

Rachel is a thirty-four-year-old homemaker with three kids under the age of six. She suffers from brutal migraines as well as severe dysmenorrhea, or menstrual cramps.

Because of the difficulties of raising three young children, as well as all of her other chores, Rachel's symptoms really get the best of her. Her husband is a surgeon and he keeps crazy hours, so she is unable to unload any of her responsibilities on him.

Never one to complain, Rachel came to me one day looking tired and weary. She had just made it through another week of migraines and menstrual cramps. "Doctor, I've tried to stay cheerful, but I have to confess that I'm beginning to get depressed. My headaches have gotten so much worse lately; I think it's the stress. And my cramps are just awful."

I conferred with her neurologist, who had seen her a few months earlier, when her headaches were much less severe. In addition, I repeated her neurological exam and she showed no abnormalities.

During the course of our conversation, I realized that Rachel's headaches seemed to coincide with her monthly cycle. When I mentioned this, she said, "You know, you're right. My worst headaches come a day or two before my period. I've often wondered why everything happens at once." This wasn't unusual, I explained to her. Many ailments seem to ebb and flow with the menstrual cycle, and migraines are high on that list. Although I understood how stressful her life was, fluctuations of estrogen and progesterone were probably playing the key role in her headaches.

I performed an acupuncture treatment utilizing the traditional cranial points, and showed her some acupressure points she could massage the next time she felt a migraine coming on. I also explained how she could fashion a warm compress steeped in the herb feverfew.

I suggested that Rachel start eating fish on a regular basis. Fish oil, rich in omega-3 fatty acids, is now being used to relieve menstrual cramps. It may also prevent the widening and narrowing of blood vessels that causes migraines.

To bolster her diet, I recommended Tums (calcium carbonate)

and magnesium supplements. These minerals work together to improve muscle tone, which can reduce cramping. And they seem to play an important, though as yet unexplained, role in reducing the frequency and duration of migraines. In addition, I told her, they would also help prevent osteoporosis. "Doctor, I'm too young and too busy to think about that, but I'll take your word for it," she laughed. Finally, I suggested that Rachel try SAMe (see page 94). I have had excellent success using this supplement. Not only does it help treat depression, there's also preliminary evidence that it relieves migraines.

If all else failed, I gave her a prescription for rofecoxib (Vioxx), which is approved by the FDA for dysmenorrhea. Rofecoxib is one of a new generation of pain relievers, called Cox-2 inhibitors, that cause fewer gastrointestinal side effects. It's also an all-purpose pain reliever, so it would help her migraines, too.

Several months later Rachel checked in with me by phone. "Things are so much better I don't need to come back," she said.

NOCICEPTORS, NERVES, AND PAIN

Although we don't completely understand pain, we've learned an enormous amount over the last few decades. And new techniques continue to stretch the frontiers of scientific exploration. We can now look at images of brain activity in awake human subjects as they perceive pain. Some researchers are revealing special pathways and chemicals involved in pain, and performing cellular analyses of the molecular signals that transmit and receive the pain message. And on every level, men and women appear to be different.

Pain occurs in response to a possibly harmful stimulus, such as a burn or a pinch. It's a complicated drama with many actors directed by the central nervous system—the brain and spinal cord. Nociceptors (from the Latin *noceo*, "hurt," and *capio*, "receive") are unique receptors in the skin and most other tissues. They are the first link in the chain of neurophysiological events that ultimately ends when you perceive pain. Some nociceptors react to several kinds of painful stimulation; others are pickier and respond to heat, perhaps, but not to a pinprick. When these small nerve endings are activated by something painful, they transmit signals through the nerves in the spinal cord to the brain, leading to pain.

Certain sharp pain signals are routed immediately. When you stub your toe, for example, your body instantaneously flashes an emergency bulletin.

Less urgent news—duller, more persistent pain—travels on an alternative, slower pathway.

Activated nociceptors also trigger the release of chemicals, such as prostaglandins, serotonin, and histamine, that are associated with pain and inflammation. And they alert the autonomic nervous system, which regulates involuntary processes such as breathing, blood flow, pulse rate, and the release of hormones like epinephrine (adrenaline).

But let's get back to the nervous system, the neurological hardwiring that allows you to perceive pain. Nerve cells, or neurons, form a highly organized, complex web of nerves throughout the body, extending to the toes and fingers as well as to the heart, liver, lung, and other inner organs. Nerves are constantly gathering information and transmitting it to control central— the spinal cord and brain.

Nerve cells are different from other body cells; they have projections on both ends. At one end is the long, thin axon, and at the other is a shorter, more branching projection called a dendrite. These are the live wires of the nervous system. Each nerve cell is a link in a chain, with its axon in close contact, but not actually touching, the dendrite of the next nerve cell in the chain.

Nerve cells transmit information through electrochemical impulses that travel in one direction only, from axon to dendrite. When an impulse reaches the gap, or synapse, between the axon of one nerve cell and the dendrite of the next, the axon secretes a chemical substance known as a neurotransmitter to bridge the gap.

The speed and complexity of the nervous system is mind-boggling. It takes only about one thousandth of a second for an impulse to jump the gap. And a single nerve cell in the brain may have 50,000 dendrites and communicate with 250,000 other neurons.

When a painful event stimulates the nociceptors, they trigger a cascade of events by sending messages through the nervous system and up the spinal cord to several places in the brain. Some of the brain regions that receive pain signals are also involved in perception, emotion, and movement. The brain responds, sending signals through a different nerve pathway back down to the spinal cord. Recall our example of a hot stove; when you touch it, your brain directs you to move your hand. Your brain's nerve cells may also trigger the release of endorphins, the body's natural painkillers. These actually reduce pain and create a temporary sense of well-being. I'll get back to endorphins shortly.

Our knowledge of gender-related differences in nociceptive, or pain, processing is still in its infancy. But thrilling new research in animals and humans indicates that men and women differ greatly. There are probably distinctions caused not only by hormonal differences but also in the actual biochemical pathways men and women use to process pain. Here are some key findings:

- Estrogen alters the receptive properties of important nerves, and there is also clear evidence that pregnancy and progesterone affect nerve conduction.
- Sex hormones influence many central nervous system pathways involved in pain transmission.
- Electrophysiological and brain imaging studies indicate that sex differences occur at many stages of pain processing.
- Hormones also affect levels of serotonin and other transmitters, as well as other biochemicals involved in processing pain.
- Hormones may affect nociceptor receptivity; for example, nociceptors may be sensitized by ovarian hormones. In addition, the central nervous system pain circuitry may vary, depending on where you are in your menstrual cycle.

OPENING AND CLOSING THE GATE

In 1965, researchers Patrick Wall and Ronald Melzack proposed a novel explanation of how pain works. Their gate-control theory suggested that whether you experience pain depends on the balance between nonpainful information traveling into the spinal cord through large nerve fibers, and the pain signals traveling on small nerve fibers. When the activity in these small nerve fibers reaches a certain level, a "gate" opens, allowing pain signals to continue on to the brain.

Wall and Melzack also speculated that the body has its own ways to suppress pain. For example, large nerves that are stimulated by nonpainful touching or pressing of the skin send signals to the brain more quickly; once they get there, they slam the gate closed, keeping out pain signals. This explains why rubbing your twisted ankle lessens your pain: rubbing excites nerve cells sensitive to touch and pressure that can suppress pain signals from other cells.

What fascinated researchers and led to a spate of important discoveries was the idea that the gate could also be closed from above. In other words, the brain might have its own ways to block pain messages.

Neuroscientists already knew that chemicals were involved in conducting nerve signals. (Recall that neurotransmitters help messages cross the gap between two nerve cells.) Now researchers began to wonder how opioids—

morphine and other highly effective painkilling drugs derived from opium — worked. When they injected morphine into experimental animals, they found that the morphine molecules fit into receptors on certain brain and spinal cord neurons just as a key fits into a lock, opening the door to pain relief.

The researchers may have figured out how morphine did its job, but their work raised an even more puzzling question: Why would the human brain have receptors for a man-made drug? Solving this mystery revealed the existence of a whole family of naturally occurring brain chemicals that behave exactly like morphine and inhibit pain. There are a number of such neurotransmitters, but we use the term *endorphins*, meaning "the morphine within," to describe them all.

Laboratory experiments have shown that painful stimulation causes the brain to release endorphins, which then circulate in the spinal cord. Receptor sites for endorphins have been found throughout the body. Endorphins do more than suppress pain. You're probably familiar with the term *runner's high*. Endorphins also affect mood and perception. And exercise is a surefire way to get your brain to release endorphins. So the brain does indeed have a built-in mechanism for closing the pain gate. In fact, it probably has more than one. Besides the opioid system I just described, we probably have another, nonopioid circuit that blocks pain information from reaching the brain. Today, we're learning that these pain-inhibiting pathways are distinct in men and women. On an intuitive level, this makes sense, since in various areas of the brain, the neurons involved in modulating pain overlap with brain receptors for sex hormones. In addition, in some studies of mice, both males and females turn on pain-inhibiting systems when they are stressed. However, it appears that females have an additional pathway for blocking pain perception. Perhaps this evolved as a way to ease the pain associated with childbirth.

Whatever the explanations of these differences turn out to be, they have important ramifications when it comes to pain medication. Already, we know that men and women respond differently to certain types of painkillers. For this reason, it's critical that we include gender in clinical research!

PAIN IN THE BRAIN

Short circuits can occur in any electrical system, and this may be what is going on if you have chronic pain. Scientists believe that nociceptors can get stuck in an "on" mode. In extreme cases, they may become so hypersensitive that even a breeze or a gentle touch to the affected area can cause pain.

We're also beginning to untangle other mechanisms of chronic pain. We know now, for example, that nerve injury may alter how nociceptors respond to noradrenaline, a neurotransmitter used by nerve cells to communicate. And we're also discovering that the body develops long-term memories of pain that can interfere with a healthy response to pain and to pain relief therapies. In some people with chronic pain, it appears that a particular part of the brain's cortex that is involved with pain gets reorganized. As one investigator puts it, in addition to pain at the original site of injury, there is "pain in the brain." Whatever the cause, chronic pain is so real and so enervating that it should probably be viewed not as a symptom but as a disease.

Understanding the basic mechanisms of pain is just the beginning. In the following chapters, I'll show you how you can take charge of your pain with remedies specifically tailored to your needs as a woman.

PART
II

THE MANY
FACES
OF PAIN

4

The Hormonal Connection

Some painful conditions are an inescapable part of the reproductive life cycle, and they can cause ongoing, recurring pain along with the great joys of childbearing and motherhood. In this chapter, you'll find information about problems related to menstruation, such as premenstrual syndrome and cramps. I'll also go into breast and pelvic pain, pregnancy, labor and childbirth, and menopause. As a physiatrist, my interest in these issues first grew out of my work with women with spinal cord injury and other chronic disabilities as they faced these challenges.

Because there is no "cure" per se for most of these conditions, my focus will be on prevention and relief of painful symptoms.

(*Note to the Reader*: If there is any chance that you may be pregnant, please consult with your doctor before trying any of these remedies. Good communication between you and your primary medical doctor or obstetrician/gynecologist regarding all medical concerns is imperative.)

PREMENSTRUAL SYNDROME (PMS)

ANNIE'S STORY

Annie, a successful thirty-four-year-old computer consultant, suffered from intense back and neck pain compounded by her full-blown premenstrual syndrome. She was referred to me by her gynecologist. At her first visit, she told me she was at her "wit's end." Although she managed to hold herself together at work, her symptoms were getting the better of her at home. During the week before her period, her back pain flared up, causing her to be irritable with her husband. And, to her intense dismay, she found herself blowing up at her two young children over trifling incidents. In addition to moodiness, she struggled with appetite changes, cravings for sweet and salty foods, and cramping. Her chronic neck and back pain worsened and she also had trouble sleeping. "Sometimes, during those last few days before my period, I feel like I'm going to jump out of my skin," she said.

Annie had tried conventional therapies but had only gotten limited relief. She was hesitant about trying the hormonal treatment her gynecologist had recommended. She was worried about possible side effects and the long-term consequences. Besides, like many women, she'd much rather use a natural remedy than a pharmaceutical one.

Because it is a recurring ailment and there is no "cure," I told Annie that we needed to attack her PMS in a holistic fashion, using diet, exercise, and other simple lifestyle changes that she could maintain over the long term. After discussing my game plan with her gynecologist, I advised her to maintain an adequate fluid intake by keeping a pitcher of water on her desk at work and making sure she drank at least eight eight-ounce glasses, every day. To ensure that she had an adequate intake of calcium, magnesium, and vitamin E, which help fight PMS symptoms, we discussed how she could include more whole grains, fruits, and vegetables as well as other nutrient-rich foods in her diet. Because there is evidence that the essential fatty acids found in fish oil may be helpful, I also encouraged her to eat salmon, tuna, or other "oily" fish several times a week. And I explained the growing evidence that the phytoestrogens in soy foods help address PMS and other hormonal ailments. I also suggested that she cut back on starchy carbohydrate-laden foods.

Irritability, insomnia, and moodiness were big concerns for Annie. We tried simple measures first—cutting back on caffeine and taking warm aromatherapy baths with a few drops of lavender oil. I also gave her a couple of relaxation tapes to try, and recommended a gentle exercise program she could do at home, using a stationary bicycle at low resistive settings.

Annie tried everything I suggested, but at her next visit she told me: "I like the relaxation tapes, but I just don't have the time to do both them and the bicycle regularly. Is there anything else I can try for the irritability and depression?" I recommended St. John's wort, a mild herbal medication that eases anxiety and depression. (Annie was not taking antidepressants, nor did she need to.)

There's a strong connection between emotions and pain, so I knew that tackling Annie's depression and moodiness would also reduce the intensity of her cramps. And for the times when she was actually in pain, I suggested some alternative pain relief strategies. Annie was a big classical music fan, so I advised her to lie down with a warm, moist towel on her belly, listen to her favorite symphonies, and do deep yoga breathing. I also showed her how to use a reflexology point (by pressing on a specific point on the hands, ears, or feet, you can affect related organs in other parts of the body) to ease cramping. At work, when some of these techniques were impractical, she could still rely on Motrin or other pain relievers.

Over time, Annie continued to have PMS, but the intensity of her symptoms decreased significantly. "The cramps are better, the neck and back pain has subsided, and I'm not nearly as ferocious," she said. "Best of all, my husband and kids have noticed the difference. They no longer avoid me one week a month."

PMS Description

This bothersome monthly malady has been recognized since antiquity. It's linked to fluctuations in hormone levels, including estrogen and progesterone. PMS is an annoying cluster of painful physical and emotional symptoms that occurs during the luteal phase of a woman's menstrual cycle—the latter half of the cycle, or the time between ovulation and the start of bleeding. Your symptoms may begin from two to fourteen days before menstruation starts and should improve shortly after you have begun to bleed. PMS symptoms are absent during the early part of the menstrual cycle.

Researchers have cataloged more than 150 different PMS symptoms. Just as the length and severity of every woman's menstrual cycle varies, PMS has a mind of its own and behaves differently in every woman. Still, it's a nearly universal problem: A recent study reported that 30 to 80 percent of women are affected to some degree by PMS.

Despite the broad array of symptoms, pain is at the heart of PMS because symptoms like breast tenderness and abdominal and pelvic cramping are often the most vexing. Moreover, PMS may also exacerbate existing musculoskeletal pain and aggravate other ailments. If you have carpal tunnel syndrome, for example, the swelling and bloating of PMS can put pressure on your nerves and make it worse. Most of the prescription medications women take for PMS are for pain.

The National Institutes of Health (NIH) and the University of California have formulated well-accepted criteria for the diagnosis of PMS. In addition, PMDS, premenstrual dysphoric disorder, is recognized as a psychiatric disorder and included in the DSM-IV, the bible of psychiatric diagnosis. Yet PMS is not always taken seriously. Many women are still told "it's all in your head," and it's the focus of a lot of jokes. What's more, PMS sufferers are all too often urged to "wait it out" or to "grin and bear it." As a result, many women—as many as 81 percent in one study—look to self-help remedies and complementary providers to ease their symptoms.

Causes

Hormones are chemical messengers produced by glands and organs that are transported through the bloodstream to target organs. They are the major drivers of physiological changes in the body. Menstrual hormones like estrogen, progesterone, luteinizing hormone, and follicle stimulating hormone play an important role in orchestrating the menstrual cycle. Although it was once considered a psychiatric condition, we now believe that PMS is caused by fluctuations in the hormone levels that occur during the menstrual cycle, specifically from a change in the ratio of progesterone to estrogen. Research has also shown that serotonin, the well-known mood modulating brain chemical, may be reduced in women during the premenstrual phase of the menstrual cycle. If you are depressed and moody before your period, this might explain why.

Signs and Symptoms

The most common PMS symptoms are:

- Abdominal cramps
- Pelvic discomfort
- Headaches
- Backaches
- Other musculoskeletal pain (joint, neck, muscle aches)
- Breast tenderness and swelling
- Weight gain and bloating
- Mood swings (irritability, anger, depression, anxiety)
- Fatigue
- Difficulty concentrating
- Sleep disorder
- Lethargy
- Appetite changes (food cravings for carbohydrates or sweets, especially chocolate)
- Acne

Keep a Pain Diary

Use a calendar to track when your symptoms begin and end, as well as their severity. If you have PMS, your symptoms will occur during the two weeks before your period *and* they will disappear after your period starts. A diary will also help you learn your body's biological timing. If you can predict when you will have the worst symptoms, you can make adjustments to your schedule, saving big projects or major social events for a better time.

Conventional Treatments

PMS is short-lived and self-correcting, but it comes back every month. Over-the-counter (OTC) drugs can improve some symptoms. You may have success using Tylenol, Advil, and other analgesics for muscle, neck, back, and joint pain. However, Tylenol can cause liver damage and Advil and other so-called NSAIDS have been linked to stomach and gastrointestinal ulcers, kidney damage, and bleeding disorders.

Despite the severity and diversity of symptoms, there are few tried-and-true "shotgun" approaches for PMS. Nor is there widespread consensus about its appropriate management, even among health professionals. Once you get beyond the OTC medications, your options are likely to include a broad array of prescription medications, each dealing with one aspect of PMS. (Bear in mind, however, that most of these drugs have side effects. For example, diuretics rob the body of potassium; antianxiety drugs may be habit forming and cause sleepiness or seizures, and antidepressants can cause weight changes. Be sure to ask your doctor about possible side effects or interactions with other drugs you may be taking.)

Your doctor may prescribe prostaglandin inhibitor medications, like Motrin, if you suffer from disabling menstrual spasms and cramps (dysmenorrhea). Recently there has been a growing body of literature on the benefits of Cox-2 inhibitor drugs, a new class of NSAIDS. Currently, rofecoxib (Vioxx) is the only Cox-2 drug that has been approved by the FDA for dysmenorrhea. Many women also report that Celebrex (celecoxib), the other drug in this class, is helpful. Other "boutique" anti-inflammatory drugs are in the pipeline.

If you get migraines (see Chapter 9), the risk of getting a headache increases in the four days before your period starts. For severe headaches, your physician may prescribe medications known as beta-blockers or calcium channel blockers.

Some doctors prescribe diuretics (water pills) to minimize water retention and bloating. If you have severe symptoms, including anxiety, your doctor may suggest an antianxiety drug such as Xanax (alprazolam). When depression or moodiness is the problem, he or she may suggest one of the SSRI (see page 316) antidepressant medications, which have been touted to address the emotional issues that so often accompany PMS. One drug in particular, Sarafem, has earned FDA approval. However, Sarafem is the same as Prozac (fluoxetine hydrochloride).

Some doctors prescribe oral contraceptives to regulate hormonal shifts. And in very severe cases of PMS, gonadotropin-releasing hormone agonists—drugs that eliminate the menstrual cycle entirely—are a radical but sometimes used strategy.

Dietary Strategies (See Chapter 14 for food sources of specified nutrients)

- Overall, a well-balanced diet that emphasizes vegetables, fruits, and whole grains is beneficial.
- Eat a diet that maintains an optimal ratio of estrogen and progesterone. Two simple measures include reducing your consumption of simple carbohydrates (sugars) and cutting back on meat and saturated fat. Simple carbohydrates may lead to fluctuations in blood sugar levels resulting in hypoglycemia (low blood sugar). Hypoglycemia can trigger adrenaline release, which can interfere with the function of progesterone. Studies have proven that there is a strong association between PMS and eating a lot of sugary food. And excessive ingestion of meat and saturated fat may raise blood estrogen levels.
- Diets high in fiber can help promote bowel regularity, thereby reducing the risk of abdominal cramping and constipation, which can worsen your menstrual cramps.
- Reduce salt, which can increase bloating, water retention, and weight gain.
- Alcohol, tea, coffee, and other caffeinated beverages increase your risk of PMS.
- Use a lot of parsley to battle bloating and fluid buildup.
- Calcium, magnesium, and vitamins E, B6, and A have all been shown to reduce PMS symptoms.

Supplements

Although we don't yet know precisely how they work, these vitamin and mineral supplements have been shown to help PMS symptoms.

Vitamin A
Vitamin A is thought to increase progesterone levels. High doses of vitamin A can be toxic; the acceptable dose range is 900 to 3,000 mcg.

Vitamin B6
By promoting the production of their building blocks (tryptophan, tyrosine, and glutamate), B6 may enhance the release of important neurotransmitters, including serotonin, dopamine, and norepinephrine. Deficiencies of these brain chemicals may influence other important chemical messengers, such as prolactin and aldosterone, causing fluid retention and breast pain. B6 may also reduce some of the effects of estrogen. The recommended range is 2 to 100 mg a day. Excessive B6 can cause neurological problems in some people.

Magnesium
A study published in *Obstetrics and Gynecology* in 1991 indicated that magnesium could help the pain associated with PMS, and several other small double-blind randomized studies also support its value in beating this ailment. We also know that women with PMS have low levels of magnesium in their red blood cells. Magnesium supplementation may have an impact on PMS through a variety of mechanisms: It is important in regulating blood vessel tone, in serotonin and neurotransmitter activity, and in cell membrane stability. The accepted range is 320 to 350 mg a day.

Vitamin E
This vitamin helps prevent breast tenderness and minimizes PMS. The accepted range is 15 to 1,000 mg a day.

Chromium
An essential trace mineral, chromium helps regulate sugar levels in the body and may reduce sugar cravings. The recommended daily intake is 25 mcg. No safe upper limit has been established.

Calcium
Calcium plays a role in skeletal and smooth muscle function, neurotransmitter release, and many other bodily processes. It can keep menstrual cramps in check by helping to regulate muscle tone. I strongly endorse the use of calcium supplements for menstrual cramps. Calcium carbonate (Tums) is the most economical commercial calcium supplement and it has the added bonus of being an antacid. A 1998 study by Dr. Susan Thy-

Jacobs in the *American Journal of Obstetrics and Gynecology* showed that women who took calcium carbonate for three menstrual cycles experienced a 54 percent reduction in PMS symptoms including abdominal cramping, generalized aches, and low back pain; women in the control group had only a 15 percent reduction in their symptoms.

Calcium supplementation is generally thought to be safe in women who may become pregnant. Since many scientific studies have shown that calcium deficiency is linked to PMS, there has been much speculation about the relationship between PMS and other calcium-related disorders, such as osteoporosis. To date, at least two studies have shown an association between PMS and reduced bone mass and osteoporosis in women, raising the possibility that low calcium may be an early warning sign of potential future difficulties. (See Chapter 6 for more information on osteoporosis.)

The acceptable daily dose range for calcium is 1,300 to 2,500 mg.

Long-chain fatty acids (Essential Fatty Acids, or EFAs)

Evening primrose oil, borage oil, black currant oil, grapeseed oil, and flaxseed oil are all high in gamma-linolenic acid, which contributes to the body's production of prostaglandin PGE1, a potent anti-inflammatory. Besides their value in PMS, EFAs may reduce the pain of fibrocystic breast disease, as well as lower a woman's risk of heart disease. Recommended dose is 3,000 to 4,000 mg a day.

B Complex

One to two tablets a day may reduce cramping and other PMS symptoms.

Manganese

This trace element (metal) is found in small amounts in human tissue. It helps create connective tissue, blood clotting factors, fats, and cholesterol. In a 1993 study, women on a diet low in manganese had increased premenstrual pain symptoms and mood changes compared to women placed on a high-manganese diet. The acceptable range is 1.8 to 11.0 mg a day. *Warning*: Manganese can be toxic in large amounts.

Herbs

Chaste tree (Vitex agnus-castus)

A study published in the April 2000 issue of the *Journal of Women's Health and Gender-Based Medicine* reported that after three months of using *Vitex* daily, 93 percent of the women studied had improvements in PMS symptoms of depression, anxiety, cravings, and breast pain. More recently, in results of a double-blind trial, published in the *British Medical Journal*, a majority of women taking *Vitex* for three menstrual cycles reported a 50 percent or more improvement in PMS symptoms. This herb is approved in Germany to reduce symptoms of PMS. The recommended daily dose is 30 to 40 mg in an aqueous-alcohol extract. Do not use chaste tree if you may be pregnant or if you are nursing.

Black cohosh (Cimicifuga racemosa)

This popular herbal remedy is thought to work by binding to estrogen receptors, thereby balancing your hormones. A native American herb, it is used extensively by women in Europe, especially Germany, to treat a variety of PMS symptoms. Although the doses of this herb are not standardized, the German Commission E recommends taking an alcohol extract of 40 percent. This corresponds to 40 mg a day.

Kava kava (Piper methysticum)

This is an herbal alternative for treating tension and anxiety, common features of PMS. The accepted dose range is 60 to 120 mg a day, when needed. CAUTION: This herb may interact with Xanax (alprazolam).

Valerian (Valeriana officinalis)

This is another useful herb that relieves insomnia and anxiety. The accepted dose is an infusion, made by adding 2 or 3 grams of herb to 150 ml of hot water, steeping for 10 to 15 minutes, and straining before use. To simplify things, I recommend commercial teas, such as Dr. Stuart's, Traditional Medicinals, or Yogi Tea. Drink one cup before bedtime.

St. Johns wort (Hypericum perforatum)

One of the best studied herbal remedies, St. John's wort is effective in the treatment of mild to moderate depression, although its value in treating severe depression has recently been questioned. Herbalists recommend drinking one cup of infusion three times a day. To make the infusion, use 2 teaspoons of herb in 150 ml of boiling water and steep for 10 minutes. Do not take this herb with other antidepressants.

Yarrow (Achillea millefolium)

This herb has been traditionally used throughout Europe to relieve menstrual ailments with its anti-inflammatory effects. We believe it's named in honor of Achilles of Greece, who used it to help his bleeding soldiers. You can drink yarrow as a tea or use it in your bath to treat menstrual spasms. To make the tea, steep 1 to 2 teaspoons in a cup of boiling water. Try several cups a day just before and during the first day or two of your period.

Do-It-Yourself

Yarrow sitz bath

A warm sitz bath is particularly helpful for painful ovaries or uterine cramps. Fill the bathtub so the water covers your hips and reaches the middle of your belly. Soak in the warm water two to three times a day for ten to fifteen minutes. To further decrease pain and cramps, add a yarrow infusion as you run the water for the bath. You can make the infusion by adding 15 grams of herb to one gallon of water. You may want to cover your upper body with a towel to stay warm.

Reflexology

In a solid, credible study, women treated with true reflexology (see page 353 for reflexology technique) had a more dramatic reduction in PMS symptoms than women who were given "sham" reflexology treatments. The difference in symptomatic relief persisted for two months after treatment.

For PMS or menstrual cramps, try these points:

- SP-1 (also known as Spleen-1 in acupuncture parlance) is located at the great toe, along the midline portion of the nail bed. This point helps relieve spasms in the uterus.
- SP-6 is located behind the tibia (shin bone) approximately four finger widths above the inner portion of the ankle. It may help to normalize menstrual flow and promote relaxation. Avoid this point if you may be pregnant.
- LI-4 (Large Intestine 4) is in the space between the thumb and second finger. It relieves uterine spasms. Avoid this point if you may be pregnant.

Contrast baths

Contrast baths relax cramps and spasms by quieting down uterine contractions. Alternate a five-minute warm-water bath (choose your own temperature comfort level) with a one-minute cold bath. To the warm water, add five drops of a fragrant essential oil such as mandarin tangerine (*Citrus reticulata*), which has a refreshing scent. Or try camomile, which is gentle, antiseptic, and relaxing. You can repeat this process four times.

Warm heat towel
Applying moist, warm heat to your belly and pelvis is a particularly soothing way to tame the spasms and contractions caused by your period. Take a thick towel and drench it in hot water. Wait for it to cool down, and then wring it dry and apply it. If you prefer the convenience of a pre-packaged, portable hot towel, you can buy a therapeutic heat wrap product called Thermacare, which uses air-activated heat discs that give off a low-level, penetrating heat lasting eight hours.

Mind/Body

Guided imagery and relaxation therapy
In a study published in the *Journal of Holistic Nursing*, researchers found that, when used for six months, progressive muscle relaxation followed by guided imagery lengthened and regulated women's menstrual cycles and diminished premenstrual distress. Other studies have also demonstrated the value of deep breathing and progressive relaxation (see page 340 for instructions).

Exercise

A considerable amount of evidence shows that regular exercise—specifically, aerobic exercise such as running, brisk walking, biking, or swimming—decreases depression. Studies dealing specifically with PMS confirm this and also show that aerobic exercise reduces fluid retention and breast tenderness. In addition, it may minimize cramping by relaxing muscles and by bringing better blood circulation and more oxygen to your pelvis. Your baseline should be at least thirty to forty-five minutes of aerobic exercise three times a week; aim to exercise daily during your period.

Seeking Help from Complementary Practitioners

Massage
One recently published study of twenty-four women with diagnosed PMS compared the effects of massage and relaxation therapy. Women in the massage group had less anxiety, depression, and pain. And in the long term, massage reduced water retention, pain, and overall PMS distress.

Red Flags

Check in with your doctor if you experience:

- Excessive bleeding
- Abdominal cramping associated with excessive discomfort
- Fever or chills
- Vaginal discharge
- Urinary frequency
- Bowel changes
- Pain during or after intercourse

DYSMENORRHEA (CRAMPS)

Description

If you get cramps with your period, you're not alone. At least half of menstruating women have dysmenorrhea, the medical term for menstrual cramps. There are two types. Primary dysmenorrhea, with its crampy abdominal pains, typically appears in adolescence and can be severe enough to affect your quality of life; it's a major cause of work and school absenteeism. In contrast, secondary dysmenorrhea occurs as a result of endometriosis or some other cause, and starts later in life.

Causes

During your period, your uterus normally has painless, rhythmic contractions. If you have dysmenorrhea, however, an excess of a certain type of prostaglandin (hormonelike substances found throughout the body) causes these contractions to become longer and tighter. This results in ischemia, or decreased oxygen going to the uterine muscles, and that causes pain.

Conventional Treatments

Since uterine prostaglandins are thought to play a role in its contractions, prostaglandin inhibitors are a logical means for decreasing cramps. The NSAIDS fill this role. Although they are expensive, the Cox-2 inhibitor-type nonsteroidals are an especially safe choice because they have fewer effects on the stomach lining, so they reduce the risk of bleeding complications.

Dietary Strategies (See Chapter 14 for food sources of specified nutrients)

- Some studies have found niacin (a B vitamin) to be helpful in relieving menstrual cramps.
- Fish oil and vitamin B12 reduce menstrual cramps. In a study published in 2000, Danish researchers gave four groups of women five capsules a day of fish oil, fish oil with vitamin B12, seal oil, or a placebo. The women were followed for three menstrual cycles. The results? Compared with the placebo group, the group receiving fish oil had less menstrual pain. And the women who took fish oil with B12 had the best results—substantial relief from pain and discomfort.
- Vitamin C is a powerful antioxidant. It decreases lethargy and fatigue and improves the supply of blood to your uterine muscles.
- Be especially careful to avoid foods to which you're allergic; food allergies can contribute to water retention, gas, and bloating, which may intensify your cramps.
- Eat enough fruits, vegetables, and other fiber to maintain regular bowel habits, which can also ease dysmenorrhea.
- Eat raspberries to crimp cramps.

Supplements

Fish oils
So significant were the results in the Danish study described above that the researchers concluded that supplements of fish oil and B12 may serve as an alternative to NSAIDS in treating dysmenorrhea. Although I believe your best bet is eating fish three times a week, you can take fish oil supplements along with vitamin B12 daily.

Calcium
Calcium helps muscle tone, which can reduce cramping. In addition, low calcium intake may contribute to water retention and increased menstrual pain. The acceptable dose range is 1,300 to 2,500 mg a day.

Vitamin E
Vitamin E can help treat menstrual cramps. It can also cut back on breast symptoms. The acceptable dose range is 15 to 1,000 mg a day.

Vitamin C

An antioxidant, vitamin C improves blood flow, nourishes the uterine muscles, and relieves fatigue. The acceptable dose range is 90 to 2,000 mg a day.

Iron

Iron helps enhance the oxygen-carrying ability of your blood. The recommended dose range for premenopausal women is 18 to 45 mg a day.

Vitamin B complex

This is a group of many different vitamins. They play a role in glucose and amino acid metabolism, cell division, and many other biochemical processes. Both B6 (pyridoxine) and B3 (niacin) may be helpful for cramps. Human needs for members of the B complex vary considerably. The best way to make sure you're getting the right amounts is to take a multiple vitamin/mineral product containing the B complex. If you have liver disease, check with your physician before taking a supplement containing niacin.

Magnesium

This mineral works synergistically with calcium, helping to regulate neuromuscular tone. The accepted dose range is 320 to 350 mg a day.

Herbs

Red raspberry (Rubus idaeus)

Red raspberry leaf can relieve menstrual cramps. Herbalists suggest trying this as a tea, brewed using half a teaspoon of herb for each cup of water, once or twice a day.

Black cohosh (Cimicifuga racemosa)

Although this herb can be taken daily to prevent PMS, it is also useful for relieving cramps. The doses of this herb are not standardized, but the German Commission E recommends taking an alcohol extract of 40 percent. This corresponds to 40 mg a day.

Valerian (Valeriana officinalis)

Used mostly as a sedative, this herb also reduces muscular contractions. To make an infusion add 2 or 3 grams of herb to 150 ml of hot water and steep for 10 to 15 minutes. Strain before use. The recommended dose is one cup before bedtime.

Do-It-Yourself

Contrast baths (See page 50)

Massage
You'll need a friend or partner to help you with this simple abdominal pain reliever. Lie on your back, flat on the floor. Your partner should kneel by your head, sliding his hands under your back so they meet at your spine; then, pull them out toward your hips. Next, he should firmly pull his hands over your waist and gently draw them back to their starting position. Repeat. Your partner now puts his hands on your belly and circles them in a clockwise direction. Repeat this action, using the fingers to go deeper as long as this isn't painful. Finally, the partner puts his hands over your navel; he should relax and send calming thoughts through his arms and hands into your body.

Aromatherapy
Use essential oils made from lavender, jasmine, or rose in your massage oil, your bath, or in a diffuser.

TENS (transcutaneous electrical nerve stimulator)
TENS — applying brief pulses of electricity to nerve endings under the skin — is a relatively new pain treatment. Although this is a conventional treatment, often performed in a physician's or physical therapist's office, you can buy home units. A Swedish study published in the *American Journal of Obstetrics and Gynecology* showed that treatment with TENS reduced pain and did not increase cramps.

Reflexology (See page 50)

Posture
Good posture may reduce your tendency to have menstrual cramps.

IUDs
Menstrual cramps can be worse if you use an IUD for contraception. You may want to consider an alternate method of birth control.

Mind/Body

Biofeedback (See page 341 for technique)
You can effectively use mind-body techniques such as biofeedback to influence subconscious (autonomic) processes. There are even computer programs and electronic devices you can buy to perform biofeedback in your own home.

Yoga (See pages 344–351 for postures)
The Locust Pose helps relieve pain.

Exercise

Aerobic exercise
Women who get regular aerobic exercise, including brisk walking, biking, running, or swimming, have reduced menstrual pain. Exercise improves blood flow to the uterus and strengthens pelvic muscles. It promotes the release of endorphins, which are natural painkillers, and also provides immeasurable psychological benefits (the "runner's high"). Aim for thirty to forty-five minutes of aerobic exercise three to five times a week.

Other exercises
Some exercises can be done around the house without special equipment. My patients find that these are energizing and bring about relaxation.

EXERCISE 1
Stand with your legs 2 feet apart and your feet directed out. Gradually bend your knees and lower your bottom until your buttocks are as low as your knees. Cycle up and down about 15 times. You may also swing your pelvis forward and backward in a regular fashion. (*Note:* Avoid this if you have knee problems.)

EXERCISE 2
Stand in an upright position. Lift one knee up and, at the same time, bend both arms up and outward. Lower your foot to the floor and bring the other knee up while bending your arms up and out again. Repeat this sequence 10 to 12 times.

EXERCISE 3

Increase the blood flow to your pelvis with this simple exercise, which involves circling your hips: Stand with your feet about hip width apart. With hands on your hips, circle your hips 5 times in one direction; then reverse. Repeat.

Seeking Help from Complementary Practitioners

Acupuncture

A study published in 1987 by the world-famous acupuncturist-physician Joseph Helms compared four groups of women who received, respectively, acupuncture, sham acupuncture, extra office visits, or no intervention. Ninety-one percent of the women who got acupuncture cut their monthly pain by half, while only 36 percent of the women in the control groups improved. In addition, the women in the acupuncture group used 41 percent less painkilling medication in the nine months following treatment.

Also, the consensus panel of the NIH has found acupuncture to be effective in the treatment of menstrual cramps and PMS.

Red Flags

- Excessive bleeding
- Abdominal cramping associated with excessive discomfort
- Fever or chills
- Vaginal discharge
- Urinary frequency
- Bowel changes
- Pain during or after intercourse

BREAST PAIN (MASTODYNIA OR MASTALGIA)

Description

In 1829, Sir Ashley Cooper attributed mastodynia to psychological factors, claiming that breast pain occurred in nervous and irritable women. Today we know differently. I have many active, healthy women patients who come to see me for sports injuries. After examining their ankles, knees, or whatever has brought them in, I usually ask, "Does it hurt anywhere else when you exercise?" And many of them mention that they have sore, tender breasts, particularly around the time of their periods.

Causes

There are three types of breast pain: cyclic, noncyclic, and nonbreast in origin. Cyclic breast pain, which is what we deal with in this chapter, is the most common, affecting as many as 67 percent of women. Sir Cooper notwithstanding, it is hormonal changes that cause cyclic breast pain. The pain fluctuates with the menstrual cycle and it affects both breasts. Typically, your breasts worsen during the luteal phase of your cycle, and the pain and soreness reach their peak as your period begins.

Noncyclic mastodynia affects only one in ten women. It bears no relationship to the menstrual cycle; the drawing, burning, achy, or throbbing pain may be constant throughout the month or intermittent with periodic exacerbations.

Mastodynia that is nonbreast in origin has several causes. Costochondritis is diffuse, localized, noncyclic pain in the mid-chest that may radiate to the underarm or back. Deep pressure on the area usually makes the pain worse. We usually treat it with lidocaine injections. Other reasons for noncyclic breast pain include cervical radiculopathy, or compression of a nerve root, angina, rib fracture, gallbladder or peptic ulcer disease.

Signs and Symptoms

· Nodularity (lumpiness) of both breasts
· Diffuse tenderness or heaviness
· Soreness
· Fluctuating severity
· Pain may radiate to underarm, arm, or elbow

Conventional Treatments

A wide range of OTC and prescription drugs are used to treat cyclic breast pain. Besides diuretics, there are a variety of hormone treatments, including oral contraceptives, hormone replacement therapy, progesterone and thyroid hormones, tamoxifen, and gonadotrophin-releasing hormone agonists. Your doctor might also prescribe bromocriptine, which treats excessive levels of prolactin, a pituitary hormone that can cause breast pain. Because of its severe side effects, danazol, a synthetic male hormone available only by prescription, is used only in severe cases.

Dietary Strategies (See Chapter 14 for food sources of specified nutrients)

- Eliminate caffeine, which can make your symptoms worse.
- Vitamins E, A, and B6 may help reduce the pain.
- There is some evidence that reducing dietary fat decreases breast swelling, pain, and lumpiness.

RECIPE

DUTCH COLLARD GREENS WITH CREAMY MASHED POTATOES

Collard greens, like other members of the cruciferous family of vegetables, are rich in the protective phytochemicals indoles and glucosinolates. In addition to their anticancer benefits, these compounds suppress free radical formation, so they are useful for joint pain and inflammation. Collards are also rich in beta-carotene, vitamin E, zinc, calcium, manganese, and iron.

2 pounds new potatoes
2 tablespoons Spectrum Spread
1 cup fortified soy milk
1 tablespoon olive oil
1 sweet onion, chopped
4 cloves garlic, chopped
1 pound collard greens, coarsely chopped
3 green onions, chopped
½ teaspoon pepper

1. Wash the new potatoes and trim off imperfections, leaving the skins on. Cut the potatoes in half and boil them in a pot of salted boiling water until they are cooked through. Drain out the water.
2. Mash the potatoes and add the Spectrum Spread and soy milk as you are mashing. Cover the mashed potatoes and set them aside.
3. Heat the olive oil in a skillet over medium-high heat, and sauté the sweet onion and garlic for one minute.
4. Add the collard greens, green onions, and sprinkle in the pepper. Sauté for 2 to 3 more minutes.
5. Stir the collards mixture into the potatoes and serve immediately.

SERVES 4

Supplements

Vitamin A

We think this vitamin alters progesterone levels. High doses of vitamin A can be toxic. The acceptable dose range is 900 to 3,000 mcg a day.

Vitamin B6

B6 may enhance the release of important neurotransmitters, including serotonin, dopamine, and norepinephrine, which in turn may affect other chemical messengers that cause fluid retention and breast pain. It may also reduce the effects of estrogen. Recommended dose range is 2 to 100 mg a day. Excessive B6 can cause neurological problems in some people.

Vitamin E

Helps prevent breast tenderness. Recommended dose range is 15 to 1,000 mg a day.

Herbs

Evening primrose oil (EPO) (Oenothera biennis)

This treatment is good because it has few side effects yet is very effective. EPO contains a large amount of polyunsaturated essential fatty acids and is considered an effective anti-inflammatory. In a 1985 study, women taking EPO supplements for three to six months experienced a significant decrease in cyclical breast pain. The recommended dose is 3 grams daily.

Do-It-Yourself

Bras

There's good evidence that one of the best things you can do for yourself is to buy a well-fitting support bra. In one study, a hundred women with breast pain were professionally fitted for bras; 75 percent of them had complete relief from pain.

Red Flags

Breast pain is not usually a sign of breast cancer, but don't make assumptions. Any pain, bumps, or lumps in your breast should be evaluated by your health care provider. In addition, be sure to practice monthly breast self-examination, have an annual examination by a physician, and a regularly scheduled mammogram.

FIBROCYSTIC BREAST DISEASE (FBD)

Description

This condition is a catch-all description of several different benign conditions of the breast that are common in younger women. Fibrocystic changes are the most frequent cause of breast lumps in women between the ages of thirty and fifty; approximately 60 percent of childbearing-age women have lumpy breasts as a result of fibrocystic breast disease. However, if you are menopausal, FBD is unlikely to occur if you are not taking hormone replacement therapy.

Although FBD is not usually serious, it can be painful, and it is a frequent cause of cyclic breast pain. The pain can be so bothersome that it prevents exercising or other activities.

If you have FBD, you've probably noticed that your breasts become painful, tender, and lumpy before your period. The condition clears up once your period begins, only to return the following month.

You must take great caution to differentiate FBD from other causes of breast lumps. If you have a breast lump, be sure to have it evaluated very carefully by a qualified health care practitioner and ultrasound, mammogram, or other appropriate diagnostic testing to be sure it is not malignant.

Causes

Your breasts respond to monthly changes in estrogen and progesterone levels by alternately swelling and shrinking. Hormonal stimulation causes the milk glands and related ducts to engorge and other breast tissue to retain water. Your breasts become swollen, lumpy, and painful. After your period, the swelling decreases. As this process repeats every month, your breasts may become firm and pockets of fluid may accumulate in enlarged, obstructed milk ducts and neighboring tissue. After a while, your breasts may contain many irregularly shaped areas of tissue that feel beady in consistency.

Signs and Symptoms

- Breast pain
- Tenderness
- One or more breast lumps
- Breast swelling

Conventional Treatments

Your doctor may suggest that you try cold compresses on your breasts. You may also be offered aspirin or other OTC pain relievers, prostaglandin inhibitors, or diuretics to reduce fluid retention. If you have severe FBD, your doctor may suggest a trial of danazol, a synthetic male hormone available only by prescription. Most of these drugs have side effects. For example, diuretics rob the body of potassium and the painkillers called nonsteroidal anti-inflammatory drugs (NSAIDS) can cause stomach and gastrointestinal problems.

Dietary Strategies

- Although there is some controversy in the literature about the effects of caffeine, it's wise to avoid excessive, long-term use of caffeinated beverages. Caffeine, known chemically as a methylxanthine, has been linked in some studies to a woman's risk of developing FBD.
- Avoid meat and full-fat dairy products. We think the saturated fat in these foods has an adverse effect on the body's estrogen levels, worsening breast symptoms. Instead, try to eat tofu, nonfat dairy products, and fish.
- Eat foods from the sea, such as seafood, kelp, and sea vegetables, to be sure you're getting enough iodine. Some research has shown that this trace element helps alleviate fibrocystic breast disease.

Supplements

Vitamin A

Vitamin A may alter progesterone levels. In addition, it helps cells reproduce, maintains healthy cell membranes, and enhances the body's use of iron. High doses of this vitamin, however, can be toxic; the acceptable dose range is 900 to 3,000 mcg a day.

Vitamin B6

B6 is thought to be the "maestro" vitamin for the metabolism of amino acids, important building blocks for neurotransmitters, including serotonin, dopamine, and norepinephrine, which in turn may affect other chemical messengers that cause fluid retention and breast pain. It may also reduce the effects of estrogen. The recommended dose is 2 to 100 mg a day, either separately or as part of a B-complex vitamin. Excessive B6 can cause neurological problems in some people.

Vitamin E
Vitamin E is a potent antioxidant that plays a role in building immunity and preventing infection. It may also have a protective effect on the breast and nipples, and helps prevent breast tenderness. It works together with selenium. The acceptable dose range is 15 to 1,000 mg a day.

Iodine
This trace element is necessary for maintaining normal breast tissue and may help relieve FBD. In one study, the authors speculate that iodine has an effect on breast cells, making them less susceptible to circulating estrogens. Although you can take it as a supplement, I suggest you take it as part of a multivitamin. Even better, you can get it through dietary sources, such as fish, kelp, dairy, and sea vegetables (dulse and nori). Excessive consumption of iodine can adversely affect your thyroid function, so use caution. The acceptable dose range is 150 to 1,100 mcg a day. Remember, iodine deficiency is rare since the introduction of iodized salt.

Selenium
This mineral, found in Brazil nuts, helps activate an antioxidant enzyme called glutathione peroxidase, which protects against cancer and is important for immune function. As an antioxidant, selenium enhances vitamin E and can help nourish breast tissue. Dose range is 60 to 400 mcg a day.

Herbs

Evening primrose oil (EPO) (Oenothera biennis)
Double-blind research has shown that daily use of evening primrose oil reduces breast pain and inflammation. Recommended dose is 3 grams daily.

Chaste tree (Vitex agnus-castus)
In a study published in April 2000, *Vitex* was found to reduce breast pain after three months. Suggested daily dose is 30 to 40 mg in an aqueous-alcohol extract. Do not use chaste tree if you may be pregnant or if you are nursing.

Black cohosh (Cimicifuga racemosa)
This herb is thought to work by binding to estrogen receptors, which balances hormones. Although the doses of this herb are not standardized, the German Commission E recommends taking an alcohol extract of 40 percent. This corresponds to 40 mg a day.

Exercise

You can reduce breast pain by exercising regularly throughout the month. In a study published in 1987, women who ran forty-five miles per menstrual cycle (or a little more than ten miles per week) had less breast tenderness and relief of other symptoms. Because exercise releases endorphins, it also provides natural pain relief when you have symptoms. My recommendation is thirty to forty-five minutes of aerobic exercise, three to five times a week.

Do-It-Yourself

Chest wall and breast massage

The pain and soreness of fibrocystic breast disease often cause a great deal of neighboring "referred" pain in the chest wall area. To decrease pain, improve soreness, and alleviate tension, try this massage: Firmly plant your thumb and fingers on the pectoral muscle (the main chest wall muscle above and to the side of your breast). Using a kneading motion, caress the muscle in an upward and outward direction, toward the shoulder. You can use the same technique on the muscles between the ribs.

Bras

Be sure to wear comfortable, well-fitted bras. One controversial school of thought holds that women who discontinue use of constrictive bras and go "bra free" have a reduced incidence of fibrocystic breast disease and other breast ailments. The theory is that the bra's constrictive effect on the breast restricts blood and lymphatic flow, causing stagnation. I haven't found good research to support this theory. On the other hand, there is some evidence that a well-fitted supportive bra can reduce breast pain.

Mammogram Pain

When it comes to medical procedures, mammograms are the quintessential "necessary evil." Although they know it's a potentially life-saving procedure, most of my women patients dread their appointments and anticipate them with trepidation, if not downright anxiety. It's not unusual to experience discomfort during a mammogram, but some women find it to be quite painful. If you are particularly sensitive, try these tips before your next mammogram:

- Schedule your exam at the time in your menstrual cycle when your breasts are the least tender. This is usually during the first two weeks of your cycle, but you know best. (According to some research, if you are premenopausal, a mammogram during this time may also be more accurate.)

- Reduce and, if possible, eliminate caffeine for a week before the exam.
- Taking vitamin E for a few weeks before your appointment may also help. The acceptable daily dose range is 15 to 1,000 mg.
- To reduce fluid retention, avoid salty foods for a few days before the procedure.
- Take an over-the-counter pain reliever about an hour before you go. Take more after the procedure, if necessary.
- Be sure to tell the technician if you're in pain. She may be able to make some adjustments to increase your comfort.

CHRONIC PELVIC PAIN

Description

Chronic pelvic pain is continuous or intermittent pain that has lasted for at least six months. It is usually severe enough to affect your daily functioning, social relationships, work, and family. The pain may fluctuate with your monthly menstrual cycle.

Pelvic pain affects one in seven women. It accounts for 10 to 20 percent of office visits to gynecologists, and 20 percent of all laparoscopies. (A laparoscopy is a surgical procedure, requiring anesthesia, that can cause uncomfortable pressure or pain for a few days afterward.) There are many possible causes, including endometriosis, pelvic inflammatory disease and other infections, ovarian cysts, fibroid tumors, ulcerative colitis, irritable bowel syndrome, spasms of the pelvic floor muscles, urethritis or other urinary tract infections, constipation, strains, and trauma. Dyspareunia (painful sex) is also sometimes associated with pelvic pain. Unfortunately, in many women with chronic pelvic pain, no identifiable organic cause can be found, even after laparoscopy.

Close communication with your gynecologist is essential if you have pelvic pain. To get a proper diagnosis, you need a thorough physical exam and history. In addition, you may have lab cultures, ultrasound, abdominal X rays, computerized tomography (CT) scans, magnetic resonance imaging (MRI) or other imaging studies, and laparoscopy. (However, bear in mind that some research shows that laparoscopy is of little value in treating endometriosis, and that attention to organic, psychological, dietary, environmental, and other factors is of more value.) Once your gynecologist has determined your diagnosis, she may send you to a physiatrist for focused pain management help.

In the following section I focus on endometriosis, a frequent cause of pelvic pain. You can effectively deal with its painful symptoms using a balanced therapeutic approach. However, do not use complementary treatments as a substitute for gynecological care.

ENDOMETRIOSIS

Description

This disease affects between 10 and 15 percent of menstruating women between the ages of twenty-four and forty. What happens is that tissues usually found in the lining of the uterus (the endometrium) grow in other parts of the body. Although these growths are most commonly found in the ovaries or elsewhere in the pelvic area, they may also occur on the bladder, in the intestines, the lungs, or in more distant places in the body. Like your uterine lining, the growths may respond to hormonal fluctuations of your menstrual cycle, building up tissue and breaking down every month. They can cause internal bleeding, cysts, the formation of scar tissue, and severe pain.

Causes

We don't yet know the cause of endometriosis. The most popular theory, yet to be proven, involves "renegade" cells from the uterine lining. It's thought that these cells spill into the abdominal cavity when menstrual blood backs up in the fallopian tubes, which connect the ovaries and the uterus. Although this may occur in all women, those with an immune or hormonal problem may develop endometriosis.

Signs and Symptoms

Common symptoms of endometriosis include:

- Severe pelvic pain, especially before and during periods or during sex
- Painful urination or bowel movements during periods
- Fatigue
- Diarrhea, constipation, nausea, or other gastrointestinal problems during periods

Endometriosis can also cause long-term problems, such as infertility or bowel problems.

Conventional Treatments

Over-the-counter pain relievers, such as aspirin, Tylenol, or the NSAIDS may help, or, if you are in severe pain, your doctor may prescribe pain medications. There are also a variety of hormonal treatments used to suppress ovulation, including oral contraceptives or Depo-Provera injections; danazol, a testosterone derivative; or medications called GhRH agonists (gonadotropin-releasing hormone drugs).

With or without hormonal therapy, your doctor may suggest surgery to remove or destroy the growths, relieve pain, and/or try to restore fertility. The options range from the conservative — laser ablation of growths — to the radical — hysterectomy, including removal of your ovaries.

Dietary Strategies (See Chapter 14 for food sources of specified nutrients)

- The liver detoxifies hormones, so it's important to keep this organ happy. Liver-friendly foods include carrots and vegetables in the cabbage family (kale, brussels sprouts, cauliflower, broccoli), beets, artichokes, lemons, and dandelion greens.
- Cut back on caffeine; it's associated with an increased risk for endometriosis.
- Limit your alcohol consumption; it stresses the liver.
- Spice up your meals with ginger and turmeric. The former helps fight inflammation and aids liver detoxification; the latter decreases inflammation and increases bile secretion.
- Make sure you get plenty of dietary fiber, which speeds food through the intestines and contributes to regular bowel movements.
- Reduce your intake of animal protein, especially red meat, which promotes inflammatory prostaglandins (i.e., inflammation and pain). On the other hand, a diet rich in vegetables, soy, nuts, and salmon increases the production of anti-inflammatory prostaglandins.
- Beta-carotene helps enhance immunity and may be protective against early stages of tumor growth.

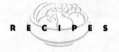

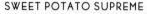

SWEET POTATO SUPREME

Try this delicious side dish, rich in beta-carotene.

> 4 *sweet potatoes, baked and peeled*
> 2 *tablespoons olive oil*
> 2 *cloves garlic, minced*
> 1 *red onion, chopped or sliced thinly*
> ¼ *cup sesame seeds*
> ¼ *cup pumpkin seeds*

1. Cut sweet potatoes into one-inch slices.
2. In a saucepan, add oil and sauté remaining ingredients for 5 minutes, until golden brown.
3. Combine the sweet potatoes and the mixture from the saucepan in a bowl. Serve warm.

SERVES 4

VEGETABLE RICE MEDLEY

This healthy dish features ginger and turmeric.

> 2 *tablespoons olive oil*
> 1 *onion, diced*
> 4 *cloves garlic, minced*
> 2 *tablespoons fresh parsley, finely chopped*
> 1 *cup raw cashew nuts*
> 2 *carrots, sliced*
> 1 *tablespoon low-sodium soy sauce*
> 2 *zucchinis, cut into thick slices*
> 1 *cup cauliflower florets*
> 1 *green pepper, sliced*
> 2 *teaspoons freshly grated ginger*
> 2 *teaspoons turmeric*
> 1 *teaspoon coriander*
> 2½ *cups plus 2 tablespoons water*
> 1¼ *cups short-grain brown rice*

1. Heat the olive oil in a large saucepan. Add the onion, garlic, parsley, nuts, and carrots. Stir over medium-high heat for 1 minute.
2. Stir in the soy sauce and rest of the vegetables and spices. Pour in the water and bring almost to boiling.
3. Stir in the rice, mix well, cover the pot and reduce heat. Simmer over a low flame for 40 to 45 minutes.

SERVES 6

Supplements

Vitamin C
This vitamin enhances your immune system and reduces fatigue. The accepted range is 90 to 2,000 mg a day. Cut back if you get diarrhea.

Vitamin E
To help correct your estrogen/progesterone ratio, try taking between 15 and 1,000 mg a day.

Essential fatty acids (EFA)
Both alpha-linolenic acid (found in flaxseed, canola, pumpkin seed, and walnut oil) and gamma-linoleic acid (in borage, black currant, and evening primrose oils) fight inflammation. Take 300 mg a day.

B vitamins
To help your liver process estrogen, take 1 B-complex vitamin tablet daily.

Selenium
This mineral is involved in the liver's detoxification processes. It also enhances immunity. Accepted dose range is between 60 and 400 mcg a day. Remember, too much causes toxicity.

Herbs

Chaste tree (Vitex agnus-castus)
This herb is showing great promise as a treatment for all sorts of ailments resulting from hormonal imbalances, although the scientific support specifically for endometriosis is lacking. The recommended dose is 30 to 40 mg daily in an aqueous-alcohol extract. Do not use chaste tree if you may be pregnant or if you are nursing.

Do-It-Yourself

Sitz baths

To ease pain by increasing blood circulation and reducing pelvic congestion, add 2 ml of an essential oil—such as clary sage, rose, nutmeg, or geranium—to your bath. Use warm water.

Mind/Body

Relaxation and imagery

Get into a relaxed state (see pages 340, 341). Visualize the inside of your uterus and other endometrial tissue shrinking. Continue to focus on this until you can imagine the painful tissues disappearing altogether. Do the exercise for fifteen to thirty minutes at least five days a week.

Yoga (See pages 344–351 for postures)

Try the modified Bridge Pose.

Biofeedback

Although biofeedback is often performed with sophisticated electronic equipment in the doctor's or therapist's office, there are many forms of biofeedback that you can do on your own. (See page 341.)

Exercise

Kegel exercises

These exercises strengthen the muscles in the pelvis and pubic floor. They involve contracting and releasing the muscles that start and stop the flow of urine. Start by contracting the muscles for a second and then releasing completely; repeat ten times. Do this exercise five times a day. It is completely inconspicuous, so you can do it during meetings, as you ride the subway, talk on the telephone, or watch TV.

Red Flags

If you develop fever, chills, bleeding, discharge, or persistent abdominal discomfort, call your doctor.

MENOPAUSE

Description

Menopause refers specifically to the cessation of the monthly menstrual cycle. According to the Massachusetts Women's Health Study, the median age for menopause is about fifty-one. However, hormonal and other changes leading to menopause take place gradually, over a period of years. During this transition, sometimes referred to as perimenopause, it's possible to start having troublesome menopausal symptoms as early as age thirty-five or forty, even while you're still getting regular periods.

Causes

As you approach menopause, your menstrual cycle may become irregular. You may skip periods or find that they are more widely spaced. On the other hand, your cycle may shorten, so you have more frequent periods. You may bleed for a shorter or for a longer time, and your flow may become lighter or heavier. All of these changes result from a natural ending of ovarian activity. Your ovaries are producing less estrogen, and there is also a significant reduction in progesterone production. Your estrogen levels eventually drop so much that ovulation, uterine tissue buildup, and menstruation all stop. These hormonal changes don't just affect your period, they influence every part of your body and your mind. As the changes occur, you may experience a variety of painful, annoying symptoms.

Signs and Symptoms

Few women experience all of these symptoms. You may, however, have at least a few:

- Hot flashes (flushing of face, neck, and/or trunk)
- Headaches
- Palpitations
- Dizziness
- Night sweats
- Cold hands and feet
- Painful sex associated with vaginal thinning and drying caused by loss of estrogen
- Vaginal pain and bleeding after intercourse

- Vaginal discomfort
- Dryness, pain, and itching of the vulva
- Urinary pain and burning due to urinary tract atrophy
- Insomnia
- Depression or anxiety
- Decreased memory
- Reduced cognition
- Reduced sex drive
- Facial hair
- Hair loss
- Acne
- Irregular bleeding
- Osteoporosis
- Heart disease

In addition, the dramatic drop in estrogen levels leads to a higher risk of osteoporosis and heart disease.

Conventional Treatments

Your doctor may prescribe estrogen replacement therapy (ERT) or hormonal replacement therapy (HRT). There are a variety of approaches. Estrogen helps relieve hot flashes, decreases vaginal atrophy, and slows the bone loss and fractures of osteoporosis. It may also prevent heart disease, although recent research casts some doubt on that finding. And although it's too soon to say this conclusively, it may also prevent Alzheimer's disease. Estrogen is frequently taken in pill form as conjugated equine estrogens (Premarin). Estradiol, in patch or a gel, facilitates the passage of estrogen directly into the bloodstream. And vaginal creams, although they may take four to six weeks to have an impact, help relieve urinary and vaginal symptoms. But taking estrogen may raise your risk of uterine cancer, as well as blood clots. And some women experience new or increased migraines when they take estrogen.

To reduce estrogen's cancer risks, progesterone (or progestin) is usually included in the treatment; it's then called hormone replacement therapy. But HRT also has side effects, including headaches, nausea, vaginal discharge, fluid retention, swollen breasts, weight gain, and abnormal vaginal bleeding. And the jury is still out on the relationship of HRT and breast cancer risk.

To decrease spinal osteoporosis and increase libido, your doctor may prescribe methyltestosterone (the "male" hormone, testosterone). We don't yet know the long-term effects taking testosterone will have on women. If you're only concerned about osteoporosis, several new drugs, such as Alendronate, have a narrower focus.

Dietary Strategies (See Chapter 14 for food sources of specified nutrients)

- Compounds called isoflavones found in soy foods may reduce menopausal symptoms. Because they are phytoestrogens, which have a chemical structure similar to estrogen, they provide weak estrogenic action. Soy isoflavones may relieve hot flashes and vaginal atrophy. In one recent study, researchers found that women eating 60 grams of soy protein had a 33 percent reduction in hot flashes after four weeks; this increased to a 45 percent reduction after twelve weeks. Aim for 25 to 50 mg of soy protein a day.
- Smoking, alcohol, caffeine, and spicy foods may increase hot flashes.
- Feed your bones with calcium-rich foods.
- Use alfalfa sprouts in your salad; this member of the pea family contains isoflavones with weak estrogenic effects.
- Eat foods rich in bioflavonoids, plant pigments that enhance absorption of vitamin C and reduce menopausal complaints.

RECIPE

The following recipe contains many healing ingredients; I recommend that you have some every day. Dulse flakes come from a sea vegetable. They are an excellent source of B vitamins, including vitamin B12. It is also an excellent source of beta-carotene, calcium, iodine, iron and magnesium. Miso, fermented soybean paste that is often prepared with barley and rice, has been a staple of the Asian diet for centuries. Miso soup is prominent in the macrobiotic diet because of its concentrated protein content and its documented anticarcinogenic properties. The phytoestrogens and calcium in tofu help to alleviate the unpleasant symptoms of menopause, such as hot flashes, and also help to prevent the onset of osteoporosis.

HEALING MISO VEGETABLE SOUP

1 tablespoon sesame oil
1 tablespoon low-sodium soy sauce

1 onion
5 cloves garlic, minced
1 green pepper, chopped
2 cups fresh spinach, chopped
3 stalks bok choy, including leaves
10 cups water
1 leek
1 parsnip, chopped
½ cup scallions, chopped
½ cup chopped carrots
8 ounces firm silken tofu, cubed
1 tablespoon dulse flakes
½ cup barley
½ cup red or green lentils
1 teaspoon coriander
¼ teaspoon sea salt, or to taste
2 tablespoons sweet miso

1. In a large, heavy stockpot heat the oil and soy sauce over a medium-high flame and sauté the onion, garlic, green pepper, spinach, and bok choy for 2 minutes, stirring constantly. Add the water and heat to almost boiling.
2. Trim off and discard the bottom and green parts of the leek. Chop the leek and add to the pot. Stir in the rest of the ingredients, except the miso.
3. Cover the pot and simmer over a low flame for 1 hour.
4. Take the pot off the flame; remove lid, stir soup, and let cool for 10 minutes.
5. In a small bowl mash the miso with 2 tablespoons hot water and then stir well into the soup.
6. Serve immediately or freeze individual portions to heat daily (do not boil as this weakens the potency of the miso) and enjoy over the week.

SERVES 6 TO 8

Supplements

Vitamin E

Vitamin E helps prevent hot flashes and protects your heart. Recommended dose is between 15 and 1,000 mg a day. Check with your physician if you have high blood pressure.

Vitamin C
This powerful antioxidant may help prevent hot flashes. The accepted dose range is 90 to 2,000 mg a day.

Calcium and magnesium
The loss of these two minerals during and after menopause contributes to the development of osteoporosis. The accepted dose range for calcium is 1,300 to 2,500 mg a day; for magnesium it's 320 to 350 mg a day. If you're not taking estrogen, aim for the higher end of the range, for both calcium and magnesium.

Flaxseed oil
Rich in omega-3 fatty acids, this oil helps prevent inflammation and contributes to healthy vaginal tissue. Take one tablespoon a day.

Rice bran oil containing gamma orzanol
This dietary supplement may relieve hot flashes. Take 300 mg a day.

Bioflavonoids
These are plant pigments thought to have a weak estrogenic effect. Bioflavonoids can decrease hot flashes, reduce muscle cramping and bleeding, ease sore joints, improve vaginal lubrication. Take 500 mg a day; it's best when combined with vitamin C.

Vitamin B6
This vitamin enhances the release of important neurotransmitters, including serotonin, dopamine, and norepinephrine. The recommended range for this nutrient is 2 to 100 mg a day as part of a B-complex supplement.

Herbs

Chaste tree (Vitex agnus-castus)
This herb is touted as helping to normalize your pituitary gland's production of hormones. It may take six months before you notice its effects. The daily dose is 30 to 40 mg in an aqueous-alcohol extract. Do not use chaste tree if you may be pregnant.

Black cohosh (Cimicifuga racemosa)
This herb, which decreases hot flashes, is available in a standardized tablet form under the name Remifemin. Several double-blind trials have shown it to be safe and effective. In addition, in a policy statement about herbal

remedies in May 2001, the American College of Obstetrics and Gynecology upheld the short-term value of black cohosh in menopausal women with vasomotor symptoms (sweating and hot flashes). The dose is 20 to 40 mg a day.

Licorice (Glycyrrhiza glabra)

This herb balances estrogen. The recommended dose is 250 mg, or one cup of tea three times a day. Use caution if you have high blood pressure.

Ginkgo (Ginkgo biloba)

To enhance memory and improve circulation to cold hands and feet, the recommended dose is 120 mg two to three times a day.

Sage (Salvia officinalis)

If hot flashes are getting you down, and particularly if you sweat a great deal, try a tea made by steeping 2 to 3 teaspoons of this herb in water for fifteen minutes. Drink 2 cups a day.

Evening primrose oil (EPO) (Oenothera biennis)

EPO reduces inflammation, helps alleviate hot flashes, and curbs breast pain. The recommended dose is 1,500 to 3,000 mg a day.

Homeopathy

A German homeopathic "cocktail" called Mulimen effectively reduces hot flashes. It contains chaste tree, St. John's wort, and black cohosh. It should be available in your local pharmacy or health food store. Otherwise, you can buy it on-line. Follow package directions.

Do-It-Yourself

Reflexology

- SP-6 is located behind the tibia (shin bone), approximately four finger widths above the inner part of the ankle. It helps normalize menstrual flow and promotes relaxation.
- SP-9 is situated in the hollow right below the top (head) of the tibia. It also helps normalize menstrual flow.

Exercise

Kegel exercises (See page 70)
Done regularly, these exercises strengthen muscle tone and prevent uterine and bladder prolapse and incontinence.

Regular exercise
Swimming, running, or brisk walking (preferably outdoors in the fresh air) triggers the release of endorphins, natural chemicals that help to diminish pain and improve your perception of well-being. In addition, regular aerobic exercise helps keep your weight under control and lowers your risk of heart disease, osteoporosis, and bone fractures. It also provides specific benefits for menopausal women. Besides alleviating pain, depression, and anxiety, a study of nine hundred Swedish women suffering from menopausal symptoms found that thirty minutes of daily aerobic exercise cut back their hot flashes significantly.

Exercise at least thirty to forty-five minutes at least three times a week. Work hard enough to achieve a 70 percent target heart rate.

Lift weights
Strength training (weight lifting) stresses and strengthens the muscles, which begin to atrophy as you age. It also stimulates bone growth. What's more, strength or resistance training helps you keep your weight from creeping up. The reason? Muscle takes more calories to sustain than fat tissue, so as you build muscle mass you burn more calories all day long, even when you're resting.

Mind/Body

Yoga
Menopause may sometimes leave you feeling drained, zapped of energy, and depressed. Yoga is the perfect exercise for you since it improves your endurance and enhances your mood. While the postures increase joint mobility and ease symptoms like hot flashes, yoga breathing and meditation quiet your nerves and ease irritability. I suggest that you try Bow Pose, the Locust, Alternating Leg Lifts, Head to Knee Pose, and Standing Forward Bend (see pages 344–351). Perform these stretching exercises slowly so you can maintain control over your body movements. And don't hold your breath!

Seeking Help from Complementary Practitioners

Massage

Getting a massage helps you relax, relieving irritability, tension, and depression. It also improves circulation, which can be especially helpful if you suffer from cold hands and feet. Use a vitamin E oil to relieve dry skin and vaginal atrophy.

Acupuncture

Besides increasing the body's production of endorphins, acupuncture may help balance hormones and relieve flushing and temperature changes.

Red Flags

Call your doctor if you have persistent hot flashes or a lot of pain. And remember, once the menstrual cycle stops, it stops. If you experience any bleeding six months or more following menopause, contact your doctor.

PREGNANCY

Pregnancy, in and of itself, is not typically painful. But a number of uncomfortable and sometimes painful ailments can occur.

Back Pain During Pregnancy

When you are pregnant, your body releases many different hormones, including relaxin. This causes slackness of some of the spinal ligaments, the pubic symphysis (the slightly movable joint at the front of the pelvis), and the sacroiliac joint. Besides, as the pregnancy progresses, your center of gravity shifts and the growing fetus puts a heavy burden on your back. For these reasons, low back pain is a common complaint during this time. For information on treating low back pain during pregnancy, see Chapter 6.

LABOR AND CHILDBIRTH

Description

One of my favorite jokes, attributed to Maurice Chevalier, is this:

WOMAN TO MAN: What is the difference between a man and a woman?
MAN TO WOMAN: Madam, I can't conceive!

Unfortunately, the pain of childbirth is no joke. Of all the pains of womanhood, those associated with labor and giving birth are the most vicious. Since biblical times, childbirth has been recognized as a major cause of pain and modern studies confirm this view. Yet contemporary medicine, despite all of its accomplishments, has not identified the optimal treatment for this pain. Controversies rage about the use of pain medications, anesthetics, and other modern treatments and technologies. I feel that the best treatment is a combination of traditional medical interventions, balanced with complementary medicine. For example, the sound of gentle music in the background or the tender caress of a spouse massaging your back can go a long way.

Causes

During labor, the muscles of the uterus, stimulated by the hormone oxytocin, stretch the cervix, or uterine opening. The cervix gradually widens enough for the baby to emerge. At the same time, uterine contractions push the baby out of the uterus and into the vagina, allowing it to be born.

Physiology and anatomy, the size and position of the fetus, and the nature and frequency of the contractions determine how painful this process will be. But cultural beliefs and customs as well as anxiety and other psychological factors have an enormous impact on pain.

Signs and Symptoms

Bloody show
The small plug that seals the cervix during pregnancy may come out as the cervix begins to open. It looks like pink or blood-tinged mucus.

Ruptured membranes/waters breaking
This is a sign that the baby's head is pressing against the amniotic sac. The "water," or amniotic fluid, may come out in a rush or a trickle.

Contractions
These pains may feel like menstrual cramps, a backache, or gas. As labor progresses, they become longer and more rhythmic; they also occur more frequently.

Conventional Treatments

Tranquilizers, barbiturates, or narcotic medications in oral, intramuscular, or intravenous form are often utilized during the birthing process. Like most medication, their use may be associated with nasty side effects. These include nausea, lethargy, drops in blood pressure, slowed contractions or respiration, moodiness and hangover for you, and slowed respiration for your baby. Besides, the effects are often short-lived. For example, many women have said that Demerol, a commonly used narcotic, didn't ease their pain much during labor and made them feel disoriented.

You can also get relief in the latter stages of labor from an epidural block, but this form of anesthesia has limitations. It is highly dependent on the skill of the person performing the procedure. In addition, it is costly and fraught with complications, technical limitations, and risks.

You can use complementary remedies instead of conventional strategies or in addition to them. By doing so, you may decrease or eliminate your need for medications. In addition, you may be able to avoid an epidural or forestall it until it matters most, when your labor is very active.

Do-It-Yourself

Besides being soothing, these techniques are distracting because stimuli such as heat and cold compete with and diminish your awareness of pain.

Superficial heat

Heat is calming and comforting. In addition, it lessens your body's fight-or-flight response to stress. During active labor, you can speed up contractions by applying heat to your abdomen over the upper uterine area. Local application of hot compresses to your perineum may be especially helpful during the second stage of labor.

As long as you are careful to avoid burning, using heat is perfectly safe. You can use hot-water bottles, heated silica packs, a warm blanket, heating pads, electric packs, warm baths or showers, or hot, moist towels or washcloths. Your pain threshold may be altered during labor so allow someone else to check the temperature before applying anything to your skin. And when using moist heat, be sure to use extra towels to protect against sudden temperature changes.

Superficial cold

The numbing effect of cold decreases pain sensation. It is particularly useful for musculoskeletal pain, so if you have back pain during labor, cold is in order.

Good methods for applying cold include ice bags, gel packs, or rubber gloves filled with ice. Always use some protection between your skin and the source of cold; what you want is a gradual increase from cool to cold. If you are chilled or shivering, do not make matters worse by using cold.

As soon as possible after giving birth, apply ice packs to your perineum to reduce swelling and relieve pain.

Bath or Shower

Hydrotherapy, or immersion therapy, is a comforting, age-old treatment. It lowers blood pressure, improves contraction efficiency, relieves pain, and helps you relax. So beneficial is this simple strategy that the British House of Commons Health Committee recommended that birthing pools be made available to women during childbirth.

During early labor, taking a bath may slow contractions, so it's best to wait until you start active labor. Consult your midwife or physician about when to take a bath, how long to stay in it, and the temperature of the water.

The effects of showers haven't been studied as thoroughly as baths, but a warm shower will help you relax and reduce your pain. Try directing the warm water over your abdomen or lower back. Go easy on yourself by sitting on a chair while you're in the shower.

Keep moving

If possible, take advantage of gravity by walking. If you are confined to a bed, changing your position frequently will help you stay comfortable and speed the progress of your labor.

Massage

If you clench your hands into fists during contractions, ask your partner to provide a soothing massage by kneading, stroking, and applying pressure and friction to your hands. Do the same with any other parts of your body that you tense during contractions. If you like, have your partner use a massage oil with a few drops of essential oil, such as lavender, clary sage, mandarin, or jasmine to enhance the effect and promote relaxation.

On the other hand, you may not want to be touched during labor. Obviously, there's no way to know this in advance, so you'll have to play it by ear.

Counterpressure

It's estimated that one-third of women suffer from terrible low back pain during labor. Narcotics and epidurals are not the only answer. Your simplest option is to have someone massage your lower back and buttocks. Bring a rolling pin with you to the hospital or buy a cold can of juice or soda while you're there. Your partner can roll it back and forth over your lower back during or between contractions.

Here are three other techniques your partner or a nurse can use during contractions. These were suggested by physical therapist Penny Simkin:

1. For the partner: Use your fist or the heel of your hand to apply steady pressure to painful spots on her back. At the same time, put your other hand in front, over her hip bone, to offset pressure on the back. Rest between contractions.

2. Sit in an upright chair with good low-back support. Your feet should be flat on the floor and your knees a few inches apart. Have your partner cup each of your knees with the heel of a hand and steadily lean toward you, pressing your knees back toward your hip joints.

3. If you can, get onto your hands and knees; if you can't, stand and lean forward. Have your partner place his hands over the meatiest part of your buttocks. He should then apply steady pressure with his palms, directing the force diagonally toward the center of your pelvis.

Reflexology

Stimulation of a variety of reflexology points can help control the pain of labor. Don't use these points before Week 38 of pregnancy, since they can induce premature labor.

- LI-4, located in the web between the thumb and first finger, helps to relieve spasm of the uterus.
- BL-60 (Bladder 60), located on the ankle's outside surface, helps quell back pain and can facilitate the baby's delivery.
- GB-21 (Gallbladder 21), found in the depression on top of the shoulders that is directly in line with the ears, helps speed the very last stages of labor and delivery of the afterbirth.

Mind/Body

Fear and anxiety about pain, loss of control, or injury to yourself or your baby during labor are common. Being in the unfamiliar environment of a hospital doesn't help matters. Unfortunately, anxiety can magnify your perception of pain, so anything you do to promote relaxation will improve your labor. Try using these techniques between contractions.

Relax
The pain and anxiety of labor can activate the fight-or-flight response, which increases muscle contractions and may intensify pain. Getting into a relaxed state lowers the heart and respiratory rates, decreases blood pressure, and reduces muscle tension. There are many ways to do it. Whatever you choose—belly breathing, progressive relaxation, or meditation—your goal is to get in to a neutral mental and physical state (see Chapter 18 for details).

Imagery
Once you are relaxed, you can further distract yourself by concentrating on positive thoughts. Think about your other children, members of your family, or the new baby. Or focus on a calming, beautiful image—a favorite vacation spot or a pleasant memory.

Autogenic training (See page 341)

Music
Music has powerful effects on emotion and mood, stress, tension, and anxiety. In relation to childbearing, researchers have found that music reduces agitation, enhances relaxation and concentration on breathing patterns, and decreases pain during labor. During your pregnancy, think about the kind of music you most like and be sure to bring CDs, tapes, and a player to the hospital. You can listen to it simply as a distraction or use it, alone or with imagery, to enhance your relaxation.

Trance
Hypnosis can reduce pain, shorten labor, and reduce the need for medication. To use this method, however, you and your labor partner must be trained before the big day comes. Ask your midwife or doctor for a referral.

Seeking Help from Complementary Practitioners

A doula is a trained professional whose only role is to provide you with emotional and physical comfort through hand-holding, massage, suggesting position changes, and continuous emotional reassurance. The doula works alone or with your partner, nurse, midwife, or doctor. Women who use doulas rely less on pain medications, have shorter first-time labor, reduced rates of cesarean section, and a generally enhanced childbirth experience.

Breast-feeding-Related Ailments

Sore nipples or engorged breasts
Here are some tips that may help:

- Reposition the baby. Turning the suckling infant so he or she is belly to belly with you is optimal.
- Nurse first on the breast that hurts less. If there's no difference between your breasts, alternate.
- Each time you start a nursing session, stimulate the suckling reflex by touching your baby's bottom lip to your breast or by expressing a small amount of milk.
- If your baby is able to put a larger amount of breast into his or her mouth, it will result in less nipple soreness and pain.
- Nurse frequently and until your baby is satisfied. The baby will suck less vigorously and this will also help prevent engorgement.
- If your breasts become engorged—full and painful—continue to nurse frequently to encourage your body to adjust your milk supply to your baby's demands. In addition, hot showers or warm water compresses, applied right before nursing, will help.
- Rub some milk on your breasts after nursing to soothe and heal.
- If your nipples are sore, exposing them to sunlight and air will help.
- Clean your breasts with warm water and avoid soap.
- For cracked or painful nipples, one of my Ob/Gyn colleagues recommends gently applying moist tea bags, geranium leaf, or ointments made from comfrey, yarrow, or marigold. Other alternatives are vitamin E oil or calendula cream.
- Change your breast pads or liners frequently.
- Avoid underwire bras or other constrictive clothing.

Mastitis

An inflammation of the breast, mastitis is usually a swollen, warm, red, and/or painful spot. The area may feel hard. Often, hot compresses, massaging the area, and frequent nursing can ease the problem. However, if you develop a fever, feel tired, achy, or fluey, or if the symptoms don't clear in twenty-four hours, call your health care provider. You may have a breast infection.

Sunflower oil

Because it is rich in vitamin E, sunflower oil may help ease sore, inflamed breasts. A recent study published in *Immunology* assessed whether dietary interventions, specifically the use of sunflower or red palm oil, had an impact on breast inflammation during late pregnancy and breast-feeding. The researchers found a beneficial role for sunflower oil. If you want to give it a shot, try incorporating it into your diet on a regular basis. It's best not to cook with sunflower oil since it loses its therapeutic potency when heated. Instead, use it in a salad dressing two or three times a week.

Reflexology

Two points on your ear may help relieve inflammation and provide some relief. One is the apex of your ear, which you can find by folding your ear flaps together and finding the topmost point. The other is the endocrine point on the lower cartilage projection in the front crease of the central hollow of the ear.

Another point to try is GB-42 (Gallbladder 42), located on the top of the foot in the space between the fourth and fifth toes.

Helpful Hints for Miscellaneous Ailments of Pregnancy and Childbirth

Morning Sickness

Ginger (Zingiber officinale)

Thanks to its antispasmodic properties, ginger effectively prevents nausea. However, its safety in pregnancy has not been conclusively proven. Check with your practitioner before trying it. Usual dose is 250 to 500 mg four times a day.

Vitamin B6

In some studies, this vitamin has been shown to prevent nausea. The safe upper limit for this nutrient is 100 mg a day.

Acupressure wrist bands

Using these bands to apply continuous pressure to your wrists effectively reduces nausea and vomiting. The bands come with instructions; however, the acupressure point you want to use is between the two central tendons of the forearm, three finger widths from the wrist crease.

Reflexology
- LU-8 (Lung Meridian 8), just above the wrist crease, on the thumb side.
- PE-6 (Pericardium 6), two thumb widths above the wrist crease, in the middle of your inner arm.

Hemorrhoid Pain

To reduce pain, take warm baths with a few drops of cypress, juniper, or lavender essential oil. Applying cool, soothing witch hazel or witch hazel ointment or slippery elm cream promotes healing.

Postpartum Perineal Pain

After birth, many women experience perineal pain, especially if they've had an episiotomy. In a randomized clinical trial published in 1994, researchers found that adding six drops of lavender oil to a daily bath for ten days after birth reduced discomfort within three to five days.

5

Tender to the Bone:
A Joint Problem

GLADYS'S TURNAROUND

Gladys is a sixty-three-year-old woman referred to me by her coworker, one of my longtime patients. At her first visit, Gladys's chief complaint was dull, aching, boring pain in her knees and hips that had steadily been getting worse. Gladys didn't usually go to the doctor unless she was really suffering. But somehow we hit it off. She reminded me of my late mom, both in appearance and in personality, and I listened intently as she opened up to me on that wintry day.

A couple of months earlier she had seen her primary care physician. All he had done was suggest Motrin, a pain reliever. He also referred her to a specialist. That's what had precipitated her visit to me. She was scared and depressed. "The specialist told me my only option was surgery. I'm just praying that you can figure out something else," she said.

Gladys's husband had died unexpectedly of a heart attack several years back. It quickly became apparent to me that Gladys loved to take care of people, sometimes at the cost of her own health. She had a stressful job working as an executive secretary at a local college. Although she was approaching retirement, she doggedly spent many hours a day on her feet visiting various administrative departments. "I want to make sure everything is just right for my boss," she explained. On weekends, she baby-sat for her grandchildren, taking them on outings to the zoo and children's museums. Meanwhile, she had let herself go, ignoring the worsening pain in her knees.

Now she could ignore it no longer. Sheepishly, she pointed to her legs: "My knees are turning in; they're so crooked you can drive a trailer truck under me," she half-joked. But her situation was serious; she was having trouble walking.

Gladys was a picture of advanced osteoarthritis in full bloom. Her right hip and knee were markedly worse than the other side. They really acted up when she climbed stairs. Occasionally, her knee buckled when she stepped off a curb. On physical examination, she showed osteoarthritic changes (bony enlargement, motion restriction, pain, and stiffness) not only in her knees and hips, but also in her fingers. Her X rays further corroborated her advanced degenerative joint disease.

While I recognized that joint replacement surgery might eventually be inevitable, my task now was to buy her time. To complement her conventional treatments, which included Tylenol and a nonsteroidal anti-inflammatory drug, I suggested a four-part plan. First, I recommended glucosamine and chondroitin, two nutritional supplements, to fortify her weight-bearing joints. To further strengthen her joints and offer her some aerobic exercise, I encouraged her to enroll in an aqua therapy program at the local community center and taught her several quadriceps exercises.

There was no way Gladys would cut back on her walking. "My grandchildren won't hear of it. They love our weekend outings and so do I!" she exclaimed. Instead, I suggested that she buy a pair of well-cushioned, impact-absorbing walking shoes to avoid stress to her joints. And since her extra weight—she needed to lose about 15 pounds—put more pressure on her joints, I gave her some general nutritional guidelines to follow, and suggested hypnosis to reduce food cravings.

To tide her over until these measures kicked in, I proposed that we start an acupuncture regimen for immediate relief and gave her detailed acupressure exercises to do at home.

Over the course of several weeks Gladys began to notice a change. She still had pain, but it had diminished considerably. Her walking was more confident, less painful, and, best of all, she was feeling good again.

The musculoskeletal system—the elaborate bulwark of bones, muscles, tendons, ligaments, and soft tissue that provides structural support and protection to the body—is a frequent source of pain for women. Among older women, musculoskeletal complaints are also a common cause of disability. Women more frequently suffer from osteoarthritis and rheumatoid arthritis as well as systemic lupus erythematosus, systemic sclerosis, and fibromyalgia. In addition, women and men sometimes describe different symptoms for the same problems.

There are a number of possible reasons for these striking disparities, including hormonal makeup, physical and anatomical differences, and genetic constitution. Social or cultural influences, such as how physically active you are or whether your job is sedentary, probably play a role. Research has also shown that women spend less time than men in organized sports and high-intensity exercises and more time in housework and caregiving activities.

In this chapter, my primary focus is pain from rheumatoid arthritis and osteoarthritis, the two predominant forms of arthritis in women. (Other ailments related to the musculoskeletal system are covered in Chapters 6 and 7.)

Over 43 million Americans suffer from the pain, stiffness, and associated anxiety, stress, and depression of arthritis. Of those, 7 million are limited in their daily activities. In fact, according to the Centers for Disease Control, arthritis disables more Americans than heart disease and stroke. By the year 2020, as the baby-boom generation ages, an estimated 60 million people will have arthritis.

Arthritis affects the joints and their surrounding structures, especially the shoulder, elbow, wrist, hip, knee, and ankle. Arthritis has many faces and forms, and each one affects different parts of the joint. Whatever shape it takes, arthritis all too often wreaks havoc. Along with pain and stiffness, it causes dramatic deformity and misalignment of joints.

OSTEOARTHRITIS

Description

Osteoarthritis (OA), a degenerative joint disease, is the most common form of arthritis, affecting nearly 21 million Americans. OA is far more common among women, who may also suffer a more severe form of the disease than men.

OA is caused by degeneration of cartilage, a jellylike material that protects the ends of many connecting bones. When it's healthy, cartilage allows bones to glide smoothly over each other without rubbing together. It acts like a shock absorber to cushion the joints and protect them from the weight and jarring of your movements. When cartilage breaks down, the bones rub together and this causes pain.

OA affects the integrity of joints, which, along with surrounding bone, become thickened and distorted. Bone spurs (osteophytes) may develop, causing more deformity, damage, and pain.

In addition, each joint is enveloped in a capsule with a lining called the synovium, which produces fluid that lubricates the joint, allowing smooth and free movement. This may also be affected by osteoarthritis.

OA worsens over time. It is linked to age-associated joint changes, and there's a dramatic increase in OA in women over the age of sixty-five. As you get older, along with the pain you may experience dysfunction and even loss in the range of motion of your joints.

Causes

Being a woman increases your chances of developing OA. So does aging, because the years of wear and tear on your joints can trigger the breakdown or wearing away of the smooth cartilage coating that protects joints and adjoining bone structures. Prior trauma to a joint from an accident, sports or work-related activity, as well as poor diet and obesity, also raise your risk.

Other contributing factors are your body mechanics, the health of your nerve and muscle structures, and stress on your ligaments—the structures that connect bone to bone. Particularly relevant in this regard are high-heeled shoes. Over time, by putting added pressure on your knees, high heels can lead to osteoarthritis. Don't fool yourself into thinking that as long as you avoid stilettos, you're safe. It turns out that shoes with chunky high heels are deceptive—they feel more comfortable, so you wear them longer. Even if they're better for your feet, they're just as bad for your knees as thinner heels, according to researchers at the Harvard Medical School.

Finally, genetics may play a role, particularly in OA of the hands. Some of these risk factors are easier to modify than others.

Signs and Symptoms

- Pain, stiffness, or decreased range of motion in your joints
- Deformity of your joints—they become bony or knobby
- Enlargement of the joints but with little inflammation
- Although OA can affect many joints, it may only strike one or two. The knees, hips, fingers, neck, and back are the most likely to be affected.

Conventional Treatments

If you're overweight, your doctor will suggest that you drop some pounds to reduce pressure on your joints. She may also recommend a hot pack. To use this, immerse it in hot water, cool it a little, and wrap it in a towel. It imparts moist heat to your aching joints. Even easier to use are electrical moist heat packs. A thermal pack is a new product that involves no electricity; you activate it by crushing and its heat lasts for twelve hours. Hot baths or showers and even heat lamps are also helpful.

There are a variety of drugs, such as Tylenol and NSAIDS, used to reduce pain and improve function.

If you have a local inflammation with swelling, warmth, and redness, your doctor may recommend injecting your joint with steroids. This will provide immediate, albeit short-term relief. And if oral medications aren't helping, another treatment option is a series of injections with synthetic cartilage (hyaluronase) to restore your body's natural shock absorber. These injections are approved for use only in arthritis of the knee; their effects on other joints have not yet been extensively studied.

Splinting or bracing a joint to stabilize and align it and redistribute weight can reduce pain and inflammation and help avoid more damage. Your physician (a physiatrist, orthopedist, or rheumatologist) can evaluate you for these devices. You can buy other aids, such as neoprene sleeves for your knees, at the pharmacy. Finally, shoe orthotics, crafted by a podiatrist or pedorthotist, can correct the way you walk and prevent damage to your joints caused by faulty biomechanics.

Topical gels, creams, and ointments are a great way to avoid the nasty side effects of oral medication. Unfortunately, they are not as readily available in the United States as they are abroad. In many other countries you can buy topical nonsteroidal products for localized relief of arthritic joints over the counter. In this country, you'll have to have your doctor ask the pharmacist to custom prepare topical analgesic formulations.

Dietary Strategies (See Chapter 14 for food sources of specified nutrients)

Lose weight
Both women and minorities are disproportionately affected by obesity and are less likely to exercise. Remember, obesity dramatically raises your risk of developing OA. It doesn't take much to improve your chances: In one study, loss of a little more than 10 pounds over a ten-year period cut the risk of OA in half.

Avocados and soybeans

Recently, French researchers have focused on the potential value of an avocado/soybean oil combination. People in their study had less pain and used fewer pain relievers. There was even a suggestion that this combination might promote cartilage growth. You can eat raw soybeans or try commercial brands of soybeans that are lightly dried and toasted to enhance the taste. You can even sample soy chocolate bars. Some of these tasty items provide a whopping 12 grams of soy protein.

Fish

Most studies of EPA and DHA, the essential fatty acids found in fish oil, have involved people suffering from rheumatoid arthritis. Still, because they interfere with chemical messengers that influence the body's inflammatory cycle, it's reasonable to use them to fight the pain and inflammation of OA. I am not a fan of fish oil supplements, because they tend to get rancid and become dangerous quite easily. What's more, you can get enough fish oil by eating fish at least two or three times a week. Besides fish, diets that include whole grains, leafy vegetables, and seeds (flax and sunflower) supply the proper ratio of omega-6 to omega-3 fatty acids likely to benefit arthritis.

Vitamin B3, or niacinamide, helps improve joint mobility.

Vitamin E and selenium may relieve pain.

Antioxidants

Antioxidants are natural chemicals that destroy free radicals, those nasty cellular renegades that have been implicated in the development of arthritis and many other diseases. Consuming antioxidants has been associated with reduced risk for OA. The best food sources for antioxidants are fruits and vegetables.

R E C I P E

RED PEPPERS WITH MUSHROOMS AND GINGER

2 *tablespoons olive oil*
2 *tablespoons low-sodium tamari sauce*
1 *teaspoon honey*

1 *tablespoon grated, fresh ginger*
3 *cloves garlic, minced*
1 *sweet onion, sliced very thinly*
½ *cup sweet snow peas*
1 *cup mushrooms, halved*
3 *red peppers, cut into strips*

1. Heat olive oil in a heavy skillet over medium-high heat. Add the tamari sauce, honey, and ginger.
2. Stir in the garlic and sweet onion, and cook for 1 minute, stirring constantly.
3. Add the rest of the vegetables and stir-fry for 4 minutes, or until vegetables are just tender.
4. Serve immediately as a side dish or over brown rice or whole-wheat pasta.

SERVES 4

Supplements

Glucosamine sulfate

Some of the most promising developments in treating arthritis come from the world of "nutraceuticals," or dietary supplements. A large-scale meta-analysis published in the *Journal of the American Medical Association* in March 2000 evaluated the use of glucosamine and chondroitin preparations for OA of the knee and hip. Overall, researchers found these supplements to be effective. Here are more specifics.

Glucosamine sulfate is a nutritional supplement that comes from seashells or seafood. It is an important building block for the manufacture and repair of cartilage. More and more scientific literature is emerging to support glucosamine's value in reducing OA pain. A 1998 double-blind study showed that glucosamine, taken for four weeks, was just as effective as ibuprofen in curbing OA symptoms, and it caused fewer side effects. So exciting is the preliminary research on this supplement that the National Institutes of Health (NIH) has embarked on a study to explore its role in cartilage restoration.

You'll see glucosamine in a variety of forms. It's often bundled with chondroitin sulfate and other nutritional supplements thought to be helpful for healthy bones. But there is no evidence that the combination product acts synergistically or is more effective. I recommend glucosamine sulfate or hydrochloride, which have been most extensively studied. Take 500 mg three times a day.

Chondroitin sulfate

A natural constituent of cartilage, chondroitin helps to provide elasticity and structure. Since cartilage lacks a blood supply, chondroitin plays an important role by allowing water and nutrients to pass to and be retained by the joints. Chondroitin also shields cartilage from destructive chemicals and enzymes, thereby slowing deterioration.

Clinical studies have shown that chondroitin supplementation helps joint function, manages joint narrowing, and reduces pain. Unfortunately, it doesn't repair already damaged cartilage.

Most chondroitin supplements are derived from the tracheal cartilage of cattle and are slow-acting, often taking two months to work. Although the side effects — indigestion and nausea — are minimal, there may be interactions with blood thinners or some herbs. The dose is 400 mg three times a day or 600 mg twice a day.

SAMe (S-adenosyl methionine)

SAMe is a natural substance produced from methionine, an amino acid, and adenosine triphosphate (ATP), a metabolic chemical associated with energy production. It can significantly improve joint function by enhancing cartilage production, increasing joint mobility, and bolstering ATP levels. It is also an antidepressant. Taken in large doses, it can upset your stomach. The dose is 200 to 400 mg two or three times a day. Do not take SAMe if you take levodopa for Parkinson's disease. This nutrient may trigger manic episodes in people with bipolar disease.

Vitamin B3

Use of vitamin B3 can lead to improved joint mobility. Although it has not been conclusively shown to reduce pain, people in one study reduced their use of NSAIDS by 13 percent when they took B3. The accepted range is 18 to 35 mg a day. It may cause flushing.

Vitamin E and selenium

A potent antioxidant, vitamin E has been shown to relieve pain better than a placebo and NSAIDS. It works well with selenium. Accepted dose range is 15 to 1,000 mg a day of vitamin E and 60 to 400 mcg of selenium.

Zinc

This mineral has been shown to be of value. The accepted range is 8 to 40 mg a day.

D-phenylalanine

The jury is still out on this synthetic form of the amino acid phenyla-lanine. Because it inhibits the breakdown of an enzyme that, in turn, breaks down enkephalins, the body's natural painkillers, it may help decrease pain. It is sometimes commercially available in a product called DLPA (D-phenylalanine with L-phenylalanine). CAUTION: Do not take this sup-plement if you have phenylketonuria (PKU), diabetes, hypertension, or panic attacks or if you are pregnant or on antidepressants.

Herbs

White willow bark (Salix alba)

The bark of the white willow tree, native to central and southern Europe and North America, contains salicin, a substance chemically related to as-pirin. This herb is a potent anti-inflammatory and pain reliever. Several studies focusing on osteoarthritis have found that willow improves function by relieving pain, especially in the knee and hip. Although its analgesic action is slow, it is quicker than aspirin. Herbalists suggest these daily doses: 60 to 100 mg in tablets; one or two cups of tea, made by steeping 1 or 2 grams of herb in 200 ml of boiled water for 10 minutes; or 1 or 2 ml of tincture, three times. Possible side effects include gastritis and ulcers. Do not use willow if you are allergic to aspirin.

Boswellia (Boswellia serrata)

Also known as frankincense and salai guggal, *Boswellia serrata* is a tree found throughout Asia. It was used in sacraments by the ancient Hebrews in the Holy Temple. Its key component, boswellic acid, has potent anti-inflammatory properties. The recommended dose is 400 mg three times a day.

Ginger (Zingiber officinale)

This herb may have anti-inflammatory as well as painkilling properties. You can make a delicious, healing ginger tea by steeping a teaspoon of grated fresh ginger in a cup of boiling water. Add sugar if you like. Drink 3 cups a day when you're in pain.

Turmeric (Curcuma longa)

This is the pungent yellow spice frequently used in curry. Its active ingre-dient is curcumin, which is an anti-inflammatory that also has antioxidant effects. While eating it in a meal is more fun, research published in Indian medical journals suggests that taking 400 mg three times a day is effective in some forms of arthritis.

Devil's claw (Harpagophytum procumbens)

This South African herb is named for its distinctive fruit, which resembles a claw because of its tiny, fruit-bearing hooks. Although it's used extensively in Europe for arthritis pain, there has been little solid research — until recently. A randomized, double-blind, multicenter trial conducted in France and published in 2000 found devil's claw to be as effective as a commonly used conventional drug for osteoarthritis. Recommended use of devil's claw is as an infusion, up to 3 times a day: Combine 1 teaspoon of herb with 300 ml of boiling water and steep for 8 hours; then strain. CAUTION: Do not take if you are on medication for heart arrhythmias, are pregnant or breast-feeding, or at risk for ulcers.

Herbal Creams and Ointments

Nature's Chemist

This product contains menthol and a copaiba extract harvested from the Amazon. It's generally thought to be a counterirritant, or a chemical that promotes the release of the body's natural pain relievers. Use it on affected areas three times a day.

Capsaicin cream (0.025–0.075 percent)

This spicy, therapeutic botanical remedy is harvested from red peppers or cayenne. It can be a potent analgesic. Capsaicin blocks pain by interfering with a neurotransmitter known as substance P. It can also trigger release of endorphins.

Capsaicin is sold under many names, including Zostrix. Use it sparingly, since it may burn. (Cap Max is a form of extra-strength capsaicin that is thought to cause less burning.) Apply it directly to the skin around affected areas three times a day. Avoid contact with your eyes, any mucous membrane, or with open or irritated skin. Do not use capsaicin with heat. Be sure to wash your hands after use.

Joint-Ritis

An all-natural topical analgesic that combines maximum strength menthol for pain relief with skin conditioners lanolin, glucosamine, and chondroitin to help prevent skin dryness. Joint-Ritis comes in a unique roll-on applicator and a pump.

Triflora Arthritis Gel

This is a combination homeopathic gel that you can use to relieve the aches, pains, and stiffness of arthritis. Its ingredients include comfrey (*Symphytum officinale*), poison ivy (*Rhus toxicodendron*), and marsh tea (*Ledum palustre*). A randomized controlled trial recently found that it was at least as effective as Piroxicam gel, a nonsteroidal anti-inflammatory drug (NSAID), in treating osteoarthritis of the knee.

Arnica (Arnica montana, leopard's bane, mountain tobacco, sneezewort)

This herb is especially helpful for the aches and pains of arthritis. Use an arnica cream or add several drops of a tincture to a cold compress and apply when your joints are swollen. Do not use on open wounds.

Aloe (Aloe vera)

The simplest, least expensive way to use aloe is to buy a plant for your house. Simply break off a leaf and apply to your sore joints the jellylike substance that oozes out.

Dimethyl sulfoxide (DMSO)

DMSO is an industrial solvent that has been a subject of great controversy. In its gel form, it may have value. In a recent double-blind placebo-controlled study, its use resulted in a 25 percent reduction in pain. The gel is a standardized dose, so rubbing it on twice daily is enough.

Do-It-Yourself

Acupressure (See Chapter 19 for technique)

Here are some important pressure points:

1. "HO KU" is located in the web space right by the base of the thumb. Using your other hand, press on this spot for several seconds at a time to relieve arthritic pain in the upper arms and shoulders.
2. For pain in the legs, apply pressure to the outside part of the calf, about four finger widths below the knee joint.
3. Pressing hard on the bottom of both feet should improve pain in the lower legs.

Heat

To reduce stiffness and pain, try applying moist heat. Heated pools, whirlpools, warm baths, and showers are helpful. But localized heat applied directly for twenty minutes to sore spots is more effective. You can use moist compresses or microwaveable heat packs wrapped in a damp towel. However, don't do this when an area is inflamed—signs include redness, swelling, or skin that is hot to the touch. Heat draws blood to the area and increases inflammation.

Mind/Body

Relaxation and meditation (See page 340)
Since there is no cure for arthritis, these techniques will help you cope and relieve stress and depression.

Exercise

Once upon a time it was felt that arthritics shouldn't exercise because of potential damage to their joints. This myth has now been replaced by widespread acceptance of the value of exercise and fitness. In fact, I was recently part of a national expert consensus panel to formulate specific guidelines for exercise in geriatric patients with degenerative arthritis.

Joints need movement to stay healthy. Exercise can help you limit impairment by increasing your joints' range of motion and your flexibility. Building muscle strength and endurance also reduces pain and helps you better manage your daily activities. Besides, exercise improves your overall fitness and health, boosts your spirits, and helps you sleep. Of course, exercise also helps you maintain or lose weight, and obesity is a major risk factor for osteoarthritis.

Before you begin, you should consult your doctor or find a physical therapist who works with people who have arthritis. Your exercise program should be individualized to work the right muscles and avoid overstressing the affected joints. A physical therapist can design an appropriate home exercise program that you can then continue on your own.

Along with the Arthritis Foundation, I recommend several forms of exercise: strength training, range-of-motion or flexibility, and endurance.

Strength training
Strengthening exercises build muscles. This helps stabilize and support the joints and reduces pain by taking pressure off weak, hurting joints. These should be done at least every other day unless your joints are swollen or very painful. There are two types. Isometric exercises work by tightening and building strength in the muscles rather than by moving joints. Isotonic exercises move the joints to strengthen them. Try Quadriceps Sets and Leg Lifts. (See page 334 for exercise.)

RANGE-OF-MOTION EXERCISES

Also called flexibility exercises, these keep your joints moving, preventing stiffness and soreness. Your aim is to systematically, one by one, move each joint. It may help to do these exercises at the time of day when you are most comfortable. Or you may try them first thing in the morning, when your joints are at their stiffest, so you can better meet the challenges of your day. But do them every day. If your joints are swollen or painful, move them gently.

These exercises, recommended by the Arthritis Foundation, focus on the three joints most commonly afflicted in OA—knees, hips, and fingers.

Hip (CAUTION: If you've had joint replacements, do not do this exercise.)
1. Lie on your back on a comfortable friction-free surface.
2. Keep your legs straight with about a 5-inch distance between them.
3. With the toes pointing to the ceiling, glide your right leg out to the side (abduction) and then back to midline. Your leg should maintain contact with the ground at all times.
4. Repeat with the left leg.
5. Do this 10 to 15 times with each leg. You can also do this while standing.

Knee and Hip
1. Lie on your back.
2. Keep one leg bent, with foot on the floor, and the other perfectly straight.
3. Bend the knee of the straight leg.
4. Grasp the back of your thigh, just above the knee, with your hands and pull it into your chest.
5. Straighten the leg up into the air (extension).
6. Lower it to the floor.
7. Repeat with the other leg.
8. Do this 5 to 10 times with each leg.

Fingers
1. Open your hand, keeping your fingers straight and spread apart.
2. Move all of your fingers toward your palm without bending the knuckles.
3. Try to touch the top of your palm with your fingertips.
4. Extend the thumb across the palm so that it touches the creased second joint of your little finger.
5. Repeat 5 to 10 times.

AEROBIC OR ENDURANCE EXERCISES

This type of exercise will help you to control your weight, which relieves pressure on sore joints. Walking, riding stationary bikes, and swimming are good options. I especially like swimming, since the buoyancy of water supports your weight. The water also provides two-way resistance: Although movement seems easier in water, your muscles are actually working harder than they would on land. Unless you have severe joint pain or swelling, aim for twenty to thirty minutes, three times a week.

Seeking Help from Complementary Practitioners

Acupuncture

Both the World Health Organization (WHO) and the National Institutes of Health (NIH) support the use of this age-old healing art for osteoarthritis. And a powerful study of acupuncture published in 1992 found that as many as 25 percent of patients with severe arthritis canceled planned knee replacement surgery because the acupuncture gave them adequate pain relief.

Massage (See page 326)

Avoid direct massage for areas that are acutely inflamed, infected, or fractured.

Red Flags

Call your doctor if you develop fever, weakness in your muscles, or extreme fatigue.

RHEUMATOID ARTHRITIS (RA)

THE STORY OF FRANCES

People with rheumatoid arthritis are often consumed with pain and fatigue. Frances, a fifty-four-year-old African-American woman, was no exception. When I first saw her she complained of stiffness, swelling, soreness, and pain in her fingers, wrists, and ankles. She was referred to me by her rheumatologist, who had helped her come a long way, but was referring her to me for holistic pain management.

Frances's pattern of pain was not unlike that suffered by many people with rheumatoid arthritis. She had morning stiffness, occasional warmth and tenderness of her joints, loss of appetite, and fatigue. She jokingly showed me "her battle scars," small bumps on the skin known as rheumatoid modules.

The bigger problem, though, was that she experienced so much pain from her RA that everyday activities of daily living were a chore. The pain and deformity in her hands made it hard to open jars or do housework or clerical tasks. Still, I sensed that she wasn't telling me the whole story; there was another cause for her distress. When I pushed a little, she confided: "I'm embarrassed to tell you this, Doctor, but just taking care of my home, husband, and children is almost too much for me. And I feel so guilty." Needless to say, work was out of the question.

Frances had tried many pain relievers, including NSAIDS (non-steroidal anti-inflammatory drugs), corticosteroids, disease-modifying arthritis agents (DMARDS), narcotics, injections, and other traditional therapies, but nothing had helped her. She was despondent.

I started giving Frances regular acupuncture treatments and I also prescribed a host of nutritional and herbal remedies. At home, she learned to use visual imagery to relax. Frances began feeling better, but I had a hunch that the key to our success would be exercise. Pain doesn't exist in a vacuum; it is highly subjective. When I treat pain, I'm treating the body and the mind, and exercise benefits both. Still, she wasn't thrilled about the idea: "Doctor, I'm fifty-four years old, my body aches, and I've never been able to stick to an exercise routine. Do I have to?" I promised that we'd begin slowly and got her started with stretching exercises, yoga for relaxation, and tai chi. In addition, I gave her some simple acupressure techniques she could do at home while she watched TV.

As she gained confidence, I pushed her to begin a regular swimming routine. As I expected, exercise rallied her endorphins and set a restorative process into motion. Her sleeping and eating improved, as did her interactions with her husband and children. Sticking with the exercise regimen gave her more confidence in her body and empowered her to take control over her pain. I knew she had turned the corner when she told me the next time I saw her: "I feel like I deal with the pain so much more effectively now; it's probably about 75 percent less intense."

Over time, Frances developed a more optimistic outlook; at each visit, she seemed less depressed and withdrawn. She told me she was thinking about expanding her horizons and doing something in the world outside her home, a prospect that had seemed far too daunting before. The real turning point came when she walked into my office with a new suit and a stylish hairdo and said proudly: "I'm taking a job as a volunteer at the local hospital. I feel so much better about myself, it's time to help others."

Description

Rheumatoid arthritis is a chronic, debilitating, inflammatory condition that causes pain, stiffness, swelling, and loss of function in the joints. The joint linings, bones, and cartilage can all become painfully inflamed.

Joints are surrounded by a joint capsule, which is lined with thin tissue called the synovium. For some reason, the body's immune system begins to attack the synovium, causing it to become inflamed. As its cells grow and divide abnormally, the synovium thickens and the joint becomes swollen. As the disease progresses, the abnormal synovial cells invade and destroy the joint's cartilage and bone. Muscles, ligaments, and tendons surrounding the joint are weakened. The result of the process is pain and deformity.

RA usually occurs between the ages of thirty and sixty. More than 2 million people in the United States suffer from RA and it affects two to three times more women than men. Making matters even worse, RA significantly increases your chances of developing osteoporosis. Risk may be twice as high for women with RA, according to recent research.

RA may also affect women more severely. In one recent study, for example, women reported more painful joints, more swollen joints, and poorer function. And the majority of studies show that RA is slightly more disabling for women than it is for men.

Still, RA varies a lot from person to person. You may have mild RA, with flares (periods of worsening symptoms) and periods of remission. Or you may have a more severe form, where the disease is active for most of the time and results in severe joint damage and disability.

Causes

We don't yet completely understand what causes RA or why it disproportionately affects women. We do know that it is an autoimmune disease in which, for some reason, the body's immune system mistakenly attacks the synovium, or the lining inside the joint.

Although the causes of RA are elusive, there are several factors that increase your risk of developing the disease:

- Genetic predisposition—Researchers think an inherited trait, combined with a bacterial, viral, hormonal, or other environmental factor, triggers RA.
- Being female—The disease affects far more women than men.
- Hormonal factors—These may influence RA frequency and severity.

For example, in up to 75 percent of women, the disease diminishes during pregnancy; it flares up in 80 percent of women once pregnancy is over. Pregnancy may also confer a long-lasting protective effect because women who have never been pregnant are at higher risk for RA.
· Psychological stress.

Signs and Symptoms

- · Pain, swelling, soreness, and stiffness of the joints
- · Morning stiffness
- · Joints on both sides of the body are usually affected
- · During a "flare," the joints may feel warm to the touch
- · Joints most commonly involved are the fingers, hands, wrists, knees, ankles, feet, and elbows
- · Loss of appetite
- · Low-grade fever
- · Rheumatoid nodules (small bumps on the skin), especially near affected joints

Conventional Treatments

The goals of RA treatment are to relieve symptoms, prevent joint degradation, and preserve joint function. Typically, doctors rely on NSAIDS, which can cause gastrointestinal bleeding or ulcers, or the new Cox-2 anti-inflammatory drugs, which don't irritate the stomach as much. If you don't respond to these medications, your physician may prescribe disease-modifying, antirheumatic drugs (DMARDs) such as penicillamine, sulfasalazine, antimalarials, and gold salts. However, these drugs have terrible side effects. Another option is corticosteroid drugs, which are anti-inflammatory and suppress the immune system. But these also have serious side effects, especially when used over a long period.

Rest, cold, and heat applications (except during a flare) are all standard treatments. And techniques to preserve joints, such as splints and other assistive devices, may allow your inflamed joints to rest.

Dietary Strategies (See Chapter 14 for food sources of specified nutrients)

Weight
Controlling or losing weight reduces the stress on the joints.

Food allergies

Diet and food may have an impact on rheumatic disease by changing the immune or inflammatory response. In addition, allergenic foods contain antigens, or substances that provoke the immune system, triggering a hypersensitivity that can make the symptoms worse.

Calcium and vitamin D

You'll have an increased risk for osteoporosis, so make sure you get plenty of calcium-rich foods.

Vegetarian diet

In some studies, a vegetarian diet has been beneficial. Be sure to include plenty of legumes, nuts, eggs, dairy products, and vitamin B12 if you go this route. You can take this further and try a vegan diet, which excludes all animal products. A Scandinavian study found that four months on a vegan diet, along with cutting back on coffee, tea, sugar, and spice, reduced joint pain and stiffness.

Foods in the nightshade plant family (Solanaceae)

Eliminating these may provide some relief. These plants contain substances that may increase pain and discomfort by causing inflammation and halting the repair of damaged joints. The family includes potatoes, peppers, eggplant, and tomatoes.

Flaxseed oil

This oil contains alpha-linolenic acid (ALA), a precursor of the EPA and DHA in fish oil. Use 1 tablespoon a day. It should not be heated, so it's best used in salads. Smaller quantities of ALA are found in soy, canola, black currant, and walnut oil.

Green tea (Camellia sinensis)

Unlike its black and oolong counterparts, green tea is not fermented. This leaves its active ingredients—vitamins, minerals, volatile oils (polyphenols), and caffeine—intact and boosts its health-giving properties. Drink three cups a day.

Pineapple

This fruit contains bromelain, an enzyme with anti-inflammatory properties. (See page 324.)

Fish

DHA and EPA, two oils found in fish, appear to reduce RA symptoms.

RECIPE

BAKED SESAME AND OAT-CRUSTED FLOUNDER

½ cup oat flour
¼ cup sesame seeds
1 tablespoon coriander
1 tablespoon garlic powder
1 tablespoon onion powder
1 teaspoon cilantro
1 tablespoon paprika
4 egg whites
¼ cup sesame oil
4 to 5 flounder fillets, rinsed and dried
Olive oil cooking spray

1. Preheat oven to 375 degrees.
2. Combine the oat flour, sesame seeds, and spices on a shallow platter.
3. Mix the egg whites and sesame oil in a bowl.
4. Dredge the flounder fillets first in the egg mixture and then in the oat-flour mixture, until coated.
5. Spray the bottom of an ovenproof baking dish with olive oil cooking spray. Place coated fillets side by side in the baking dish and bake for 40 to 45 minutes.

Supplements

Calcium and vitamin D

These will help reduce your risk of osteoporosis. The accepted daily dose range for vitamin D is 15 to 50 mcg. The range for calcium is 1,300 to 2,500 mg. Pay special attention to calcium if you are pregnant, breast-feeding, or postmenopausal.

Fish oil

A study published in the January 2000 issue of the *American Journal of Nutrition* again corroborated the growing evidence that omega-3 fatty acids are a wise strategy. Patients who took two fatty acids—eicosapentaenoic (EPA) and docosahexaenoic acids (DHA)—for twelve weeks had less morning stiffness and fewer tender joints. These fatty acids, found in fish oil, interfere with chemical messengers that contribute to the inflammatory cycle of RA. Consuming fish oil regularly may also help you reduce your dependence on NSAIDS. Fish oil may be particularly useful if you are pregnant or breast-feeding as it may help you avoid toxic medications.

While my personal preference is that my patients get their dose of EPA and DHA from eating fish two to three times a week, those who are unable to consume fish may take supplements of fish oil; the dose is 3 grams. Be sure to keep them refrigerated because they go rancid, becoming potentially dangerous, quickly. Consuming flaxseed oil may also be helpful.

Evening primrose (EPO), borage, and flaxseed oil

These oils help elevate concentrations of a fatty acid called gamma-linoleic acid (GLA), which has potent anti-inflammatory properties. The recommended dose is either 45 mg of EPO or 1,800 mg of borage oil daily. Make sure these supplements are refrigerated.

Antioxidants

People with low antioxidant levels have a higher risk of developing rheumatoid arthritis. Take 900 to 3,000 mcg of vitamin A (retinol and beta-carotene), and 15 to 1,000 mg of vitamin E (alpha tocopherol) each day. You should also take vitamin C (ascorbic acid). The accepted range for C is 90 to 2,000 mg a day.

Herbs

Boswellia (Boswellia serrata)

Boswellic acid, a key component in this tree's bark, has pain relieving and antirheumatic properties. The jury is still out as to its absolute effectiveness but research by Dr. Deepak Chopra has demonstrated that boswellia reduces arthritis pain, especially when used with other Ayurvedic herbs, such as ginger and turmeric. The recommended dose is 400 mg three times a day.

Turmeric (Curcuma longa)

This is the pungent yellow spice frequently used in curry. Its active ingredient is curcumin, which is an anti-inflammatory that also has antioxidant effects. While eating it in a meal is more fun, research published in Indian medical journals suggests that taking 400 mg three times a day is effective in some forms of arthritis.

Ginger (Zingiber officinale)
This herb is used in both traditional Indian healing and Ayurvedic medicine. It works by inhibiting the body's production of inflammatory substances called prostaglandins. You can make a delicious tea by steeping a teaspoon of grated fresh ginger in a cup of boiling water. Add sugar if you like. Drink three cups a day when you're in pain.

Ashwaganda
Known as "Indian Ginseng," this herb in the pepper family is part of the Ayurvedic medicine chest and is also used in Africa to treat inflammatory conditions. One teaspoon of powder twice a day is the recommended dose. Use caution if you are on sedative drugs.

Valerian (Valeriana officinalis)
If pain is disturbing your sleep, you can make an infusion by adding 2 or 3 grams of herb to 150 ml of hot water and steeping for 10 to 15 minutes. Strain before use, and drink a cup 30 to 45 minutes before bedtime. I recommend that you obtain a commercially prepared infusion tea, called Dr. Stuart's "Vesper Tea," which blends valerian with limeflower, hops, passionflower, and fennel.

Ginseng
This popular herbal remedy will lessen your fatigue and improve your stamina. The suggested dose is 500 to 1,000 mg of powdered root once a day or 100 mg in standardized extract twice a day.

Herbal Creams and Ointments

Aloe (Aloe Vera) (See page 97)

Joint-Ritis (See page 96)

Do-It-Yourself

Smoking
A recent study of more than thirty thousand women found that smokers have nearly twice the risk of developing early-onset rheumatoid arthritis as do nonsmokers. So *stop smoking!*

Heat (See page 97)
Do not use heat during an acute flare.

Cold
Cold packs may be helpful after exercising especially if you get muscle spasms.

Mind/Body

Relaxation
Using progressive relaxation (see Chapter 18) to release tension in your muscles reduces pain. It also relieves the depression, anxiety, and feelings of helplessness you may feel as you try to cope with daily joint pain.

Tai chi
Tai chi is a traditional Chinese martial art that combines deep breathing with slow, gentle movements and good postures. It is also a weight-bearing exercise, so it has the potential advantage of stimulating the bones and strengthening connective tissues, which may be helpful for RA. It is often prescribed for arthritis sufferers in China. Recent research has shown tai chi to be safe for people who have RA.

Exercise

While it's important to rest, especially during periods of flares, the days of no exercise for RA patients are long gone. Lack of exercise results in weak muscles and loss of joint mobility, only causing more problems. You can use the same exercises I recommend in the osteoarthritis section. However, avoid active exercise as well as range-of-motion work when your joints are acutely inflamed.

Seeking Help from Complementary Practitioners

Acupuncture
By encouraging your body to release endorphins, acupuncture helps relieve pain.

Massage with healing oils
Swedish massage involves stroking or kneading the muscles, using lotion or oil. Nature's Chemist, a topical pain reliever, works well. So do essential herbal oils, such as eucalyptus, rose, lavender (a good stress reducer), rose-

mary, tea tree, and St. John's wort. Many essential oils can irritate the skin in their unadulterated form, so it's best to dilute them in wheat germ, almond, or sunflower oil. Using a medicine dropper, mix five to ten drops of essential oil with one tablespoon of the "carrier" oil. Because arthritic joints are sensitive, be sure your therapist is familiar with the disease.

Red Flags

Contact your doctor if you have a fever or develop spasms, weakness, or generalized fatigue.

6

Your Spine, the Body's Backbone

Eileen was a forty-three-year-old woman who managed a busy party goods store in an affluent part of town. She was frustrated and unhappy because she had chronic back pain. "My first bout took me by surprise nineteen years ago, several months after my oldest son was born," she told me. Back then, she recalled, her family doctor simply suggested that she keep off her feet for a couple of days.

But her problem never really went away. When Eileen came in, her back had troubled her for years, although she described her pain as sporadic. When it flared up, she felt a sore, aching sensation and spasms in the small of her back. Her internist had treated her with nonsteroidal anti-inflammatory medications and told her "not to overdo it." When that didn't do the trick, she referred Eileen to me.

As we talked, I realized that Eileen was a dedicated and conscientious worker. She pitched in at the store, frequently bending and lifting heavy boxes of party favors, which didn't help her achy back. Neither did her worn-out shoes, which affected the way she walked, giving her, in medical parlance, an "altered gait pattern." Making matters worse, she had gained twenty pounds over the past couple of months, thanks to refrigerator raids driven by her pain and by the stress of her job.

After reviewing her medical records, completing a thorough physical examination, and personally viewing her X rays and MRI studies, I decided that Eileen's back pain did not come from a damaged disc. It was largely mechanical in nature, although it was exacerbated by the extra weight she was carrying. I recommended a program of complementary treatments that would address the mechanical, postural, and lifestyle factors that were causing her pain.

Because it is effective for both weight control and pain management, I suggested acupuncture as a logical starting point. Of course, different acupuncture techniques are used for each problem. Usually, we use auricular (ear) acupuncture points for weight management and traditional meridian points for pain control. For an added measure of help with food cravings, portion management, and weight loss, I referred her to a hypnotist colleague.

I also gave Eileen a personalized formula for pain relief. This included postural exercises as well as a specific regimen to strengthen and tone her abdominal muscles, which would help support her spine. To mobilize her endorphins, I suggested a program of regular aerobic exercise. She balked at first, but she eventually began to take brisk daily walks, using a new, comfortable pair of impact-absorbing walking shoes. At one visit, she told me that she now looked forward to her walks. The secret of her success? "What really did it, Dr. Young, was listening to Yanni, my favorite singer, while I walk," she confided. Eileen also started a yoga class; besides the physical benefits of strengthening her muscles and increasing spinal flexibility, it also helped her unwind after work.

Over time, Eileen appeared stronger—and thinner—at her periodic visits. And her mood improved as the back pain that had plagued her for nearly twenty years gradually got better.

LOW BACK PAIN

Description

We all live with aches and pains. But low back pain is another story—it's a daunting ailment that has been around for centuries. As many as 60 to 80 percent of Americans experience low back pain at some point in their lives, with as many as 50 percent suffering from it every year. The annual cost to society, including direct medical expenditures and indirect costs, such as lost time from work, is estimated at a staggering $60 billion.

The jury is still out as to whether women actually suffer low back pain more often than men at all ages. A study of more than a thousand patients enrolled in an HMO found that women experienced more low back pain than men at young ages, but that the frequency of back pain increased significantly in men as they got older. However, in another study, women older than sixty years of age more frequently reported spine pain, possibly due to the rising incidence of osteoporosis. Other research has produced mixed results.

It may be that differences in the occurrence of low back pain have more to do with occupation than with gender. Still, it does appear that hormonal distinctions play an important role. And women bear the brunt of the astronomical human costs of low back pain, which frequently leads to time away from daily responsibilities and pleasures—working, child-rearing, recreation, and sexual activity.

There are several times during your life when you are uniquely susceptible to developing low back pain or aggravating an already-existing problem.

- During pregnancy, the burden of the baby you're carrying shifts your center of gravity forward, which may result in back pain. You also weigh more and have added breast tissue, which exacerbates the problem. Loosening of ligaments due to the hormones relaxin, estrogen, and progesterone, as well as pelvic widening, a normal physiological preparation for delivery, can increase lumbar lordosis, or normal curvature of the spine. (Typically, your spine has a curve or concavity in the back. The curve may become exaggerated when you're pregnant, creating "hollow back," "saddle back," or "sway back.") This dramatically alters body mechanics and puts stress on the lower back. These physical changes can also soften and loosen the ligaments that stabilize the pelvis.
- When your monthly menstrual period rolls around, cramps, pelvic discomfort, and bloating may aggravate existing low back pain.
- During menopause and the ensuing postmenopausal years, you may develop osteoporosis of the spine, placing you at risk for painful spinal compression fractures.

All back pain is *not* created equal. Back pain can take on many faces and can be mild or very severe. Besides, we need to distinguish between acute and chronic back pain, two sides of the same coin. Unlike acute low back pain, which is short-lived and temporary, chronic pain of the low back is protracted. It lasts three months or more and often demands a more innovative approach to treatment.

When I treat women with chronic low back pain, I like to keep in mind these words from the famed twelfth-century physician and philosopher Maimonides, who extolled the value of a restrained, middle-of-the-road, compassionate approach to dealing with medical illness, including low back pain: "To recognize the frailty of the human body and to effect a gentle cure is virtuous." I believe that if Maimonides were around today, he'd embrace the therapeutic value of complementary medicine for managing low back pain.

John Sarno's book *Mind Over Back Pain: A Radical New Approach to the Diagnosis and Treatment of Back Pain* (Berkeley Publishing Group, 1999) offers an intriguing and innovative approach to back pain that many of my patients find helpful.

Causes

To get a handle on the causes of back pain, a brief anatomy lesson about the spine, also known as the backbone, vertebral column, or spinal column, is in order. I tell my residents and medical students that the spine is a structural bulwark. It's composed of twenty-four "building blocks" or individual bones called vertebrae. These include seven in the neck or cervical area, twelve in the chest or thoracic area, and five in the low back or lumbar area. In addition, there are five sacral bones fused together to form the sacrum, the large triangle-shaped bone at the top of the pelvis, and three smaller coccyx bones at the base of the spine. Other key elements of the spine include muscles and ligaments, which play a structural and supportive role.

The spinal cord is a critically important cablelike structure that sends and receives electrical impulses between the brain and the nerves. It passes through the vertebrae by means of the spinal canal, a tubelike passageway made up of a series of interconnected holes located within each vertebra. The spinal cord terminates in the upper lumbar spine and sends nerve projections to the sacral regions.

The causes of low back pain in women are many and diverse. Some are more severe than others. The mind-boggling list includes degenerative, inflammatory, infectious, and metabolic ailments; cancer and traumatic injury; and developmental, musculoskeletal, vascular, psychological, organ-based (e.g., kidney pain), and postoperative conditions. In addition, there are many external factors that contribute to back pain, including postural problems, obesity, menstrual and pelvic disorders, and improper lifting techniques.

For the convenience of classification and simplicity, I divide back pain into three very broad categories: muscular and soft tissue, structural, and organic.

Muscular and Soft-Tissue Causes

The most common source of back pain lies in soft tissue structures — muscles, tendons, and ligaments. This pain is often mechanical in nature; in other words, it is nondisc pain that is relieved by rest and worsened by activity. Typically, it occurs because you put too much stress on your back's supporting structures when you improperly bend, twist, or lift.

In your lower back, there are several major groups of muscles that stabilize, protect, support, and aid movement. Sometimes referred to as the paraspinous muscles, these key spine muscle groups include the erector spinae (from the Latin for spine extenders, they span the entire length of the vertebral column), the semispinalis muscles, the multifidus muscles, and the interspinales muscles.

Besides the spine muscles, other muscle groups including the psoas, or limb muscles, and the quadratus lumborum play an important role in buttressing and moving the spine. In addition, the abdominal muscles provide support from the front.

Many different things can go wrong with these spinal muscles, including sprain, strain, and outright injury. Back strain can develop over time from faulty posture, or it can happen suddenly. You know this if, for example, you have ever twisted the wrong way and felt it immediately. Back strain can also result from automobile accidents or other trauma.

Spasm of the spinal muscles can lead to stiffness and aching in the low back and difficulty bending. After pregnancy and childbirth, slack belly muscles can contribute to back strain. And tight hip flexor muscles (the psoas) tilt your pelvis backward, placing added strain on the back.

Myofascial pain

This is back pain caused by inflammation and irritation of muscles and their supportive tissue, or fascial, lining. Myofascial pain, often an important component of the myofascial pain syndrome (MPS), can lead to pain in a specific region on one side of the back. MPS is often confused with fibromyalgia syndrome because of the presence of "tender pointlike areas" called trigger points, but it is *not* associated with fatigue, stiffness, or generalized aching. I organized a symposium at Johns Hopkins University Medical School in 1992 with the late Dr. Janet Travell (JFK's physician). She explained myofascial pain this way: "acute strain to the back muscles can result in localized tissue and muscle (myofascial) damage." This may injure the body's calcium storehouse (called the sarcoplasmic reticulim) and lead to muscle contraction and fatigue. Together with other metabolic changes, this causes amplified pain in the muscles of the back. (See Chapter 12 for information on fibromyalgia and MPS.)

Fibromyalgia
This syndrome is the most frequent rheumatic cause of chronic widespread pain and it is certainly a leading cause of back pain. More than 75 percent of people with fibromyalgia are women. Symptoms include fatigue, sleep disturbances, and stiffness. It also causes generalized aching with multiple tender points, as opposed to myofascial pain syndrome, which results only in localized lower back pain. Tender points occurring in fibromyalgia and myofascial conditions can be treated with local injections as well as myofascial "spray and stretch." This technique uses a prescription-only vapo-coolant spray, called ethyl chloride or fluori-methane, to chill the muscle before and during stretching.

Structural Causes

Back pain caused by abnormalities in bone and disc structures comprise this category.

Herniated disc
The intervertebral disc (disc located between vertebra) is a jellylike protective shock absorber that cushions adjoining spinal vertebrae. If the inner core of the disc (the nucleus pulposus) moves or "herniates" out of its tough, fibrous outer envelope (the annulus fibrosus) it may place pressure on neighboring nerves and/or spinal structures. There are several variations of this ailment. Ranging from the mildest to the most severe, they are:

- Disc bulge—a slight dislocation or abutment of the disc associated with weakening of the annulus.
- Disc protrusion—migration of the disc, along with partial tearing of the annulus.
- Disc extrusion—the disc pushes through or tears the full thickness of the annulus. This may even result in a "free fragment," where a part of the nucleus pulposus completely separates or is dislodged from the disc.

Disc rupture is the general term used to signify a severe form of herniation.

Many factors contribute to disc damage, including bone degeneration, poor posture, weak muscles, obesity, and stretched ligaments. Because of the burden of the added weight on the lumbar (lower) spine, pregnancy increases the risk.

A herniated disc often leads to numbness and tingling as well as shooting pain down the leg or in the buttocks or back. It may also cause pinching of neighboring nerve structures (radiculopathy) or squeezing of the sciatic nerve, the body's thickest and possibly most painful nerve.

Sciatica

This dreadful condition often results from pressure on the sciatic nerve from a herniated disc or other lumbar abnormalities, such as spinal stenosis (see below). It causes sharp, shooting pains down the thigh and leg that get worse when you walk, run, cough, sneeze, or even laugh. Because of its enormous size and its location, the sciatic nerve is especially susceptible to pressure from the growing uterus during pregnancy. If you have referred pain down your leg (pain whose source is elsewhere in your body) it does not necessarily mean you have sciatica. It could be referral from myofascial trigger points, or sacroiliac or facet dysfunction. There are also other nerves that run from the spine down the leg that can elicit similar symptoms.

Compression fractures

With age, and particularly after menopause, you may lose key bone minerals, including calcium and magnesium. This decreases bone density and places the spine at risk for fracture (see page 137). As the spine becomes less dense and more fragile, portions of the vertebrae may disintegrate and collapse onto one another. On an X ray this looks like a wedge. Loss of height, pain, stiffness, spasm, and a deformity known as dowager's hump are often the result.

Spinal stenosis-lumbar

Although it is sometimes the result of a birth defect, this condition, common in older women, more often occurs when the spinal canal and/or existing nerve roots become narrowed from degenerative arthritis or trauma (often superimposed on a congenitally narrowed spinal canal). If you have X rays or other imaging studies your doctor will probably see evidence of an enlarged disc, bone spurs, or thickened ligaments. Symptoms include pseudoclaudication, or cramping in the legs and feet, weakness, numbness, and pain radiating down the leg. Your doctor will need to differentiate this pain from hardening of the arteries in your leg.

Spondylolisthesis

Sometimes, a malfunction of the spinal stabilizing ligaments causes slippage of one vertebra over a neighboring one, resulting in spinal instability. A small fracture, a prior trauma history, a birth defect, or another abnormality of the bones may be associated with this ailment. While most cases of spondylolisthesis are inconsequential, severe slippage (more than 50 percent) can threaten the spinal cord or nerves.

Spondylosis

This is a common condition that does not necessarily produce symptoms. It is caused by degenerative joint disease (osteoarthritis) and loss of flexibility of the spine. As a result, you may feel stiff and sore.

Scoliosis, kyphosis, or exaggerated lordosis

These are different types of abnormal curvature of the spine. They may be present at birth and worsen with age or they may occur during adulthood.

Other causes

Other structural causes of low back pain include rheumatoid arthritis and ankylosing spondylitis, or AS, a genetic condition where the vertebral bones fuse to one another. (AS is three times more common in men than in women.) It's not unusual to have these conditions along with osteoarthritis of the spine. (For more information on arthritis, see Chapter 5.)

Occasionally, a combination of mechanical and structural problems may cause back pain. Examples include an imbalanced or rotated pelvic bone (pelvic obliquity), ligament abnormality, facet joint arthritis, or myofascial pain.

Organic Causes of Low Back Pain

Low back pain is sometimes the result of infection or disease. Some of the more common causes are: infections of bone or disc; kidney stones or infections; gynecological, intestinal, or pancreatic diseases; cancer that originates in (myeloma or leukemias) or spreads to the spine (breast, lung, prostate, and colon cancers); and aneurysms.

Signs and Symptoms

These vary, depending on the specific problem. However, common symptoms include:

- Stiffness
- Pain
- Muscle spasms
- Pain shooting down to the buttocks or legs
- Numbness or tingling in the buttock or groin
- Numbness or tingling in the feet, legs, or toes

Conventional Treatments

Because there are so many possible causes for back pain, it is important for a medical professional to sort through them and diagnose your pain. Physiatrists, medical doctors who specialize in physical medicine and rehabilitation, are specially trained in this area. They are the best medical doctors to evaluate and treat acute and chronic back and neck pain without surgery. If you consult a physiatrist, you can expect to undergo a thorough physical examination that focuses on your neurological and musculoskeletal systems, in addition to other important organ systems. Your functional status (how well you walk, work, and perform basic activities of living) will be evaluated. It may be necessary for your doctor to order additional diagnostic testing including X rays, MRI, or electrodiagnosis (nerve conduction studies and electromyography to pinpoint nerve injury). The physiatrist will carefully assess your body mechanics and suggest a customized, conservative (i.e., nonsurgical) strategy for dealing with your back pain, depending on its cause. If necessary, she will refer you to a physical therapist for a customized home exercise regimen or she will provide one herself.

Several classes of medications are used for back pain:

Analgesics

Pain relievers are a first line of treatment. These include everything from Tylenol (good for pain relief but not for battling inflammation) and other over-the-counter drugs (e.g., aspirin, Motrin, Aleve) to prescription nonsteroidal anti-inflammatory drugs (NSAIDS), Cox-2 selective inhibitor NSAIDS (Vioxx and Celebrex), and narcotics, such as codeine. Bear in mind that narcotics can cause constipation, breathing difficulty (in large doses), sedation or drowsiness, or addiction. Tramadol (Ultram), another type of analgesic, acts on your central nervous system and may act as a weak opioidlike drug. However, this drug can lower your seizure threshold. Also, use caution if you take St. John's wort or 5-HTP. (See page 304.)

Topical pain relievers

Recent developments include topical forms of nonsteroidals. Because they can be applied locally, topicals do not cause stomach upset or other forms of organ damage that may be associated with NSAIDS in pill form. As I travel all over the world for visiting lectureships and scientific symposia, I marvel at these rub-on prescription pain relievers that are readily available in other countries, and I regret that they are not available in the United States. Over-the-counter topical creams that can help include Arthromax, Ben Gay, Icey heat, and similar formulations.

There is some good news, however. Complementary topical pain relievers, such as Nature's Chemist and Joint-Ritis, are starting to appear in the American marketplace. They've proven to be effective for many of my patients (see page 96).

Other medications

If you suffer from muscle spasms, your doctor may prescribe muscle relaxers, such as Valium, baclofen, Flexeril, Skelaxin, and Robaxin. For severe conditions, to improve your mood and help you sleep, she may suggest Elavil or another antidepressant, an antianxiety drug, such as Valium or Xanax, or sleeping pills, like Ambien or Sonata.

When you see your physiatrist or musculoskeletal physician, she will determine forms of treatment best suited for your particular situation. If your pain comes from compression fractures due to osteoporosis, improving your bone stock is a priority, and calcitonin or Fosamax may help.

Injections or nerve blocks

Depending on the cause of your pain, your doctor may recommend the following:

- Fibromyalgia and myofascial pain frequently involve trigger points or tender points in individual muscles. Lidocaine injections or a lidoderm patch may help.
- If you have an extremely severe case of structural pain, and your doctor determines that true nerve root irritation is the cause, a spinal block (epidural injection) may be indicated. Other types of blocks include facet joint blocks and paravertebral blocks.
- Prolotherapy, or injections of concentrated sugar water and alcohol, stimulate the body to produce connective tissue. This can strengthen ligaments and tendons, thus stabilizing the spine or pelvic joints.

TENS

Applied over the painful site, a transcutaneous electrical nerve stimulator (TENS) unit uses electrical impulses to help block the pain signals before they enter your spine.

Mechanical strategies

Your doctor may recommend a back brace, lumbar supports, switching to a comfortable mattress, using new shoes, getting shoe orthotics, or correcting a leg length discrepancy.

Hydrotherapy

Swimming is an excellent choice since it improves flexibility of the spine and extremities in a low impact, soothing environment. Other types of hydrotherapy include the whirlpool or Jacuzzi.

Supplements

Melatonin

This is a natural hormone that modulates sleep. If you have trouble sleeping take 1 or 2 mg, thirty minutes before bed.

SAMe (S-adenosyl methionine)

This nutritional supplement is composed of two amino acids. It is useful in many types of pain syndromes, including back and neck pain. Studies of SAMe in patients with osteoarthritis have found that it is as effective as NSAIDS. SAMe is also an antidepressant. Dose is from 200 mg twice a day up to 400 mg three times a day, if you can tolerate it. Large doses may upset your stomach. Do not take SAMe if you take levodopa for Parkinson's disease. This nutrient may trigger manic episodes in people with bipolar disease.

Herbs

White willow bark (Salix alba)

Used in China for centuries as a treatment for pain and fever, white willow bark has become a popular mode of treating back pain. A study published in *Rheumatology Diseases of North America* demonstrated its benefits and, best of all, found that it caused minimal gastrointestinal discomfort, an advantage over other anti-inflammatory drugs. Do not take willow concurrently with aspirin or NSAIDS. Use caution if you take blood thinners, diuretics, or blood pressure medications. Recommended dose is 60 to 120 mg a day.

Valerian (Valeriana officinalis)

Since sleep may be difficult for you when you are experiencing back pain, you may be able to catch some "Zs" with the help of valerian, a plant that is on the FDA's list of herbs generally recognized as safe (GRAS). It's best taken as a tea, one cup before bedtime. Some people complain of the odor, so if you prefer a tincture, the recommended dose is 1/2 to 1 teaspoon (1–3 ml).

Chamomile (Chamaemelum nobile or Matricaria recutita)

This sweet-smelling herb helps fight inflammation and promotes relaxation. To help you sleep, make a double-strength tea by using two tea bags or steeping 2 teaspoons of dried flowers in one cup of boiling water. Avoid contact with your eyes; chamomile may cause irritation. It may also cause an allergic reaction.

Herbal Creams and Ointments.

Nature's Chemist (See page 96)

Joint-Ritis (See page 96)

Dimethyl sulfoxide (DMSO)

DMSO is an industrial solvent that has been a subject of great controversy. It has not been approved by the FDA despite its popularity as a remedy for musculoskeletal pain, arthritis, and neck and low back pain. However, I believe the gel may have value. In a recent double-blind placebo-controlled study, using it led to a 25 percent reduction in pain. Rubbing it on twice daily is enough.

Arnica

Rub Arnica cream or ointment into the affected area. Don't use this herb on broken skin.

Capsaicin cream (0.025–0.075 percent) (See page 96)

Spine Injections and Interventional Procedures

Some physiatrists, orthopedists, and anesthesiologists perform interventional pain procedures, including epidural blocks, paravertebral blocks, facet blocks, and others. These may decrease your pain.

Do-It-Yourself

Everyday things

- Back pain is linked to smoking, so here's one more reason to stop if you haven't already.
- Avoid sleeping on your stomach. Instead, curl up on your side with a pillow between your knees, or sleep on your back. And stay away from soft, sagging mattresses.
- If you have to lift something from a height above your shoulders, stand on a sturdy, steady ladder or stool to bring your shoulders above the object. Test the weight of the object by pushing against it before picking it up; if it's too heavy for you, ask for help.
- When lifting heavy objects, start with your legs bent and your feet apart. Take a deep breath and tighten your stomach muscles to support your back. Lift with your legs; as you straighten your legs and return to a vertical position, hold the object close to your body. Bend your legs to set the object back down.

Acupressure (See page 353)

This is a convenient way to use your fingers to exert pressure over acupoints, which stimulates the flow of *qi* through the key bladder and gallbladder meridians.

1. With your knees bent, lie on your side.
2. Take the pulpy surface of your thumb and place it on your sacrum (tailbone).
3. While applying firm pressure, glide your fingers upward along your spine until you can reach the topmost reachable vertebra.
4. Repeat this process 5 times.
5. After the fifth time, take the pulpy surface of your thumb and place it on the top of your spine, near your neck.
6. Using your other hand, follow the contour of your ribs, applying pressure in an outward direction.
7. Repeat this process, following the path of your ribs.
8. Turn over and repeat for the opposite side.

Reflexology
Several potent reflexology points can reduce discomfort in your back.

- *Bl-60 (Bladder 60)* is located around the outer ankle bone and is a good point for severe lumbar and neck pain. CAUTION: Avoid if you are pregnant.
- *SP-3 (Spleen-3)* is located at the inner arch near the front of the foot, at the very end of the first foot bone, this point fortifies the spine.
- *KI-1 (Kidney 1)* Pressing on this point, situated on the sole of the foot, between the second and third foot bones (metatarsal bones), relieves low back pain.

If you are in public and don't want to remove your shoes and socks, try some of these points instead:

- *GV-26 (Governor Vessel 26)* To strengthen the spine, try this point, which lies within the vertical depression in the midline under the nose.
- *SI-3 (Small Intestine 3)* For back pain, apply pressure to the outer edge of the knuckle below the little finger (pinky).
- *SI-4 (Small Intestine 4)* For back pain, try the point near the wrist, at the base (bottom) of the pinky.

Mind/Body

Yoga
Cat Pose, Cobra, and Spinal Twist will help increase strength and flexibility in the spine. (See pages 344–351.)

Exercise

Strengthening Exercises
Try the Pelvic Tilt, Half Sit-up, and Leg Raises. (See pages 331–338 for exercises.)

Flexibility Exercises
Try the Seated Low Back Stretch, Knee to Chest Raise, and the Lower Back Piriformis Stretch. (See pages 331–338.)

Seeking Help from Complementary Practitioners

Acupuncture

The value of acupuncture in treating back pain was recognized as far back as the late 1800s by the legendary Sir William Osler of Johns Hopkins Hospital. More than a hundred years later, study after study has provided contemporary corroboration for his early insight, culminating in an endorsement from the Consensus Group of the National Institutes of Health. Although no one knows for sure how acupuncture works, we believe it promotes the release of endorphins, thereby curbing pain and spasms and reducing anxiety.

Chiropractic and osteopathic manipulation

A substantial body of research supports the use of spinal manipulation for relief of low back pain, including several large analyses of studies that show it to be at least as effective as most standard medical treatments. Besides, in 1994, the federal Agency for Health Care Policy and Research, after reviewing thousands of studies on low back pain, concluded that spinal manipulation does provide relief. Chiropractic is more effective for acute, rather than chronic, back pain.

Massage therapy

There's plenty of anecdotal evidence for the effectiveness of massage therapy for low back pain, but until recently there haven't been many solid studies. However, an article published last year in the *Canadian Medical Association Journal* is convincing. The study compared the effectiveness of comprehensive massage therapy and a "sham" laser therapy placebo for low back pain lasting between one week and eight months. The comprehensive massage therapy group had significantly improved function and less pain. One month later, 63 percent of the people in the massage therapy group were still reporting no pain.

Red Flags

Call your doctor if you experience:

- Pain shooting down to your legs or buttocks
- Loss of control of your bladder or bowels
- Numbness or tingling in your buttocks, groin, feet, legs, or toes
- Muscle weakness in your legs or feet

- Inability to raise your foot or big toe
- Protracted night pain, when you are lying still
- Night sweats, loss of significant weight over time

LOW BACK PAIN IN PREGNANCY

Description

You are not alone if you have back pain during pregnancy. More than half of pregnant women suffer from this problem. It occurs most frequently after the sixth month of pregnancy and often lasts well after the baby is born. If you have had other episodes of back pain or if you have given birth before, you are more likely to have back pain.

Causes

When you are pregnant, a number of factors change your body mechanics, leaving you vulnerable to back pain. Obviously, you're carrying a lot of extra weight, which shifts your center of gravity forward. As your abdominal muscles stretch to accommodate your growing belly, they provide less support to your back. Your body significantly ups its production of hormones, especially relaxin, which increases tenfold. This hormonal adaptation, courtesy of Mother Nature, allows your pelvis to widen in preparation for delivery by loosening key pelvic joints, including the sacroiliac joint and the pubic symphysis (the slightly movable joint at the front of the pelvis). Rising relaxin levels also affect the anterior and posterior longitudinal ligaments, which normally act as critical guide wires for the spine. As they loosen, it significantly weakens the spine's ability to resist stress, strains, and shear forces. You may experience pain from the discs as well as other important mobile disc structures, like the facet joints.

Signs and Symptoms

- Spasms or other pain, especially in the lower back
- Tenderness
- Feeling achy
- Stiffness
- Pain that shoots down your legs

Conventional Treatments

If you suffer from lower back pain while you're pregnant, it's likely your obstetrician will recommend Tylenol and hot packs. However, be careful about bathing in hot tubs; hot water raises your body temperature, which can injure the developing fetus.

Do-It-Yourself

Cold

Applying ice bags, rubber or plastic gloves filled with ice, or frozen gel packs can numb sore areas, slowing transmission of pain signals. Keep a thin towel between your skin and the cold pack; apply for twenty minutes at a time.

Massage

Here are two easy techniques that may help. First, have your partner apply as much pressure as you can tolerate to the center of the middle of your back. Or if you prefer, try effleurage: Have your partner use a "feather touch," a very soft, tender application of the fingers to your back.

A sacroiliac corset

This maternity corset surrounds the pelvis, helping you to maintain proper position and preventing structural damage.

Bra

Be sure to wear a good, comfortable bra, preferably with nonelastic straps. This will stabilize and support your breasts and decrease low back and neck pain.

Everyday things

- Avoid strain and injury by learning and using good body mechanics. Simple movements to avoid include sitting for long periods, bending from the waist, and lifting and carrying heavy objects far away from your body's center of gravity.
- Maintain a neutral spine position. Prevent excessive curvature of the spine (lordosis) or excessive reversal of lordosis by avoiding shoes with high heels.
- To improve your comfort while standing, avoid bringing your shoulders back too far, since this increases lordosis. You can decrease strain on your lumbar spine and paraspinal muscles by putting your foot on a

chair; this relaxes the iliopsoas muscle and tilts your pelvis forward. Take frequent sitting breaks so you don't stand for long periods of time.
· Rest one foot on a chair when you are sitting.

Mind/Body

Relax
Put on some soothing music and take a warm aromatherapy bath using a few drops of essential oil made from citrus (mandarin, orange blossom) or flowers (rose, lavender, jasmine, or geranium). Just make sure the water isn't too hot.

Breathe
Deep breathing with or without progressive muscle relaxation (see Chapter 18).

Meditation (See Chapter 18)

Exercise

As long as you don't overdo it, physical activity and exercise throughout pregnancy will help keep your back muscles in shape. Walking briskly, yoga, dancing, and even running are options. I find swimming to be an excellent exercise for my pregnant patients, since it dramatically reduces the effects of gravity and relieves pressure on the back. Check with your physician before starting any new exercise program.

In addition, you can do the Pelvic Tilt (see page 331) to strengthen abdominal and low back muscles. However, do it very cautiously after the third month of pregnancy.

Seeking Help from Complementary Practitioners

Chiropractic
Chiropractic is an effective method for dealing with low back pain, and it is safe to use during pregnancy. Two manipulative techniques in particular may be helpful: the "shotgun," which eliminates asymmetry in the pubic symphysis and the "pelvic rock," for relief of lower back pain.

Acupuncture
According to an expert panel convened by the National Institutes of Health, acupuncture is an effective treatment for low back pain. More to the point,

a recent study supported the value of acupuncture for low back and pelvic pain in pregnancy. However, you should still exercise caution and discuss your condition with your acupuncturist. Certain acupuncture points are off limits during this time of your life.

Massage

Professional massage is safe during pregnancy as long as it is done gently, avoiding pressure on your belly and uterus. If possible, look for a masseuse who has had special training in pregnancy massage.

Red Flags

Call your doctor if you experience bleeding, sustained pains, or contractions, fever, or discharge.

NECK PAIN

Description

The neck performs three major functions: it provides stability and a base of support for the head, it protects the spinal cord and nerve roots, and it permits you to move your head in all directions. Of the many areas of the spine, the neck (also known as the cervical part of the spine) is the most mobile. It is also relatively fragile, given that the head is a heavy load. These factors combine to make the neck especially vulnerable to strain or injury.

Throughout history, cervical neck pain and dysfunction have been recognized as major medical concerns. In ancient Greece, the philosopher-physician Hippocrates pioneered the use of cervical traction; he was also the first to recognize the relationship between neck injury and paralysis. And a bit later, in the second century, the Roman emperor Marcus Aurelius was cared for by the celebrated physician Galen, who also proudly served as a "neck surgeon" to injured gladiators.

Today, neck pain and dysfunction are common problems. About one-third of us experience neck pain at some point in our lives, with the problem even more frequent among physical laborers. Neck pain without associated arm pain is more common in women than men.

Causes

To better understand the causes and types of neck pain, we need to digress for a brief anatomy lesson. Your neck is made up of a series of seven bones (numbered C1 through C7, with the C standing for cervical), or vertebrae, which can be conveniently divided into two sections, the upper neck and the lower neck.

The upper neck bones

The top two bones in the upper portion of the neck are unique in appearance and are called the Atlas (C1), an appropriate name because this ring-like bone holds up the weight of the head, and the Axis (C2). These two bones have a special relationship; they are connected by a structure called the odontoid process, which is bound by a transverse ligament. If disease, such as rheumatoid arthritis, or trauma disrupt this joint, the neck may become unstable. The Atlas and Axis permit flexion and extension (nodding) and rotation (saying no).

The lower neck bones

All of the lower neck bones (C3 through C7) are similar in dimension and function. They are suited for flexion, extension, and sideways flexion.

Soft tissue structures of the neck

Sandwiched between each of the cervical vertebra, except the Atlas and Axis, is an intervertebral disc. These discs facilitate motion; they are also shock absorbers that protect the spine. Degenerative changes or herniation in these discs can cause nerve root damage or even spinal cord injury.

Attached to the cervical vertebrae are a series of ligaments that lend stability and strength to the neck. In addition, the neck muscles help facilitate movement and give additional support to the cervical spine and head. The muscles in the front of the spine are flexors; they bring the head forward. Those in the back are extensors, which move the head backward.

Some of the same muscles in the lumbar spine (see page 113) are also present in the neck. Deep beneath them are the rotator muscles. Certain shoulder muscles—the trapezius, rhomboid, and levator scapulae—are attached to the cervical spine, so some shoulder injuries may cause neck pain.

The causes of neck pain are as diverse as they are numerous. Frequently it's a simple, correctable habit, such as:

- An uncomfortable sleeping position, especially if you have neck pain in the morning

- Poor posture or sitting in the same position for long periods
- Cradling a phone between your ear and shoulder
- If you already have a neck injury, leaning your head back over a sink for a shampoo in a hair salon can aggravate it
- Emotional stress

But your distress may be more than a simple "pain in the neck." Causes of neck pain include this mind-boggling list: degenerative, inflammatory, infectious, and metabolic ailments, cancer and traumatic injury; as well as developmental, musculoskeletal, vascular, psychological, organ-based (e.g., kidney pain), and postoperative conditions. I like to distill these causes into three broad categories: muscular and soft tissue, structural, and organic.

Muscular/Soft-Tissue Causes

Whiplash, which affects a million Americans every year, is the most common type of neck injury in this country. It is the result of sprain or strain injuries to the muscles, tendons, or ligaments of the neck. The most common scenario for whiplash is an overextension injury. For example, your car is rear-ended, and you first flex and then hyperextend your neck. It's not surprising, then, that epidemiological studies have shown that whiplash is far more common in major cities, where there are more cars. Women have a higher incidence of this ailment than men. About one-third of whiplash victims develop pain within twenty-four hours.

Structural Causes

Herniated disc

The disc is a jellylike protective shock absorber that cushions adjoining spinal vertebrae. If the inner core of the disc (the nucleus pulposus) moves or "herniates" out of its tough, fibrous outer envelope (the annulus fibrosis) it may place pressure on neighboring nerves and/or spinal structures. There are several variations of this ailment. (See page 115.)

Many factors contribute to disc damage, including bone degeneration, poor posture, weak muscles, obesity, and stretched ligaments. A herniated disc in the neck often leads to shooting pain as well as numbness and tingling that extends down to the fingers (radiculopathy). It may also cause painful pinching of neighboring nerve structures. Depending on which nerve roots are affected, you may also get numbness in your thumb and second finger or in your ring finger and pinky.

Cervical spondylosis
This condition is caused by degenerative joint disease (osteoarthritis) of the spine, which causes it to lose its flexibility. As a result, you feel stiff and sore.

Cervical stenosis
Although it is sometimes the result of a birth defect, this condition, common in older women, more often occurs when the spinal canal and/or existing nerve roots become narrowed from degenerative arthritis or trauma. (A congenitally narrowed canal often predisposes you to narrowing from other causes.) If you have X rays or other imaging studies, your doctor will probably see evidence of an enlarged disc, bone spurs, or thickened ligaments.

Organic Causes

Neck pain is sometimes the result of infection or other disease. Rheumatological conditions that may cause neck pain include ankylosing spondylitis, psoriatic arthritis, degenerative arthritis, and polymyalgia rheumatica (PMR). Infectious diseases, such as meningitis, influenza, German measles, mononucleosis, osteomyelitis, discitis, Lyme disease, and herpes zoster may also cause neck pain. Neurological causes of neck pain include cervical dystonias, which are involuntary, spasmodic contractions of neck muscles that lead to abnormal neck and head positioning and pain. Finally, neck pain may result from endocrinological and metabolic disorders, such as osteoporosis, osteomalacia, Paget's disease, parathyroid gland abnormalities, and pituitary tumors.

Signs and Symptoms

- Pain, spasm, or deep ache in the neck, shoulder, or arm
- Limited range of motion
- Stiffness of the neck and shoulder muscles
- Headache

Neck pain is often a temporary condition. However, you may need medical diagnosis and treatment if it persists or is associated with shooting pains, numbness, tingling, loss in strength, or abnormal reflexes.

Conventional Treatments

Analgesics, or pain relievers, are a first line of treatment. These include everything from Tylenol (good for pain relief but not for battling inflammation) and other over-the-counter drugs (e.g., aspirin, Motrin, Aleve) to prescription nonsteroidal anti-inflammatory drugs (NSAIDS) and Cox-2 selective inhibitor NSAIDS (Celebrex and Vioxx). Narcotics, such as codeine, are sometimes prescribed but they can cause constipation, breathing difficulty (in large doses), sedation or drowsiness, or addiction. Tramadol (Ultram), another type of analgesic, acts on the central nervous system and may act as a weak opioidlike drug. This drug, however, can lower your seizure threshold. Also, use caution if you take St. John's wort.

Recent developments include topical (rub-on) forms of nonsteroidals, available abroad but not yet in the United States. Because they can be applied locally, they do not cause stomach upset or other forms of organ damage that may be associated with NSAIDS in pill form.

If you suffer from muscle spasms, your doctor may prescribe muscle relaxers, such as Valium, baclofen, Flexeril, Skelaxin, and Robaxin. For severe conditions, to improve your mood and help you sleep, she may suggest Elavil or another antidepressant, an antianxiety drug, such as Valium or Xanax, or sleeping pills, like Ambien or Sonata. Be sure to ask your doctor about side effects; some of these drugs may be addictive.

If there is significant evidence of tender points or trigger points on examination, injections can be helpful. Occasionally, spinal interventional procedures are useful.

If you have neck pain emanating from cervical dystonia, injection with Myobloc (botulism toxin), along with oral medication and exercise may be the answer.

In some instances, your doctor may recommend a soft collar. This won't immobilize your neck, but it will provide cushioned comfort and remind you to keep your neck straight. The Philadelphia collar and other more rigid forms of immobilization may also be used.

Supplements

Take calcium carbonate to slow down osteoporosis. The accepted dose range is 1,300 to 2,500 mg a day.

Vitamin E

This is a potent antioxidant that may reduce muscle damage from free radical activity. The dose range is 15 to 1,000 mg a day.

Vitamin C
To promote tissue healing and cut down on soreness, take from 90 to 2,000 mg a day. Combining your vitamin C with pantothenic acid may improve the strength of healing tissue.

SAMe
A nutritional supplement composed of two amino acids, SAMe is useful in many types of pain syndromes, including back and neck pain. In some studies, it's been as effective as NSAIDS. SAMe is also an antidepressant. Dose is from 200 mg twice daily up to 400 mg three times a day, if you can tolerate it. Be aware, however, that in large doses it can upset your stomach. Do not take SAMe if you take levodopa for Parkinson's disease. This nutrient may trigger manic episodes in people with bipolar disease.

Herbs

Meadowsweet (Filipendula ulmaria)
This herb contains flavonoids and salicylates and has anti-inflammatory properties. Use caution with this herb if you are sensitive to aspirin. Meadowsweet may also cause diarrhea. Herbalists suggest that you make an infusion by steeping 1 or 2 teaspoons of dried herb in one cup of boiling water for 10 minutes. Drink up to 3 cups a day.

Kava kava (Piper methysticum)
If neck pain is making you anxious, try kava kava, a widely used natural solution. Although its effects are not always immediate, this herb's key chemical, kavalactone, has calming, sedative, and pain-relieving properties. In some cases it may also alleviate spasms. Kava kava's mechanism of action seems to be similar to that of the conventional drugs Xanax and Valium. A six-month double-blind study of a hundred people found that kava kava reduced general anxiety levels significantly more than a placebo. The recommended dose is 70 mg three times a day.

White willow bark (Salix alba)
Long used by Native Americans for pain and fever, white willow bark is now a popular mode of treating back pain. A double-blind, randomized, controlled study published in the *American Journal of Medicine* in 2000 showed that 39 percent of treated patients were pain-free after five days, compared with 6 percent in the nontreated group. Do not take this herb with aspirin or NSAIDS. Use caution if you are on blood pressure medi-

hinners, or diuretics. The recommended dose is 60 to 120

Do-It-Yourself

There are many effective techniques you can use to prevent and relieve neck and shoulder pain.

For Prevention

- Practice good posture. Keep your head up and your chin somewhat tucked in. Your ear, shoulder, and hip should be in a straight line when sitting, standing, or lying down. Don't hunch your shoulders.
- Sleep on a firm surface using a thin pillow, a specially contoured foam cervical pillow, a rolled-up towel, or no pillow at all.
- Do not cradle the telephone between your neck and shoulder. Use a headset.
- Avoid sleeping on your stomach — this can twist your neck.
- When carrying a heavy shoulder bag or luggage, try to carry the weight equally on both sides. If you can't, use a backpack.
- Move your seat up or use pillows when you're driving to help you maintain good posture. Do not drive leaning forward.
- Try not to tip your head back.

For Pain Relief

Improvement is slow and may take several weeks. Be patient.

Cold

For neck pain and most musculoskeletal problems, it's best to apply cold during the first twenty-four hours. This helps decrease inflammation and cramping. Apply ice, a cold pack, or a bag of frozen vegetables for ten to fifteen minutes every few hours.

Heat

After the first twenty-four hours, switch to heat. To relieve spasms and pain, take hot showers or apply hot compresses or a heating pad for fifteen to twenty minutes every few hours.

Herbal rubs

- Rub arnica tincture or ointment into the affected area to ease any bruising. This is especially effective if your neck pain develops after a car accident.
- Wintergreen liniment, ointment, or cream contain methyl salicylate (aspirin), which helps mask pain because of its analgesic, counterirritant effects. Use cautiously if you are pregnant, breast-feeding, or taking anticoagulants.

Posture

For acute pain relief, try:

1. Lie on your back with your head on a soft feather pillow and a small towel, rolled up and propped under your neck. Keep your knees bent and supported by large pillows.
2. Lie on your side with a soft feather pillow and a small towel rolled under your neck.
3. When sitting, use pillows so you can rest your head back comfortably, with pillows propping up and supporting your arms.

Reflexology

Apply pressure to these points:

- GB-20 (Feng Chi point), above the hairline on the nape of the neck. There are two, one on each side.
- Bl-10 (celestial pillar), at the hairline, two finger widths outside of the spine.
- LI-4 (Large Intestine-4), (He GU), on the back of your hand in the web space between the thumb and first finger. This is one of the four most potent acupressure/acupuncture points in the body.

Massage

1. Take your arm and wrap it around your neck from the front.
2. Place your fingers on the back of your opposite shoulder and squeeze and knead the muscles.
3. Work your way toward the spine and up and down.
4. Using both hands, grasp the back of the neck on each side and squeeze in a circular motion.
5. Move up the back of your neck and skull.

Pressure

Use a tennis ball to apply pressure to "hot points." Hold a tennis ball cupped in your palm. With your head and neck on a pillow, apply it to the following spots:

1. Just under the skull on the upper neck.
2. Above the shoulder blade, 4 to 5 inches from the spine or the base of the neck.
3. At the back of the shoulder, 2 to 3 inches above the crease of the arm against the body.
4. In the deltoid muscle area, 1 to 2 inches below and to the side of the top of the shoulder.

Mind/Body

Relaxation (See Chapter 18)

Because tension and stress often lodge in your neck and shoulders, relaxation techniques are particularly useful.

Tai chi and yoga

With their emphasis on gentle stretching, good posture, and deep breathing and relaxation, these techniques are excellent for neck and back pain.

Exercise

Gently stretching the neck loosens stiff muscles and relieves tension. Stop these exercises if the pain increases or moves to your arms. Try Side Stretches and Chin Tucks. (See pages 331–338.)

Seeking Help from Complementary Practitioners

Acupuncture

A three- to four-week course of acupuncture may reduce your pain and help you cut back on pain medications.

Body manipulation

A variety of techniques, including massage, will speed your recovery, reduce pain, release spasms, and promote circulation.

Red Flags

Call your doctor if:

- Your pain is associated with fever and headache, or your neck is too stiff to touch your chin to your chest; these symptoms are associated with meningitis.
- The pain travels down your arm, or you have numbness or tingling.
- You have painful or swollen glands in your neck that persist for several days.

OSTEOPOROSIS

Description

Osteoporosis is the most common metabolic bone disease, and one of the most important age-associated disorders in Western societies. In the United States it affects more than 25 million people, 80 percent of whom are women.

This skeletal disease causes reduced bone mass and deterioration of bone leading to weakness, brittleness, and an increased tendency to fracture. Typically occurring during the first or second decade after menopause, osteoporosis is the leading cause of fractures in postmenopausal women. In fact, half of all women develop osteoporosis-related fractures. The most common fracture sites are the spine, hip, and forearm. Osteoporosis can also lead to changes in posture and spinal deformities, such as the "dowager's hump," or hunchback. It is potentially a disabling disease.

Causes

Contrary to what most people believe, bones are not dead; we are constantly making and losing bone. Depending upon the type of bone involved, we replace anywhere from 5 to 25 percent each year. This normal bone metabolism depends on heredity, nutrition, lifestyle, hormones, and liver and kidney function. In childhood, we build far more bone than we lose, so our bone mass increases steadily. And during our young adult years, total bone mass is relatively stable.

But after about age thirty, both men and women start to lose bone. Until women reach menopause, the pace at which this occurs is about the same for both sexes because female reproductive hormones, especially estrogen, play a major role in maintaining the density and integrity of bone.

As your estrogen levels drop, however, you go through a period of accelerated bone loss, and your skeleton begins to deteriorate. Your bones may become more "porotic" as you age—they have more holes and are thinner and weaker. You are at a higher risk of dropping below an imaginary line called the fracture threshold, which means that you are more prone to fractures from even relatively normal behaviors. Men reach this threshold, too, but not until they are significantly older.

A number of factors increase your chances of developing osteoporosis. Some of them can't be changed; unfortunately, you're stuck with them:

- Being a woman
- Age (postmenopausal women are at highest risk)
- Caucasian race
- Heredity—both a maternal history of hip fracture and a family history of osteoporosis
- Previous vertebral fracture
- Early menopause—either naturally occurring before age forty-five or surgical- or drug-induced
- Erratic periods
- Late onset of menstruation
- Absence of ovulation
- A history of anorexia nervosa, diabetes mellitus, Cushing's disease, hyperthyroidism, or hyperparathyroidism (an overactive parathyroid)
- Medications, such as glucocorticoids (steroids), water pills, anticonvulsants, and heparin, which increase bone loss

The good news is that there's a lot you can do to lower your risk.

Signs and Symptoms

Unfortunately, the first symptom of osteoporosis is frequently a bone fracture. You may also experience:

- Loss of height
- Spinal deformity (neck hump)
- Severe bone pain

Conventional Treatments

Since prevention is the best treatment, it's important to identify your risk factors early. In addition to recommending that you exercise, take calcium and vitamin D, stop smoking, and avoid heavy alcohol use, your doctor may want to assess your calcium metabolism and bone density to help guide treatment.

A variety of drugs may be prescribed for osteoporosis:

Estrogen
Alone or in combination with progestin, estrogen is used for prevention and treatment. It slows bone loss and preserves and increases bone density. In one study, women taking estrogen increased calcium in their bones by 7 percent; they also had 50 percent fewer fractures. However, estrogens are associated with a slightly increased incidence of breast and uterine cancer; if you've had breast cancer, they are not recommended. Combining estrogen with progestin greatly reduces the risk of uterine cancer. You'll need to discuss this complicated decision with your doctor and carefully weigh the risks and benefits.

Tamoxifen (Nolvadex)
This was the first hormone-blocking drug. If you're postmenopausal it helps you maintain bone mass, but it has an estrogenlike effect on the endometrium (the lining of the uterus) and therefore raises the risk for endometrial cancer.

Selective estrogen receptor modulators
SERMs are a relatively new class of drugs that produce estrogenlike effects on select tissues without affecting the breasts or uterine lining. An example is raloxifene (Evista), which decreases bone resorption (breakdown) and increases bone mineral density but does not stimulate other tissues.

Bisphosphonates
These are nonhormonal inhibitors of bone breakdown. The first of these drugs is called aldendronate (Fosamax). Although it slows bone resorption and increases bone mineral density, it may cause gastrointestinal irritation. To prevent problems, you must follow the instructions carefully by taking it on an empty stomach with 8 ounces of water and then remain upright for thirty minutes. A newer bisphosphonate is risedronate (Actonel).

Calcitonin
Another conventional treatment is calcitonin, a naturally occurring hormone found in salmon that inhibits bone resorption and results in a slight increase in bone mineral density. It is administered by injection or in a nasal spray. However, it may cause nausea, flushing, or diarrhea.

Fluoride

Not just for teeth anymore. When combined with calcium, it appears to promote bone growth, increase spinal bone density, and reduce the occurrence of spinal fractures.

Dietary Strategies (See Chapter 14 for food sources of specified nutrients)

Soy foods

A study published in the January 2001 issue of *Obstetrics and Gynecology* reported that a group of postmenopausal Japanese women who ate a diet high in isoflavones, plant-derived estrogens found especially in soy foods, including miso and tofu, had increased bone mass. Asians eat significantly more isoflavones, which might explain why osteoporosis-related fractures are far less common in Asia than in the West.

Vitamin D

Vitamin D is essential for healthy bones.

Calcium

This is especially important if you have breast-fed your babies. The body regulates serum calcium levels very carefully and stores extra calcium in the bones. If levels get too low, the body will rob calcium from the skeleton. The daily requirement for calcium is 1,000 mg a day before and 1,500 mg a day after menopause. The average adult in this country consumes between 500 and 700 mg a day, so you may have to take supplements to achieve this level (see page 143).

Silicon

We now think this trace mineral is important for bone formation in animals.

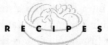

R E C I P E S

BROWN RICE WITH TOFU AND MUSHROOM SAUCE

This dish emphasizes soy, which is linked to increased bone mass.

> 2 *tablespoons olive oil*
> 1 *onion, chopped*

2 *cloves garlic, minced*
1 *cup mushrooms, thinly sliced*
2 *tablespoons chopped parsley*
1 *cup diced firm tofu*
¼ *cup unbleached white flour*
2 *tablespoons Spectrum Spread*
1 *cup water*
¾ *cup soy or rice milk*
¼ *teaspoon each pepper and salt*
4 *cups cooked brown rice*

1. Add olive oil to a saucepan and sauté the onion, garlic, mushrooms, and parsley for 3 minutes. Add the tofu and sauté for 3 more minutes.
2. Stir in the flour and Spectrum Spread. Mix in the water and milk, salt and pepper and stir until the flour is dissolved and the liquid is smooth.
3. Place the rice into a round serving dish and pour the tofu mushroom sauce over it.

SERVES 4

SALMON BURGERS

Canned salmon, with its thin, white bones, is a concentrated source of calcium. It is also high in omega-3 essential fatty acids. This recipe is a tasty way to get these vital nutrients. A salmon burger, served on a whole-grain bun with green lettuce and tomato, makes a bone-building, powerhouse sandwich.

2 *14-ounce cans, Red Sockeye Salmon*
5 *egg whites, beaten*
½ *cup bread crumbs*
½ *cup sweet onion, finely chopped*
¼ *cup carrot, finely grated*
2 *teaspoons garlic powder*

1. Preheat oven to 375 degrees.
2. Mash the salmon—*with* its fine white bones—in a mixing bowl, discarding the large central bones and skin.
3. Add the rest of the ingredients to the bowl and mix well.
4. Spread olive oil on the bottom of a nonstick baking pan or cookie sheet with a basting brush.

5. Form six patties with the salmon mixture and place on the pan. Bake for 20 minutes, turn once, and bake for 10 more minutes.
6. Serve hot or cold.

SERVES 6

ROOT VEGETABLE CASSEROLE

Root vegetables contain silicon, which is linked to the formation of healthy bones.

> 1 butternut squash, cut into chunks (1 to 2 cups)
> 1 parsnip, diced
> 2 potatoes, cut into chunks
> 1 cup large lima beans
> 2 tablespoons Spectrum Spread
> 1 tablespoon flour
> 1½ cups soy or rice milk
> ½ teaspoon nutmeg
> Salt and pepper, to taste
>
> TOPPING
> 1 cup fresh whole-grain bread crumbs
> ½ cup cashew nuts, chopped
> ¼ cup almonds, ground

1. Preheat oven to 350 degrees.
2. Cook the squash, parsnip, potatoes, and lima beans in a pot of boiling water for 10 minutes. Drain and place the vegetables and beans in an oblong baking dish.
3. Melt Spectrum Spread in a pan over low heat. Stir in flour, mixing until smooth.
4. Slowly stir in the milk, remove from heat, and mix in the nutmeg, pepper, and salt.
5. Pour the sauce over the vegetables.
6. Mix together the topping ingredients and sprinkle them over the vegetables and sauce.
7. Bake for 30 to 35 minutes until top is golden brown.

SERVES 4

Nutritional "No-Nos"

- Limit your alcohol consumption. Drinking alcohol promotes bone loss and, through its effects on estrogen, increases your risk of fractures. (Along with a colleague, I published research in the *New England Journal of Medicine* in 1988 that documented a link between alcohol consumption and bone fractures in men, as well.)
- Cut back on salt and salted, processed foods. Although a definitive link hasn't yet been made, salt increases the amount of calcium you lose in your urine and may lead to bone loss over time.
- Reduce your intake of caffeine, which also increases urinary loss of calcium and has been linked to fractures of the hip. In addition, if your calcium intake is less than 800 mg a day, two to three cups of coffee per day may speed bone loss.

Supplements

Calcium

You can take calcium supplements to make up the difference between what you get from your diet and the recommended daily intake (between 1,300 and 2,500 mg a day). This is likely to be between 500 and 700 mg a day. The FDA advises limiting calcium supplements made from dolomite or bone meal because of potentially high levels of lead.

Vitamin D

If you don't get out into the sun and don't eat many dairy products or fish, you may want to take a multivitamin that includes vitamin D. The accepted range is 15 to 50 mcg a day.

Magnesium

This mineral is essential for parathyroid function and release, which is in turn critical for activating vitamin D. In addition, magnesium depletion stops bone growth. The dose range is 320 to 350 mg a day.

Manganese

Deficiency of this mineral reduces calcium in your bones, leading to an increased risk of fracture. Recommended dose range is 1.8 to 11 mg a day.

Boron

A trace mineral, boron limits how much calcium and magnesium you lose in your urine. The upper limit is 20 mg. The RDA has not been established.

Zinc

This mineral is essential for normal bone formation. It also enhances vitamin D activity. Recommended dose range is 8 to 40 mg a day.

Copper

A deficiency of this mineral has been linked to abnormal bone growth in growing children. It has also been shown to inhibit bone breakdown. The accepted dose range is 900 mcg to 10 mg a day.

Folic acid

This nutrient is involved in the breakdown of homocysteine, an amino acid that builds up to harmful levels in some individuals. Increased levels of homocysteine may promote osteoporosis. Recommended dose range is 400 to 1,000 mcg a day.

Vitamin B6

This vitamin also plays a role in the metabolism of homocysteine. In addition, in animal studies, a deficiency of B6 has been linked to increased fracture healing time, impaired cartilage growth, defective bone formation, and more rapid development of osteoporosis.

The recommended dose is 2 to 100 mg a day.

Vitamin C

This important nutrient promotes formation and cross-linking of protein structures in bone. In animal research, vitamin C deficiency causes osteoporosis. The accepted dose is 90 to 2,000 mg a day.

Herbs

Phytoestrogens

Although technically not herbs, these compounds originate in plants or are derived by your body's metabolism from precursors found in plants. The most important class, phenolics, includes isoflavones and lignans. You have two choices:

- Isoflavones found in soybean protein, while not as effective as estrogen, do produce positive effects. The two forms of phytoestrogen isoflavones with the strongest scientific support are genistein and daidzein. The recommended dose is 25 to 60 mg a day.
- Ipriflavone is a synthetic derivative of isoflavones. It inhibits the activity

of osteoclasts, cells that break down bone. The recommended dose is 200 mg, three times a day.

High-mineral herbs

Nettles, oat straw, red raspberry leaves, chamomile, and dandelion greens have a high mineral content, so they are a good way to build your mineral stores. I suggest that you purchase commercially prepared teas which have these ingredients. (Dr. Stuart's and Traditional Medicinals are two brands that are readily available.)

Black cohosh (Cimicifuga racemosa)

Although not yet studied for this purpose in humans, this popular women's herb, used for many hormonal ailments, does improve bone mineral density in animals. The recommended dose is 1 or 2 pills a day of a standardized extract.

Alfalfa (Medicago sativa)

A member of the pea family, this herb contains isoflavones with weak estrogenic effects. The recommended dose is 1 or 2 ml of tincture three times a day.

Do-It-Yourself

- Stop smoking. Smokers have lower bone mass and lose bone more rapidly.
- Get out in the sun, since it's the best natural source for vitamin D.
- Talk to your doctor about your risk factors.
- If you're older, make your home safer to reduce your risk of falls. Install handrails for stairs, bathtubs, showers, and toilets. Put nonskid suction mats in your tub and showers and on slippery bathroom floors. Remove loose throw rugs and keep your rooms and hallways well lit.
- Don't be a couch potato—get some exercise.
- Try homeopathy. The remedies don't reverse bone loss but they may be helpful for aching bones and for preventing and healing fractures. Besides, they ensure that your body uses minerals and other nutrients efficiently. Follow instructions on the package.
  - Calcarea carbonica is helpful if you are easily fatigued, feel anxious and stressed, and experience cravings for eggs and sweets.
  - Calcarea phosphorica is useful for stiffness, soreness, and weakness of your bones and joints.

- Phosphorus is indicated for spinal weakness and burning pain between your shoulders. If you are easily tired, weak, and crave refreshing foods (such as ice cream) and cold or carbonated drinks, this remedy may be for you.
- Silicea (silica) may be helpful if you are often chilly or nervous, tire easily, or if you have night sweats, injuries that are slow to heal, and a low resistance to infection.
- Comfrey (*Symphytum officinale*) strengthens and heals bones, so you can use it to ease the pain from earlier fractures.

Mind/Body

A steady, long-term yoga practice is a wise choice if you have or are at risk for osteoporosis. Yoga not only reduces stress, but it also includes weight-bearing postures for your lower *and* upper body and spine. This is important because spinal fractures are a major cause of disability in women with osteoporosis.

For an excellent all-around pose, try Downward Facing Dog. (See pages 344–351 for postures.)

Exercise

Perhaps more than any other part of the body, bone gives meaning to the phrase "use it or lose it." That's because bone cells, when stressed, respond by building more bone. The more you use your bones, the larger and stronger they get; bones literally alter their architecture in response to mechanical loading or weight-bearing.

But the opposite is also true; decreased stress, or not using bones, leads to profound and rapid bone loss. For example, after six months of immobilization from prolonged bed rest, you can lose as much as 50 to 55 percent of your bone mass. Studies of astronauts are enlightening in this respect, because the no-gravity atmosphere of space replicates the effects of not using bone. After five months on MIR, Russian cosmonauts typically lost around 40 percent of their bone mass. And once lost, bone is very hard to replace.

If you exercise regularly, you are more likely to have a greater peak bone mass, maintain bone mass as you age, and have a significantly lower risk of fractures. Weight-bearing exercises—those that work against gravity—increase muscle mass and bone formation. After consulting with your physician, develop this or a similar regular exercise program:

- Begin slowly
- Warm up for five minutes before each session and stretch for five to ten minutes afterward.
- Train with weights, with particular emphasis on your hip, spinal, and scapular (shoulder) muscles, every other day for six weeks.
- Add an aerobic exercise component. I recommend at least thirty minutes of weight-bearing activities on most days of the week. You want to stress your bones. In addition to weight-training, good activities include brisk walking, jogging or running, gymnastics, and basketball.

Red Flags

Call your doctor if you develop:

- Pain in a bone that is severe and/or getting worse; you may have a fracture.
- Any visible deformity in a bone.
- Sudden pain in your back that wraps around in a bandlike fashion. You may have an osteoporotic compression fracture.

7

Are You Well-Connected?

Your musculoskeletal system is a complex array of structures that provide movement, support, and protection. In Chapters 5 and 6, I described painful ailments that affect the "stars" of your musculoskeletal system—the bones, joints, muscles, and spine. In this chapter I will go into problems of the supporting actors—the tendons, ligaments, bursae, and menisci. These structures play a yeoman's role in stabilizing and aligning the movement of the body's bony framework.

BURSITIS

Description

Bursitis is an inflammation of the bursa (plural is bursae), which is a small, fluid-filled sac that allows friction-free motion of muscles and tendons over bones. The bursal sac is lined with a membrane that, much like the synovial lining of the joints, produces a lubricating fluid.

There are eighty bursae on each side of the body. Each one has its own special protective role. You can develop the swelling and pain of bursitis in the upper or lower extremities, but it usually occurs in the bursae around the elbows, shoulders, hips, knees, and other large joints.

Bursitis is a very common ailment, affecting between 5 and 10 percent of people over age sixty-five. Women suffer more frequently than men from bursitis at most ages.

Common forms of bursitis include:

Upper Extremities

Subacromial bursitis

Shoulder pain is one of the most common musculoskeletal complaints for people over age forty. Your shoulder is a complex ball and socket joint that facilitates arm movement in all directions. Normally, many types of structures, including muscles, bones, ligaments, and tendons, effortlessly come together at the shoulder, allowing it to function properly and coordinating pain-free motion. The bursae protect these structures and facilitate frictionless movement.

Several "sister" bursae in the shoulder are potential pain culprits, but the most common type of shoulder bursitis is subacromial bursitis, which is often associated with another condition—rotator cuff tendinitis, also known as impingement syndrome (see page 161).

Subacromial bursitis causes pain and aching in the front or side of the shoulder. If it's severe enough, the shoulder may also swell or feel warm. Because it hurts when you lift or rotate your arm, or raise it above your head, your shoulder's range of motion may be limited. Subacromial bursitis is sometimes the result of repetitive shoulder motion, such as overhead lifting. Arthritic conditions can also contribute to this ailment.

Olecranon bursitis

Because it often results from chronic and prolonged pressure on the elbow, such as leaning on a table or desk for long periods of time, this ailment is sometimes called "student's elbow." It may also occur after a blow or other sudden injury.

Inflammatory conditions such as gout, pseudo-gout, or rheumatoid arthritis may play a role in the development of student's elbow. Less frequently, it may be the result of infection (septic bursitis) or it may develop if you are undergoing kidney dialysis.

Whatever the cause, the elbow reddens, feels warm, or becomes tender. You may also develop a fluid-filled sac around the joint.

Lower Extremities

Prepatellar bursitis

Also known as "housemaid's knee," this ailment can result from prolonged kneeling on a hard surface. It causes redness, swelling, and pain around the front of the lower portion of the kneecap. It is especially painful if you apply pressure to the knee.

Infrapatellar bursitis

A relative of prepatellar bursitis, this condition involves the bursa right below the kneecap, between the patellar ligament and the shinbone.

Pes anserine bursitis

Pes anserine bursitis is a common ailment in obese middle-aged or elderly women. If you take your fingers and place them on the medial, or inner, portion of your knee about 2 inches below the kneecap and press, prepare to yelp! Walking up steps can also be painful.

Ischial bursitis

The ischial bursa is strategically located on top of the "sitting bone," the ischial tuberosity, and below the gluteus maximus, the large muscle in your buttock. Ischial bursitis may be caused by trauma, but it is more often the result of sitting on a hard surface for long periods of time. This accounts for its common name, "Weaver's bottom."

The pain of ischial bursitis can be excruciating. And because this bursa is situated so close to the gluteus maximus, you may also experience "referred" pain (pain not precisely at the site of injury) throughout the back of your buttock and thigh.

In addition to the standard conventional and complementary treatments (see below), you may get relief from sitting on a special gel-filled cushion.

Trochanteric bursitis

The trochanter is a large, flat, expansive portion of the thigh bone, or femur. Since it is an anchor for many hip muscles, the trochanter is especially susceptible to injury.

More common in middle-aged and older people and in women, trochanteric bursitis causes aching pain and tenderness in the upper, outer part of the hip and the outer thigh. A good way to confirm this ailment is to apply deep pressure to the trochanteric area (over the side of your hip) and see if it hurts. You may also feel multiple tender points throughout the outer thigh muscle. It typically hurts more when you move your hip outward with your knee flexed at 90 degrees.

Besides traumatic and overuse injuries, rheumatoid arthritis, lumbar spine disease, leg-length discrepancy, and scoliosis may cause this problem. Your risk of developing trochanteric bursitis rises if you spend a lot of time on your feet, putting pressure on your hips, or if you are bedridden for long periods because of illness.

Iliopectineal/iliopsoas bursitis

Inflammation in the bursa located between your iliopsoas muscle and the inguinal ligament in the groin may cause tenderness and pain in that area. You may feel it when you bring your hip back (extension). Don't be surprised if you notice that your stride length is shorter; that's because you may be unconsciously taking smaller steps to avoid triggering pain when you extend your hip.

Bursitis of the Feet *(See Chapter 11 for more foot ailments)*

Retrocalcaneal bursitis

This condition causes pain at the back of the heel, behind the Achilles tendon and in front of your calcaneus, or heel bone. It hurts most when you bring your foot and toes up (dorsiflexion). Common causes include bad shoes, walking too much, and trauma to your foot. In addition, certain diseases such as arthritis, gout, spondylitis, and Reiter's syndrome can contribute to its development.

Achilles bursitis

Also known as "pump bumps," this condition is all too common in women, thanks to tight, foot-damaging, high-heeled shoes. It occurs in a bursa located next to the lower portion of your Achilles tendon, right above the spot where your tendon attaches to the back of your heel bone. Sometimes, Achilles bursitis is the result of inflammatory diseases like gout, arthritis, and ankylosing spondylitis. (However, ankylosing spondylitis, or AS, is three times more common in men than in women.)

Causes

In addition to the specific causes I described above, infection, injury, overuse, and prolonged pressure may all lead to inflammation and increased fluid in your bursae. Rheumatic disease or calcium buildup on the tendons connected to your joints may also contribute to the problem.

Signs and Symptoms

- Loss of motion due to swelling
- Dull pain and tenderness
- Fluid accumulation

Conventional Treatments

P.R.I.C.E.M.M is a handy mnemonic I teach my residents to remember for standard bursitis treatment:

Protection—Place a foam pad, pillow, or other cushioning over the inflamed bursa to prevent outside pressure or trauma that will worsen the pain.

Rest—To help inflamed tissues heal, limit weight-bearing on the joint, and avoid aggravating activities or anything that stresses neighboring bursae.

Ice—Apply ice to the area for fifteen to twenty minutes at least once a day, or as often as necessary, until the swelling goes down. I tell my patients to put the ice in a plastic sandwich bag, cover it with a cloth, and apply it to the inflamed area.

Compress—Put on an elastic bandage to limit motion and reduce swelling. If you prefer, you can wrap the area a few times, add an ice bag, and wrap it in place.

Elevate—Reduce the swelling by using pillows, a sofa back, or a chair to elevate the affected area, making sure it is higher than the joint above it. For example, if your elbow is inflamed, keep it higher than your shoulder.

Medication—You can use a variety of pain relievers, including acetaminophen, aspirin, and over-the-counter or prescription nonsteroidal anti-inflammatory drugs (NSAIDS), such as ibuprofen or Mobic. The new drugs, called Cox-2 inhibitors, may be a bit easier on your gastrointestinal tract. NSAIDS work particularly well since they have analgesic as well as anti-inflammatory properties. Topical application of aspirin-containing creams or rubs is another option.

Modalities—Use ice at first, when you are in the acute stage and the bursa is hot, tender, and inflamed. Once it has cooled down and swelling, tenderness, and inflammation have subsided, you've entered the chronic phase, when it's okay to use heat or ultrasound.

Gentle stretching exercises can help restore range of motion. You can follow them with strengthening exercises.

If these conventional treatments fail, your doctor may recommend a steroid injection, which will provide immediate relief. However, it can cause local trauma, bleeding, or black-and-blue marks. I discourage repeated (more than three times a year) injections with steroids, since they can damage surrounding tendon structures.

Should the inflamed area become infected, your doctor may need to prescribe antibiotics and drain the fluid.

Dietary Strategies (See Chapter 14 for food sources of specified nutrients)

In general, it's important to stick with a well-balanced diet that emphasizes whole grains, fruits, and vegetables. Use sugar, alcohol, and salt only in moderation.

As I mentioned in Chapter 5, there are several emerging, scientifically proven nutritional and dietary strategies that reduce inflammation, curb pain, and decrease the swelling of arthritis. Since bursitis and tendinitis share some common inflammatory features with arthritis, some of the strategies mentioned earlier will help here as well. They include:

Bromelain (See page 324)

Avocados and soybeans
In 1998 French researchers focused on the potential value of an avocado/soybean oil combination. People in their study had less pain and used fewer pain relievers. There are many ways to eat soy. You can eat raw soybeans or try commercial brands that are lightly dried and toasted to enhance the taste. You can even sample soy chocolate bars. Some of these tasty items provide a whopping 12 grams of soy protein.

Vitamin B3
A 1996 study by Wayne Jonas, M.D., the former chief of the National Institutes of Health Office of Alternative Medicine, demonstrated in double-blind placebo-controlled fashion that taking niacinamide can improve joint flexibility and reduce inflammation. It also helped osteoarthritis patients use smaller doses of pain relievers.

Vitamin E and selenium
These nutrients may relieve pain.

Fish oils
Eating cold-water fish containing the essential oils known as omega-3 fatty acids blocks inflammation.

Vitamin C
A powerful antioxidant, this vitamin speeds repair of damaged tissue by fortifying collagen, an important biological protein within tendon, cartilage, and connective tissue. There are advantages to getting vitamin C from your food because it is bundled with carotenes, bioflavonoids, and other nutrients.

Beta-carotene
Another nutrient that speeds healing.

RECIPE

PINEAPPLE SMOOTHIE

Besides bromelain, pineapple contains small amounts of vitamin C and fiber. Bromelain helps digest protein, so it's beneficial to eat it after consuming a heavy meat meal.

1 cup orange juice
1 cup frozen berries (strawberries, blueberries)
2 kiwis
1 fresh, ripe pineapple

1. Pour the orange juice into a powerful blender and add the berries.
2. Peel the kiwis and add them to the blender.
3. Trim the top and bottom off the pineapple and cut it into quarters lengthwise. Remove the peel, cut the pineapple quarters into chunks, and add to the blender.
4. Blend on high for 2 minutes or until well blended.
5. Drink immediately and enjoy!

SERVES 1

Supplements

Calcium
Calcium builds bones, thereby fortifying neighboring bursae and other supportive structures. The accepted dose range is 1,300 to 2,500 mg a day.

Magnesium
Magnesium balances calcium and promotes muscular function. The accepted dose range is 320 to 350 mg a day.

Vitamin A
Vitamin A is an antioxidant that protects the body against damage from free radicals. The accepted dose range is 900 to 3,000 mcg a day.

Vitamin C

Vitamin C, another powerful antioxidant, plays a role in reducing inflammation and promoting tissue healing. The accepted dose range is 90 to 2,000 mg a day.

Vitamin E

Vitamin E is a worthwhile antioxidant with anti-inflammatory properties. The recommended dose range is between 15 and 1,000 mg a day.

Vitamin B

Vitamin B complex is important for cellular repair. Take 1 tablet daily.

Glucosamine sulfate

This is a nutritional supplement that comes from seashells or seafood. It is an important building block for the manufacture and repair of cartilage and the formation of connective tissue. Although its main use is for osteoarthritis, you can also use it for bursitis, since it improves joint motion and decreases pain and swelling. Take 500 mg three times a day.

Methylsulfonylmethane (MSM)

This is a chemical compound that contains sulfur. It is found naturally in vegetables, fruits, milk, and meat. Early evidence from a study of people with osteoarthritis indicates that it reduces pain. Use as directed on the package label.

Herbs

Meadowsweet (Filipendula ulmaria)

This flowering plant of the meadow acts as an anti-inflammatory and contains flavonoids as well as salicylates (the active ingredient in aspirin). The recommended dose is up to three cups a day. Avoid meadowsweet if you are allergic to aspirin.

White willow bark (Salix alba)

The bark of willow trees contains an anti-inflammatory compound similar to aspirin. You can use it to reduce your need for pain relievers. Unlike other anti-inflammatory drugs, willow may be less likely to upset your stomach because it is converted into its active ingredient (salicylic acid) after it is absorbed by your gut. The recommended dose is one cup of infusion, 3 to 5 times a day. Do not use this herb if you are allergic to aspirin or other

NSAIDS, when pregnant or breast-feeding. Use caution if you take blood-thinning medications.

Devil's claw (Harpagophytum procumbens)

Despite its scary name, Devil's claw, which comes from the underground tuber of a South African plant, stood up as an effective herbal anti-inflammatory in a randomized, double-blind, multicenter study in France. Researchers compared the herb to a standard, slow-acting drug used to treat osteoarthritis. The two drugs relieved pain similarly, but the people in the group using Devil's claw used fewer NSAIDS and other analgesics and had significantly fewer side effects. Recommended use of Devil's claw is as an infusion, up to 3 times a day. Do not use Devil's claw if you are pregnant. Because it may aggravate your stomach, avoid it if you have gastritis or ulcers.

Herbal Creams and Ointments

Slippery elm (Ulmus fulva) and chamomile (Chamaemelum nobile or Matricaria recutita) poultice

Slippery elm, from the inner bark of a tree, and chamomile, a small, daisy-like flower, are both useful for fighting local inflammation. Mix 1 table-spoon of dried slippery elm with an equal amount of dried chamomile, and add hot water to make a paste. Spread it on a piece of clean cotton and apply to the affected area for forty-five minutes. You can do this three times a day.

Comfrey (Symphytum officinale) liniment

Also known as knitbone or boneset, this common wild plant has large bristly leaves and purple flowers. It promotes healing because it contains allantoin, which assists in repairing damaged tissue, and rosmarinic acid, an anti-inflammatory. Because comfrey also contains pyrrolizidines, chemicals that are potentially toxic to the liver, it is best used externally.

Aloe (Aloe vera)

A common house plant, aloe cools, soothes, and relieves inflammation. Creams are readily available; be sure to buy one with a high aloe content (it should appear as one of the first listed ingredients). To make your own medicated oil: Slice up the leaves of an aloe vera plant and put them in a glass jar. Cover with vegetable oil. Let the mixture steep for sixty days. Strain and store in a dark-colored container. Spread the oil on sore joints as necessary. If skin irritation occurs, discontinue.

Joint-Ritis

An all-natural topical analgesic that combines maximum strength menthol for pain relief with skin conditioners lanolin, glucosamine and chondroitin to help prevent skin dryness. Joint-Ritis comes in a unique roll-on applicator and a pump. You can conveniently use it when bursitis flares up.

Do-It-Yourself

Baths

Add cider vinegar or ginger (mix ½ teaspoon of ginger powder and 1 cup of hot water) to a bath or foot bath to fight inflammation.

Compresses

Hot or cold compresses can reduce swelling. Use cold initially, when the bursa is warm, red, and tender. Once this has subsided, you can use heat.

Self-massage for the knee

1. Sit on the floor or in a chair.
2. Put one hand on your thigh above your knee and the other hand on the side of your leg.
3. Move the hand on top of your leg in a circular motion that goes over the knee, along the side of the knee, and back to the starting position.
4. Make a similar motion with the other hand.
5. Continue to massage with alternating hands for 10 to 15 minutes.

Aromatherapy

- Juniper oil (*Juniperus communis*)—Add 3 to 4 drops of oil to the water for a cold compress. Do not use while pregnant, or if you have kidney disease.
- Soothing bath—Add 3 drops of lavender oil, 3 drops of chamomile oil, and 2 drops of neroli oil (made from bitter orange blossoms) to a warm bath.
- Pain relief massage—Add the preceding mixture to 3 teaspoons of grapeseed or sweet almond oil and use it to massage the sore spots.
- Rosemary (*Rosmarinus officinalis*)—To fight inflammation and relieve pain, add a few drops of rosemary oil to the water for a compress. Or add it to a neutral oil or lotion and use it to massage the sore area.

You might also enjoy this after-sport shower formula: Add 2 drops of rosemary oil, 2 drops of pine oil, and 4 drops of lemon oil to a small dollop of unscented shower gel. Work it into a lather with a sponge and use it in the shower.

Avoid rosemary if you're pregnant or if you have epilepsy or high blood pressure.

Homeopathy

There are many homeopathic remedies for specific symptoms of bursitis. A good all-purpose homeopathic ointment is Traumeel, which contains twelve ingredients, including: *Calendula officinalis* (marigold), *Arnica montana*, *Hamamelis virginiana* (witch hazel), Millefolium (milifoil), Belladonna (nightshade), *Aconitum napellus* (monkshood), Chamomilla, *Symphytum officinale* (comfrey), *Bellis perennis* (daisy), *Echinacea angustifolia* (coneflower), and *Hypericum perforatum* (St. John's wort).

Reflexology (See page 353 for techniques)

Try these points:

- Shoulder and Neck
    - SI-3 (Small Intestine-3), "Black Ravine"—along the outer side of the fifth metacarpophalangeal joint base of the pinky.
    - SI-9 (Jian Zhen), "True Shoulder"—at the border of the scapular (the bone at the back of the shoulder) and the deltoid muscle.
    - SI-11 "Celestial Gathering"—on the scapular, just below the infraspinatus muscle, right in the middle of the spine.
- Forearm and Wrist
    - On the outer side (ulnar side) of the base of the pinky.
- Elbow or Knee
    - On the outer foot, approximately mid-foot, behind the bony prominence (toward the heel).
- Hip
    - On the foot, at the base of the padded part of the heel.

Mind/Body

Yoga

Try Sankatasana (Contracted Posture) and Garudasana (Eagle Posture). (See pages 344–351 for postures.)

Exercise

Use gentle, controlled movements to feel better and maintain mobility.

PENDULUM FOR SHOULDER INJURIES AND TO KEEP THE
SHOULDER MOBILE
1. Stand or sit in a chair.
2. Bend slightly at the waist toward your injured side, and reach out with
   your arm a few inches from your body.
3. Slowly make small circles, forward and then backward, 5 times each
   way.
4. Do this for 5 minutes, twice a day.

SCAPULAR RANGE OF MOTION
FOR SHOULDER BURSITIS
1. Shrug your shoulders up and hold 5 seconds, then release.
2. Squeeze your shoulder blades together, hold 5 seconds, then release.
3. Relax for 5 seconds.
4. Repeat 10 times.

WAND EXERCISE
FOR SHOULDER BURSITIS
1. Hold a stick or a lightweight broom in both hands.
2. Keep your arms straight and lift them up over your head. If you feel
   pain, lower your arms slightly. Hold 5 seconds.
3. Lower your arms completely.
4. Repeat 10 times.

HIP STRETCH
FOR TROCHANTERIC BURSITIS
1. Stand sideways, one arm-length away from a wall, with your injured hip
   toward the wall.
2. Rest your hand on the wall, with your arm straight out.
3. Push your hip toward the wall.
4. Repeat 5 times.

Seeking Help from Complementary Practitioners

Massage (See page 326)
Avoid direct massage for areas that are acutely inflamed.

Red Flags

Call your doctor if you experience:

- Repeated pain or discomfort in a joint
- Fever, increased swelling, oozing, or other signs of infection
- Sweating

TINA'S STORY

Tina is a successful thirty-two-year-old account executive for a dot-com start-up. Her job calls for a great deal of traveling, since she represents her company at national trade shows throughout the United States. Today, she is trim and fit, and she enjoys playing tennis whenever she has the time.

When I first met her, though, her tennis game was in serious trouble. Over the course of three months she had developed a dull, aching pain in her elbow and forearm. The pain was annoying at best, and it really flared up when she was whacking forehands on the court. "I take Advil, which provides some relief, but it only lasts for a little while," she said. Tina's boyfriend, a third-year medical student, suggested that it might be tennis elbow, and sent her to see me.

I had already noticed that Tina winced when I gently shook her hand and introduced myself. I wasn't surprised; when you have tennis elbow, movements that extend your wrist irritate an already sore, inflamed outer elbow. As I examined her, I noted that she had pain and tenderness in her elbow and throughout her forearm. In spite of her elbow pain, however, her neck and back were fine. Nor did she have any loss in strength or changes in her reflexes or sensations.

Recognizing the important impact of mechanical stressors on her pain, I described for Tina the biomechanics of her arm and elbow, and how she might be exacerbating her pain with her tennis game. I could see the disappointment in her eyes when I advised her to ease off for a while: "I was afraid you were going to say that. Tennis is the one thing I do to stay fit and keep my weight down," she said. I suggested she start a swimming program at the local Y, at least for the short term.

I had also noticed another nonmedical problem during the course of our visit. When I took Tina's history, she joked that her computer was her lifeline: "I'm tethered to it, Doctor; I carry a briefcase with a fully equipped laptop wherever I go." Since traveling without her computer was out of the question, I suggested that she buy a backpack-style carrier for it.

To ease her pain, I prescribed a tennis elbow splint and started her on acupuncture. And for home benefit, I provided her with a diagram of acupressure points as well as a technique for self-massage, and a sample of a topical rub, called Joint-Ritis.

Although Tina loved her job, the constant traveling and presentations were stressful. And stress makes pain worse, so I taught her an easy-to-use relaxation and meditation technique.

Several weeks later, Tina came back for a follow-up. Her pain wasn't entirely gone, but it had improved significantly. She had found a stylish backpack for her laptop and was doing relaxation exercises while enduring the inevitable delays at airports: "It makes the waits bearable and it keeps me away from the fast-food stands," she said. And she was staying only at hotels that had swimming pools. "Swimming isn't so bad, after all," she confessed. Then, she laughed: "But when can I get back to tennis?"

TENDINITIS

Description

Tendons are fibrous, cordlike structures that attach the muscles to the bones. They are strong, but not particularly elastic. Overuse or sudden, abrupt movement may inflame tendons, causing tendinitis. More common in women than in men, tendinitis can happen in many areas of the body. The most common types of tendinitis are:

Upper Extremities

Rotator cuff tendinitis (also called supraspinatus tendinitis or impingement syndrome)
This ailment, clearly the most frequent cause of shoulder pain in both women and men, can be extremely painful. In its chronic form, it causes dull, aching pain on the side of the shoulder, over the rotator cuff muscles. Typically, you suffer most when you raise your arm to the side (abduction) between 60 and 120 degrees, and when you lower it. So putting on your blouse or brassiere becomes a grueling exercise. In severe cases, all shoulder motion is painful.

Acute rotator cuff tendinitis is more frequent in younger women. It can cause sudden, sharp pain in the shoulder. Usually, this is the result of calcium deposits that form in the supraspinatus tendon. Again, it really hurts to reach over your head or behind your back. And your pain may be worse at night. Sometimes subacromial bursitis (see page 149) exacerbates rotator cuff tendinitis pain.

Rotator cuff tendinitis may develop for many reasons. Excessive overhead shoulder and arm motions such as lifting a baby over your head to play, clearing the top shelves of the pantry, or loading and unloading bookshelves are frequently a source of the problem. Sometimes, trauma or a blow to the shoulder is the offender. Chronic diseases like rheumatoid or osteoarthritis can play a role. So can getting old; as you age, bony outgrowths called osteophytes may form under your acromioclavicular joint, the hinge between the collarbone and the shoulder blade, and they can cause tendinitis.

Bicipital tendinitis

This ailment causes pain in the front of the shoulder, right where the biceps tendon originates. Sometimes, the pain radiates down to the forearm. Bicipital tendinitis commonly occurs when the acromion — the outer, upper edge of the shoulder blade — pinches its neighboring biceps tendon. In medical lingo, the symptoms get worse when you "supinate your forearm against resistance." In plain English, it hurts to use a screwdriver to turn a tight screw or twist a corkscrew to open a bottle of wine.

Lateral epicondylitis

This overuse injury, commonly known as "tennis elbow," affects not only tennis players but also anyone who repeatedly performs activities that involve bending the wrist up against resistance (forcible wrist extension). You'll notice pain and tenderness on the outside of the elbow and sharp pain when you grip something or twist your hand and forearm. Bending your wrist up often makes the pain worse. Even simple actions, such as lifting a tote bag or portfolio, shaking hands or gardening, can make you wince (see Chapter 10 for more information).

Medial epicondylitis

Tenderness on the inside of the arm is the hallmark of this type of tendinitis, which is also called "golfer's elbow." It's especially painful when you flex your wrist (bend it down) against resistance (see Chapter 10 for more information).

Tenosynovitis

This is an inflammation of a tendon that extends to the synovium, or joint lining. It usually occurs in the hands, feet, and other areas that have many small joints.

- De Quervain's tenosynovitis—Repetitive tasks using thumb and wrist motions cause this ailment, which involves pain, swelling, and tenderness along the thumb. It also affects the tip of the radius bone, which goes from the wrist to the elbow. De Quervain's tenosynovitis is common in pregnant women. If you're a new mom, you may find that lifting your baby up, diapering her, or closing safety pins makes it hurt more. You can confirm that you have this problem by gently folding your thumb into your palm, wrapping your fingers around it, and deviating your wrist downward, to the ulnar, or outer side.
- Flexor tenosynovitis—Rest is usually sufficient treatment for this complaint, which causes pain in the palm of the hand that worsens when you move your fingers.

Lower Extremities

For more about foot and ankle ailments, see Chapters 10 and 11.

Patellar tendinitis

"Jumper's knee" causes pain, tenderness, and swelling of the tendon that connects the kneecap and the leg. Repetitive jumping, running, volleyball, basketball, and high-impact aerobics are likely to make your symptoms worse. Kickboxers and cheerleaders beware!

Achilles tendinitis

A common complaint among runners, Achilles tendinitis causes inflammation and pain in the tendon that connects the heel bone and the calf muscle (see Chapter 10 for more information). Discomfort and swelling can also occur over the spot where the tendon attaches. Overuse, tight calf muscles, uphill running, or a too rapid or sudden increase in sports activities can lead to Achilles tendinitis. It is often worsened by diseases like gout, rheumatoid arthritis, and Reiter's syndrome.

Causes

Although its possible causes are numerous, tendinitis is usually the result of overuse or overtraining. It develops when repeated motions cause tiny tears, inflammation, and thickening in the tendon.

Signs and Symptoms

- Sharp or dull pain, which is worse when you use the tendon
- Limitation of motion

· Tenderness
· Swelling

Conventional Treatments

P.R.I.C.E.M.M is the mnemonic I teach my residents to remember for standard tendinitis treatment. Refer to page 152 for specifics.

Your doctor may refer you for shoe supports, orthotics, or other shoe corrections. If you have Achilles tendinitis, a heel cup, a cushioned orthotic made of rubberized material that you insert into your shoe, may be helpful. It absorbs impact, relieves heel pain, and may reduce the load on your Achilles tendon.

Speaking of shoes, you should probably take a skeptical look at yours. Often, the wrong types of shoes or poor-fitting shoes can exacerbate tendinitis.

If these conventional treatments fail, your doctor may recommend a steroid injection. It will provide immediate relief but it can cause local trauma, bleeding, or black-and-blue marks. I discourage repeated (more than three times a year) injections with steroids, since they can cause damage to surrounding tendon structures.

Dietary Strategies (See Chapter 14 for food sources of specified nutrients)

Vitamin C
A powerful antioxidant, this vitamin prevents free radical damage and is a critical player in the manufacture of collagen, which is an important biological protein found within tendon, cartilage, and connective tissue. Getting your vitamin C from citrus carries a bonus because it's also rich in quercetin and other bioflavonoids that appear to play a role in wound healing and tendon recovery after injury. One study of forty collegiate football players showed that taking vitamin C and citrus bioflavonoids before competition can reduce athletic injuries.

Vitamin E and selenium
For pain relief.

Beta-carotene

Bromelain (See page 324)

Turmeric (Curcuma longa)
An integral part of Indian cooking, this spice has anti-inflammatory properties. Do not use turmeric if you have hepatitis or if you are pregnant or trying to conceive.

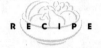

RECIPE

COUSCOUS WITH TURMERIC

4 cups water
2 cups couscous
3 teaspoons olive oil
¼ teaspoon cinnamon
¼ teaspoon saffron
¼ teaspoon cumin
1 teaspoon turmeric
½ cup chopped green pepper
1 cup grated carrots
1 teaspoon pure maple syrup
2 cloves garlic, minced
1 can chickpeas, rinsed and drained

1. Bring the water to a boil.
2. Add all the ingredients, reduce heat and simmer, covered, for 10 minutes.
3. Remove from heat and let stand for 5 minutes.
4. Fluff with a fork.

SERVES 6

Supplements

Vitamin C
This vitamin speeds healing. The acceptable daily dose range is 90 to 2,000 mg. It's best to break up the dose throughout the day. Excessive amounts may cause kidney stones, gout, cramps, or diarrhea.

Vitamin E
The recommended dose range for this antioxidant is between 15 and 1,000 mg a day.

Zinc
Zinc is a nutrient that encourages healing. The acceptable range is 8 to 40 mg a day.

Selenium
Selenium is a trace element and antioxidant. The acceptable range is 60 to 400 mcg a day.

Vitamin B
Vitamin B complex is important for cellular repair. Take one pill a day.

Calcium
Calcium helps to build bones and fortify joints and connective tissue. You can take between 1,300 and 2,500 mg a day.

Magnesium
Magnesium balances calcium and promotes muscular function. The recommended dose range is between 320 and 350 mg a day.

Vitamin A
Vitamin A is an antioxidant that prevents free radical damage to tissue. The recommended dose range is between 900 and 3,000 mcg a day.

SAMe (S-adenosyl methionine)
This compound occurs naturally in the body and is a key player in many biochemical reactions. SAMe has proven itself a helpful supplement for arthritis pain relief. It also helps tendinitis pain. Multiple scientific studies and many of my patients vouch for its effectiveness, with some reporting that it is as effective as NSAIDS. The starting dose is 200 mg twice daily. In large doses, SAMe can upset the stomach. Do not take SAMe if you take levodopa for Parkinson's disease. This nutrient may trigger manic episodes in people with bipolar disease.

Glucosamine sulfate and chondroitin
Used to bolster bones and cartilage, these can fortify the joints, potentially making them less susceptible to bursitis and tendinitis. Take 500 mg of each, three times a day.

Creatine and HMB
Although creatine and HMB (beta-hydroxy-beta-methylbutyric acid) have been touted as a possible remedy for tendinitis, I don't recommend these

supplements since there is insufficient scientific evidence to back up their use.

Herbs

White willow bark (Salix alba)

If you want to reduce your dependence on pain relievers, try white willow. This tree's bark contains an anti-inflammatory compound much like aspirin. And willow is less likely than other anti-inflammatory drugs to upset your stomach because it is converted into its active ingredient (salicylic acid) after it is absorbed by your gut. The recommended dose is one cup of infusion, three to five times a day. Do not use willow if you are allergic to aspirin or other NSAIDS, when pregnant or breast-feeding. Use caution if you take blood-thinning medications.

Horse chestnut

Classically used to treat varicose veins and swelling, horse chestnut may cut down swelling from tendinitis. It's too soon for me to make a recommendation, but this is one I'm following; future research will tell the full story.

Grapeseed oil, pine bark, and bilberry

These all contain OPCs (oligomeric proanthocyanidins), which help to decrease inflammation and nourish elastin and collagen. OPCs are safe and nontoxic but can interact with blood thinners. Follow package instructions for dosing.

Herbal Creams and Ointments

Capsaicin cream (0.025–0.075 percent) (See page 96)

Arnica (Arnica montana)

Easy-to-find ointments made from this well-known herb are useful for tendinitis, bursitis, joint problems, swelling, and bruising.

Joint-Ritis (See page 96)

Turmeric infused oil

Apply a turmeric-infused oil externally to fight inflammation around sore areas.

Do-It-Yourself

Compress and wrap
- Apply a vinegar compress to reduce inflammation.
- Wrap a wet plantain leaf around the affected area to reduce swelling and stiffness and encourage healing.

Aromatherapy
- Lavender (*Lavandula angustifolia*)—This herb calms and soothes your spirits and reduces pain. Add four drops of the essential oil to a bath or the water for a cold compress. Or try adding three drops of lavender oil, three drops of chamomile oil, and two drops of neroli oil to a warm bath. If you prefer, you can add this mixture to 3 teaspoons of grapeseed or sweet almond oil and use it for a massage. Be careful with lavender if you have hay fever or asthma; it could cause an allergic reaction.
- Rosemary (*Rosmarinus officinalis*)—To fight inflammation and relieve pain, add a few drops of rosemary oil to the water for a compress, or put it in a neutral oil or lotion and use it to massage the sore area.
- Chamomile (*Chamaemelum nobile* or *Matricaria recutita*)—Make a soothing compress by adding four or five drops of chamomile oil to a bowl of ice cold water. Soak a cloth in the bowl, wring it out, and apply to the painful area. Avoid contact with your eyes; it may cause irritation. Do not use chamomile oil during the first three months of pregnancy.

Reflexology (see Bursitis, page 158)

Seeking Help from Complementary Practitioners

Acupuncture
I use acupuncture frequently for my patients with tendinitis. My personal experience is buttressed by reports issued by both the World Health Organization and the National Institutes of Health Consensus Panel, which support acupuncture's effectiveness for this ailment.

Red Flags

Call your doctor if you experience:

- Prolonged pain
- Persistent swelling
- Fever

- Loss of muscle strength
- Numbness or tingling

INJURIES OF THE LIGAMENTS AND MENISCI

Joints are formed where bones come together. To keep joints stable, their connecting surfaces must be firmly reinforced. Two key structures perform this role. Ligaments serve as guide wires that allow the joints to move in a particular direction without deviating. They actually connect bone to bone. Menisci are made of fibrous cartilage; they protect the connecting bones. When you injure menisci or ligaments, you may also harm your joint.

Unlike injuries to the tendons and bursae, injuries of the ligaments and menisci, especially tears, are frequently severe enough to require surgery. And they also cause major-league pain.

There are many joints that benefit from the structural support of ligaments and menisci, but these injuries usually involve the knee and ankle. (For more information on treating specific ligament injuries, see Chapter 10.)

The Knee

The knee is vulnerable, especially if you run or play contact sports. Ligament injuries are common and problematic, since they can trigger additional damage to other structures of the knee joint, including the menisci. The knee may start to wobble or buckle, making it difficult to walk. And you may also become predisposed to early degenerative arthritis.

Four ligaments are most frequently affected. The lateral and medial collateral ligaments, located on each side of the knee, connect the upper outer portion of the lower leg bone (fibula) to the bottom portion of the thigh bone (the femur) and stabilize the knee. They also prevent the knee from moving side to side. In addition, you have two ligaments inside the knee— the anterior cruciate and posterior cruciate ligaments. They also provide stability and prevent the knee from overextending or rotating too much.

Meniscal injuries

A meniscus is a tough, rubberlike piece of cartilage in the knee that acts as a shock absorber. It cushions and protects the joint surface. In each knee, you have a medial meniscus and a lateral meniscus. The most common injury is a meniscal tear. You'll need a positive MRI to clinch the diagnosis, but symptoms may include one or more of the following:

- You cannot flex the knee or extend it beyond resting position.
- The knee is locked in full extension.
- You have tenderness along the joint line.

The first line of treatment for meniscal injury is to apply ice to the knee for twenty to thirty minutes every three or four hours for two or three days. You can use an elastic bandage around the knee to keep down the swelling; it also helps to elevate your knee with a pillow beneath it for support. You may need to use crutches to relieve pressure on the joint and anti-inflammatory drugs for the pain.

The Ankle

The ankle is also prone to ligament injuries. Sprains often happen after a sudden twisting or turning motion that stretches or tears the ligament. Running, wearing improper shoes, or walking on uneven terrain can result in a sprained ankle.

8

You've Got Nerve

Pain—that unpleasant sensory feeling that signals damage to your body or a perceived threat to your existence—could not be possible without an elaborate communication infrastructure, known as the nervous system. Here's a brief primer on how it works.

Neurons (nerve cells) are the basic building block of the nervous system. There are an estimated 100 billion throughout the human body and each is composed of a cell body, an axon for sending messages, and a receiving device known as a dendrite. Neurons interconnect with each other in complex ways to form nerves. Faster than the highest-speed modem, almost too fast to comprehend, nerves transmit messages in the form of electrical signals from the axon of one neuron to a neighboring neuron's dendrite.

Each axon is surrounded by myelin, an insulation material that enables efficient nerve transmission. As they travel, the electrical impulses encounter synapses, strategically positioned between the neurons, which release neurotransmitters. These specialized chemicals, such as serotonin and dopamine, help facilitate message delivery.

Nerves are essential for detecting pain. Throughout your body, you have specialized pain receptors that convey messages along the nerves to the spinal cord and then to the brain.

Two components, the central nervous system and the peripheral nervous system, comprise the nervous system. The central nervous system includes the brain and spinal cord.

The peripheral nervous system is made up of all the nerves outside of the central nervous system. This includes the cranial nerves, which connect the nose, eyes, and ears to the brain, and the many nerves that link the spinal cord to the arms, legs, and torso.

The peripheral nervous system serves as an "electronic bridge" between the central nervous system and the rest of the body. There are thirty-one pairs of spinal nerves that come off of the spinal cord. Each pair has one in the front (motor nerve), which transmits information from the spinal cord to the muscles, and one in the back (sensory nerve), which moves sensory information to the spinal cord. The spinal nerves form "plexuses," or networks, in the neck, shoulders, and pelvis. These networks divide, forming peripheral nerves that supply the outer reaches of the body.

Made of bundles of nerve fibers, peripheral nerves vary in diameter, depending on the type of information they carry. They are insulated by multiple layers of a fatty material called myelin, which facilitates the transfer of impulses. The smaller fibers carry sensory information, such as temperature and pain, from the body to the spine, whereas larger fibers transmit motor information from the spine outward to power the muscles. Larger fibers also carry some information on touch and position.

Many very painful conditions derive from nerve dysfunction, especially in women. The first part of this chapter deals with three ailments caused by nerve compression: carpal tunnel syndrome, cubital tunnel syndrome, and thoracic outlet syndrome. I use the same dietary strategies, supplements, and herbal treatments for all three, so I'm putting those recommendations right up front. You'll find other, specific information on each of these conditions in the sections that follow.

The remainder of the chapter covers two long-term, chronic nerve problems — reflex sympathetic dystrophy and peripheral neuropathy — and briefly touches on shingles (herpes zoster) and trigeminal neuralgia (tic douloureux), an excruciating ailment that affects the trigeminal nerve in the face.

Dietary Strategies (See Chapter 14 for food sources of specified nutrients)

- Cut back on salt, since it increases water retention that may aggravate swelling.
- Eat pineapple, which contains bromelain (see page 324).
- Cook with turmeric or ginger, which may enhance bromelain's anti-inflammatory effects.
- Green tea contains a number of chemical constituents with anti-inflammatory properties, including polyphenols and apigenin. Besides the great reputation that green tea has earned for its overall health benefits, it may also protect against osteoporosis, cancer, and heart disease. According to the U.S. Department of Agriculture Phytochemical Database, green tea contains many phytonutrients that may help prevent ulcers. If you frequently take NSAIDS, green tea may give your GI tract some extra protection. Try to drink three to four cups a day.

- Vitamin B2 (riboflavin) enhances the effectiveness of B6.
- Vitamin B6 plays a role in the production of neurotransmitters, specialized chemicals that transport signals between nerve cells. It may be of help for all types of nerve pain conditions.

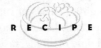

R E C I P E

SAVORY SPINACH BARLEY

2 tablespoons olive oil
2 cloves garlic, minced
1 onion, chopped
¼ cup chopped fresh parsley
8 ounces frozen chopped spinach, thawed and drained
2 cups water
1 cup barley

1. In a saucepan, sauté in the olive oil the garlic, onion, parsley, and spinach for 3 minutes.
2. Add water and bring to a boil.
3. Stir in the barley, lower heat, cover pot, and simmer on low heat for 35 minutes.

SERVES 4

Supplements

Vitamin B6
Although you may have to wait several months to see the effects, this vitamin may ease nerve-related symptoms. Start with 50 mg a day and gradually increase the dose. Or you can take a B complex that contains B6.

If your symptoms get worse, stop taking the vitamin and consult your physician. Excessive, long-term, daily doses of vitamin B6 can cause nerve damage. Do not use vitamin B6 if you are taking anticonvulsants for epilepsy or levodopa for Parkinson's disease. You may need to take more if you are taking: isoniazid, penicillamine, theophylline, MAO inhibitors, or hydralazine. The acceptable range for this vitamin is 2 to 100 mg a day.

Vitamin B2 (Riboflavin)

To increase the effects of B6, the acceptable dose is 1.1 mg a day. The upper limit has not been determined. You can also take it as part of a B complex.

Bromelain

This also helps to supplement the effects of vitamin B6 and turmeric (see below). Bromelain is best consumed in its natural form—pineapple. Still, if you wish to supplement, a dose of 40 mg, taken two to three times a day, has been used in several studies. Do not take bromelain if you are on anticoagulant medications.

Green tea

Green tea may help reduce your pain. If you prefer pills to tea, take 100 to 150 mg of green tea extract, three times a day.

Herbs

Ginger (Zingibar officinale)

To enhance the effects of bromelain (see above), the suggested dose is 100 to 300 mg of this anti-inflammatory herb three times a day. Even better, use it to spice up your meals. Other options include ginger tea and ginger candy. Ginger may cause mild heartburn; avoid it if you have gallstones.

Chamomile (Chamaemelum nobile or Matricaria recutita)

Dating back to biblical times, chamomile is a mild stress reducer and re-laxant. It also helps fight inflammation. To make chamomile tea, pour 150 ml of boiling water over 3 grams of chamomile, cover for ten to fifteen minutes and strain. (Note: one teaspoon equals one gram.) Drink three cups a day.

Turmeric (Curuma longa)

Turmeric helps reduce the inflammation associated with nerve compression syndromes. It is available in capsules, tablets, and liquid extracts. Be sure any product you buy contains at least 95 percent curcumin, the active ingredient. The recommended dose is 400 to 600 mg of curcumin, three times a day. Avoid turmeric or check with your doctor if you have gallstones or blood clotting or fertility problems. Prolonged use or higher doses may cause stomach upset or ulcers.

rnata)

at night, try this herb, which helps you relax
The recommended dose is one cup of tea twice
ake sedative medications. This herb is on the
on's list of herbs "generally recognized as safe"

ts

e 158)

75 percent) (See page 96)

E has approved arnica as a topical agent with
, and antibacterial properties. It reduces pain,

Joint-Ritis (See page 96)

Sports gel
You can rub on this homeopathic gel, made from *Bellis perennis* (daisy),
Hypericum perforatum (St. John's wort), *Rhus toxicodendron* (poison ivy),
and *Ruta graveolens* (rue), up to four times a day.

Nature's Chemist (See page 96)

CARPAL TUNNEL SYNDROME (CTS)

Description

The carpal tunnel is a narrow passageway in the wrist through which the
median nerve travels. This is the major peripheral nerve supplying the
thumb side of the hand. When it is compressed, carpal tunnel syndrome,
a common, painful disorder of the wrist and hand, is the result.

The pain of carpal tunnel syndrome ranges from minor and tolerable to
truly miserable. My patients describe it in many ways—"electriclike," dull
and aching, lacerating, burning. Particularly bothersome is the numbness,
tingling, and pain in the first three fingers of the hand. At night, in certain
sleeping positions, it may hurt more; you may even find yourself waking up

to shake your hands out. As the syndrome advances, the hand muscles may weaken and atrophy (thin).

This annoying ailment seems to favor women; in one study, three times as many women as men suffered from CTS. Why this is so is the subject of several theories:

- Anatomical—women are simply made differently from men. Because they have smaller wrists, their median nerve must travel through a narrower space.
- Vocational—women are more frequently employed in jobs that require repetitive movements of the hands and wrists.
- Recreational—many women are involved in recreational pursuits like gardening, ceramic work, and needlecrafts that also involve repetitive motion and take a toll on the wrist.
- Hormonal—CTS is sometimes associated with hormonal changes due to the menstrual cycle, birth control pills, pregnancy, and menopause.

CTS is often job-related. It is well known as an ailment of people who do data entry or other jobs with heavy use of computers. But it can affect anyone who performs repetitive hand motions—illustrators, carpenters, assembly-line workers, knitting workers, and guitar players, for example. People with rheumatoid arthritis, diabetes, and hypothyroidism are also prone to developing CTS. This condition usually occurs between forty and sixty years of age.

Causes

A large percentage of CTS cases are idiopathic, meaning that we don't know the cause. When we can figure out why CTS has occurred, it's usually due to one of two reasons. Sometimes the ligaments and tendons passing through the carpal tunnel have gotten bigger because of swelling, caused by repetitive motion. Or, the tunnel has gotten narrower, thanks to fluid retention, fat deposition, carpal synovitis, tenosynovitis, a fracture, arthritic spurs, or tumor. Either way, the net result is the same: compression of the median nerve, pain, and discomfort.

Signs and Symptoms

Carpal tunnel syndrome usually strikes the dominant hand, but it may occur in either or both. Symptoms include:

- Tingling and numbness in the thumb, index finger, middle finger, and half of the ring finger
- Numbness, tingling, and/or burning in the wrist, palm, and forearm
- More pain when you bend your wrist
- Loss of strength in the affected hand(s)
- Clumsiness and inability to hold or feel objects
- Symptoms are often worse at night
- Shaking or rubbing your hand(s) provides relief

Conventional Treatments

Your doctor may recommend a special test, called a nerve conduction velocity study/electromyography examination, to electrically troubleshoot the median nerve. Usually, a physiatrist or a neurologist performs this assessment.

If you have carpal tunnel syndrome, you'll want to avoid activities that overuse the affected hand. You can also support your wrist by wearing a splint when sleeping or during physical activity.

Depending on your job, one of the key treatments may be making changes in your work habits. An occupational therapist can help you figure out how to modify your regular tasks to prevent carpal tunnel syndrome or reduce the likelihood of a recurrence. It's important to pay attention to proper ergonomics. If you work at a computer, repositioning your workstation to better support your arm and wrist is at the top of the list. Adjust the height of your chair so that your arms and wrists are in a straight line with your elbows at a 90-degree angle. And when you type, your arm, wrist, and thumb should be in a straight line, with your fingers lower than your wrist. Do not rest your hand on the keyboard or mouse pad and take frequent breaks, as often as every hour.

NSAIDS, such as ibuprofen or naproxen, are the first line of treatment for pain and inflammation. You can also try topical analgesics. Neuropathic pain agents (drugs that act on nerves), like Neurontin, are sometimes used. If these treatments don't help, your doctor may recommend corticosteroid injections. I believe a steroid injection into the carpal tunnel can sometimes help, but it should not be done repeatedly. If conservative treatments fail and your pain continues to worsen, or you develop muscle atrophy and hand weakness, you may need surgery.

Do-It-Yourself

Ice

When your symptoms are acute, apply a flexible ice pack (or a bag of frozen peas) to your wrist for ten minutes every hour. Cold constricts blood vessels and will reduce swelling.

Every day

Use these simple techniques to take care of your wrists:

- Elevate your arm with pillows when you lie down.
- Avoid resting your wrists on hard or ridged surfaces for prolonged periods.
- Take regular breaks from repetitive motion. At least once an hour, flex your fingers and shake your hands.
- Try to keep your wrists straight. Flexing or twisting stresses the carpal tunnel.
- To reduce strain on your wrists, use both hands to lift objects.

Magnet therapy

Although I haven't seen solid research, there is anecdotal evidence that magnet therapy provides relief for some people with CTS. The idea is that the magnets create a mild electric current that stimulates nerve endings and blocks pain sensation. To try this treatment, buy magnets that have at least 250–500 gauss (the unit for magnet strength); button-sized magnets are best for this ailment. Position the magnets above and below the wrist crease and hold them in place with adhesive tape. You can also buy wristbands with magnets.

Acupressure (See page 353 for technique)

This treatment may lessen swelling and numbness. To decrease pain, promote relaxation, and reduce stress associated with carpal tunnel and other disorders, try:

- LI4 (Large Intestine 4), located at the top of the web space between the thumb and second finger. Do not use it when you are pregnant.

Mind/Body

Yoga

I recommend yoga to my carpal tunnel syndrome patients because it is an effective treatment for this condition, in addition to its general health benefits. According to a study published in the *Journal of the American Medical Association*, patients who did yoga twice a week for eight weeks had less pain and more flexibility and strength than those using a splint, a conventional treatment for CTS. Try Overhead Arm Extension and Trunk Extension. (See pages 344–351 for postures.)

Exercise

Doing gentle exercise every day may relieve your pain and improve function. It will also prevent further injury.

THERAPEUTIC EXERCISES
Try these simple exercises three to four times a day.

- Lift your arms above your head, and rotate them inward and outward.
- Extend your arms straight out in front. Move your hands in a circle, using your wrists. Repeat in the opposite direction.
- Hold your hands out in front of you with palms up. Close your fingers into your palms and open slowly until you feel a pull in the muscles. Close your hands and repeat.
- With your palms together, press your fingertips against each other. Hold, release, and repeat.
- Wrap a rubber band around all of your fingers. Spread your fingers, hold, and release.

ACTIVE RANGE OF MOTION
- Flexion: Gently bend your wrist forward. Hold 5 seconds. Relax. Repeat 10 times.
- Extension: Gently bend your wrist backward. Hold 5 seconds. Relax. Repeat 10 times.
- Side to side: Gently move your wrist from side to side (a handshake motion). Hold 5 seconds at each end. Relax. Repeat 10 times.
- Stretching: With your uninjured hand, bend your injured wrist down by pressing the back of your hand. Hold for 15 to 30 seconds. Relax. Then, stretch your injured hand back by pressing the fingers in a backward direction. Hold 15 to 30 seconds. Relax. Repeat.

- Tendon glides: Extend the fingers of your injured hand. Gently press down on the middle joints of your fingers, toward your palm. Hold 5 seconds. Relax. Repeat 10 times.
- Wrist flexion: Hold a full soda can or the handle of a hammer, with your palm facing up. Bend your wrist upward. Hold 5 seconds. Relax. Repeat 10 times. Gradually increase the weight you are holding.
- Wrist extension: With your palm down, hold a full soda can or similar object. Bend your wrist up. Hold 5 seconds. Relax. Repeat 10 times.
- Grip strengthening: Squeeze a rubber ball and hold 5 seconds. Relax. Repeat 10 times.

Seeking Help from Complementary Practitioners

Acupuncture
In one recent study, thirty-five of thirty-six patients had symptomatic relief from acupuncture, and two-thirds of the individuals reported long-term results—from 2.5 to 8.5 years of pain relief. The Consensus Panel of the National Institutes of Health has endorsed acupuncture as a treatment for CTS, and I've found it to be successful with many of my patients.

Red Flags

- Development of muscle wasting or weakness that limits function
- Numbness or tingling that persists or worsens

CUBITAL TUNNEL SYNDROME (ULNAR NEUROPATHY)

Description

The cubital tunnel is found below the "funny bone" (medial epicondyle), on the inside of the elbow. It is the passageway through which the ulnar nerve passes as it goes from the upper arm to the forearm and hand. This nerve is the culprit responsible for the odd sensation you feel when you hit your funny bone.

Cubital tunnel syndrome is a compression of the ulnar nerve at the elbow. It leads to numbness, tingling, or "pins and needles" in the ring finger and pinky. If damage to the ulnar nerve is severe enough, you can develop muscle atrophy and a claw-hand deformity.

Cubital tunnel syndrome is not as common as carpal tunnel syndrome. What's more, the extra padding women tend to have may, in this instance, be advantageous. Why? Because more fat around the elbow protects the cubital tunnel from damage.

Causes

Direct trauma to the cubital tunnel may damage the ulnar nerve. More commonly, though, this ailment is the result of overuse. When you repeatedly bend and straighten your elbow, your ulnar nerve may become irritated and inflamed. This may happen if you lean on your elbow frequently or for long periods of time, or if you do a great deal of typing, data entry, or assembly-line work.

Sometimes the nerve actually shifts position and rubs against the funny bone, snapping every time it passes over the bone. This repeated snapping further stretches and irritates the nerve.

Arthritis, diabetes, and thyroid problems raise your risk for developing nerve compressions, as does consuming large amounts of alcohol.

Signs and Symptoms

- Weakness of the ring and little fingers
- Pain in the elbow
- Weakness when pinching the thumb and index finger together
- Numbness on the inside of the hand
- Loss of hand strength, so you drop things or have difficulty opening jars
- The hand and arm become cold or numb when gripping the top of a steering wheel or other objects
- The symptoms worsen when you hold a telephone, rest your head on your hand, or cross your arms over your chest
- Pain may be worse at night

Conventional Treatments

If you have cubital tunnel syndrome, you'll want to avoid or modify activities that cause irritation. You can do this by cutting back on tasks that require repeated bending and straightening of the elbow.

Depending on your job, a key treatment may be making changes in your work habits. It's important to pay attention to proper ergonomics. If you work at a computer, repositioning your workstation to better support your arm and wrist is at the top of the list. Adjust your chair and desk so that your elbow is flexed no more than 30 degrees, and your wrist is in a neutral position. For more extensive help, your doctor may refer you to an occupational therapist, who can help you figure out how to modify your regular tasks to prevent cubital tunnel syndrome, or reduce the likelihood of a recurrence.

NSAIDS, such as ibuprofen or naproxen, help decrease pain and inflammation. Because they are easier on your stomach and GI tract, the Cox-2 inhibitor NSAIDS, Celebrex or Vioxx, are safer for long-term use.

Your doctor may want to use immobilizing therapies, such as splints, wraps, or casts to protect and allow inflamed tissue to heal. To increase circulation and soothe muscles, she may also recommend hydrotherapy and electrotherapy. Finally, physical therapy may also be an option.

Do-It-Yourself

- When your symptoms are acute, apply a flexible ice pack (or a bag of frozen peas) to your elbow for ten minutes every hour. Cold constricts the blood vessels and will reduce swelling.
- Aromatherapy: Add a couple of drops of lavender oil to your bath. It will curb any spasms and help you relax.
- Take frequent breaks—five minutes every half-hour—from repetitive activities.
- If your pain worsens at night, wrap your elbow with a towel or thin pillow to keep it straight.
- Avoid crossing your arms across your chest.

Exercise

To relieve pain, improve function, and prevent further injury, try this gentle exercise:

FINGER SQUEEZE
One by one, squeeze a sponge or pen between the individual fingers of your hand. Hold for 10 seconds, relax, and repeat 5 times for each finger.

Mind/Body

I recommend yoga to my patients. (See carpal tunnel syndrome, page 175, for specifics.)

Seeking Help from Complementary Practitioners

Acupuncture relieves the pain of cubital tunnel syndrome by triggering a massive outpouring of endorphins. I've found it to be a successful treatment.

Red Flags

· Development of muscle wasting or weakness that limits function
· Numbness or tingling that persists or worsens

THORACIC OUTLET SYNDROME
(NECK, SHOULDER, ARM, AND HAND PAIN)

Description

The thoracic outlet is a passageway located at the top of the rib cage, in the area between the base of the neck and the armpit. Thoracic outlet syndrome (TOS) can affect the neck, shoulder, arm, and hand.

Although we don't always know its cause, TOS is often related to a compression of the nerves and arteries that pass through the thoracic outlet. Sometimes, because of overcrowding, blood vessels or nerves get crunched between a rib and an overlying muscle. The result is pain, numbness, and tingling. Less oxygen may get to the hands, shoulders, and arms, causing them to swell or turn blue.

Thoracic outlet syndrome is more common in women than in men. It usually strikes between the ages of thirty-five and fifty-five. You may be especially prone to developing this condition during pregnancy because of the significant postural changes that occur. An increased thoracic curve, with rounded shoulders and a head-forward position, tightness in your middle and anterior scalene muscles, and a tendency for the clavicles (collarbone) to depress into the first ribs, may all contribute to thoracic outlet syndrome.

If you have TOS symptoms, try the ADSONS test: Take a deep breath and hold it in, while tipping your head back and turning it toward the other side. If your pulse slows down during this maneuver, you may indeed have TOS. Of course, you should see your doctor to confirm the diagnosis.

Causes

Sometimes it's not possible to figure out why you have thoracic outlet syndrome. But the usual causes are:

- Repetitive activities that require you to hold your arms overhead or extended forward. Weight lifting or loading and unloading shelves are examples.
- TOC may be associated with poor posture and rounded shoulders, large, pendulous breasts, and regular use of heavy handbags.
- Any condition that leads to swelling or movement of the tissues of, or near, the thoracic outlet. This includes muscle enlargement, injuries, and, in rare cases, tumors at the top of the lung.
- Some people are born with an extra rib in the neck (cervical rib) that can cause problems in the thoracic outlet.

Signs and Symptoms

- Pain, weakness, numbness and tingling, swelling, fatigue, or coldness in the arm and hand
- Discoloration caused by impaired circulation

Conventional Treatments

For relief of pain, your doctor may suggest a trial of NSAIDS or neuropathic agents (drugs that act on nerves). Seeing a physical therapist for postural exercises may help relieve pain. It's also important to take frequent breaks during any activities that aggravate your condition. If you get no relief, surgery may be necessary.

Do-It-Yourself

Every day
- Limit how long you stretch your arms out or overhead.
- Avoid lifting or carrying heavy objects.
- Decrease the tension on the shoulder straps of your seat belt.
- Take frequent breaks during any activities that aggravate your pain.
- Carry your purse or briefcase with the unaffected arm.
- Avoid sleeping on your stomach with your arms above your head. Instead, sleep on your side or back with your arms below chest level.

- If you have to lift a heavy object from anything over shoulder height, use a step stool.
- Heavy breasts can cause strain on your shoulders; be sure to wear a supportive brassiere. (In some cases, breast reduction may be in order.)

Aromatherapy
- Lavender (*Lavandula angustifolia*) — This herb is a strengthening tonic for your nervous system. Use it by boiling 100 grams of lavender with 2 liters of water and then adding it to your bath. Otherwise, you can buy a commercial preparation.
- Rosemary (*Rosmarinus officinalis*) — This herb may decrease pain and regional muscle spasms associated with thoracic outlet syndrome. To prepare a bath, add 50 grams of herb to 1 liter of hot water and add to your bath. Alternatively, use several drops of a commercial preparation. Do not use rosemary during pregnancy.

Mind/Body

Tai chi, a twelve-hundred-year-old, gentle form of martial arts, has gained a tremendous amount of popularity throughout China. It involves deep breathing, accompanied by slow, fluid movements through a series of body postures. The aim is to achieve balance between mind and body, and to focus *chi*, or vital energy. Although there isn't a great deal of literature on the subject, I believe tai chi enhances balance and coordination. Because it also improves poor posture, which is sometimes associated with thoracic outlet syndrome, it may be an effective treatment.

Red Flags

Call your doctor if you develop:

- Muscle weakness or wasting that limits function
- Persistent numbness or tingling
- Swollen or blue hands, shoulders, or arms

REFLEX SYMPATHETIC DYSTROPHY (RSD)

Also known as reflex sympathetic dystrophy syndrome (RSDS) or complex regional pain syndrome.

CAROL'S STORY

Carol, a woman in her thirties, had been a gardener until an awful accident with a lawn mower mangled her entire leg. That was two years before she came to see me. The obvious injuries had long since healed, but she was still in excruciating pain. She couldn't put any weight on her leg and needed a cane to walk. She described herself as "trapped in a prison of pain," unable to sleep, work, or even socialize with friends. And she was in a state of constant anxiety.

After I examined her and reviewed the necessary testing, I explained that she was suffering from complex regional pain syndrome, more commonly known as reflex sympathetic dystrophy (RSD), a painful disorder that can occur after a nerve injury or other trauma to an extremity. The pain is intense, chronic, and unremitting. But that's only the first stage; RSD is a progressive disorder. I told Carol that, without treatment, her leg would eventually become red, inflamed, swollen, and begin to lose its hair. When she responded: "Then let's get going. We have to take care of it before it gets worse," I knew I had a motivated patient on my hands.

In the office, Carol responded minimally to conventional modes of treatment. She did get an added measure of relief from nerve blocks. But she benefited more from complementary strategies, including electrical stimulation and hypnosis. I also used acupuncture, accessing what's called the "Valium point" of the ear to reduce her anxiety. Many of our most effective interventions were techniques she could use on her own at home. Carol learned to elevate and compress her leg to fight the swelling, and to use contrast baths — alternating cold and hot water — to address some of the blood vessel changes that occur in RSD. She was particularly successful with guided visual imagery. By learning to couple an unpleasant stimulus (her pain) with a pleasant thought, she was able to relax. "I think about a beach on Maui and the pain and anxiety just disappear," she laughed.

In time, Carol was able to give up her cane. She has started to go out again and has gone back to work. Today she swears by these treatments and even appeared in a local television news story about acupuncture. "I have my life back," she says.

Description

Reflex sympathetic dystrophy (RSD), known in academic circles as complex regional pain syndrome, is a potentially devastating disorder thought to be driven by the sympathetic nervous system. Among other things, this network of nerves controls the opening and closing of blood vessels and sweat glands.

RSD evolves in phases. The pain, typically accompanied by blood flow and soft tissue changes, swelling, and sweating, is intense, and has an awful, burning quality. Because the disease also leads to muscle weakness and wasting, you may suffer dystrophy, or weakness, in the affected area, in addition to severe pain. Your joints may become stiff from disuse and your skin, muscles, and bone may atrophy.

This ailment may occur as a result of injury, or from damage to nerves. It most often affects the hands, arms, feet, or legs but it may involve the knee, hip, shoulder, or other sites.

RSD occurs most frequently in women over age fifty. It is difficult to treat. Still, your chances of success are best if you start aggressive treatment early—within the first three months.

Causes

Unfortunately, in nearly a third of RSD cases, the cause is unknown. However, it often follows a sprain, fracture, or injury to nerves or blood vessels, particularly in upper or lower extremities. It can also occur after surgery.

Signs and Symptoms

You may experience the following in the area affected by RSD:

- Severe pain and burning
- Pallor (paleness) or redness
- Shiny red skin that turns bluish
- Increased or decreased sweating
- Swelling
- Skin atrophy or tightening of the skin
- Hypersensitivity to touch
- Muscle spasms
- Changes in skin temperature
- Difficulty moving
- Loss of hair in the involved extremity

Conventional Treatments

This condition is a real challenge. Almost 60 percent of patients don't respond well to conventional treatments. Medications, such as corticosteroids, which are potent anti-inflammatories; vasodilators, which open blood vessels and enable blood flow to the extremity; and alpha- or beta-adrenergic blocking compounds, which affect the sympathetic nervous system, are commonly used. Your doctor may also inject you with a local anesthetic, such as lidocaine or bupivacaine, which provides a temporary respite from pain. Somewhat longer lasting relief may come from a nerve block. In this procedure, the doctor injects a substance, usually alcohol, near the involved nerves to block transmission of pain signals.

Physical therapy may help you regain some range of motion and motor control, as well as strengthen the limb. Your PT may also do "spray and stretch," where she stretches your muscles after applying a vapocoolant spray.

A physical therapist or an occupational therapist can also do desensitization. RSD causes hypersensitivity to touch and allodynia, a condition where normally neutral or even pleasant things, such as clothing, wind, cold or a light touch to the skin, cause pain. The goal of desensitization is to help your painful skin gradually adjust to rougher textures. It will help you tolerate the touch of clothing, bed sheets, and towels, for example. To do it, your skin will be rubbed with different materials, beginning with soft, light textures and proceeding to rough, irritating surfaces.

Your doctor may suggest that you try TENS (transcutaneous electrical nerve stimulation). To utilize this therapy, you carry a small, box-shaped device that sends brief electrical impulses through electrodes into nerve endings under your skin. The pulses of electricity interfere with your body's pain signals.

If all else fails, surgery is the last resort. This involves cutting nerves; so while it may stop your pain, it may also affect other sensations.

Dietary Strategies

In one study, taking 500 mg of vitamin C for fifty days prevented the development of RSD in people who had sustained wrist fractures. Further research on this treatment is needed, although I can see no harm in trying it. In the meantime, I also recommend that you emphasize foods rich in vitamin C. (See Chapter 14.)

Herbs

St. John's wort (Hypericum perforatum)
This well-studied herb is a sedative, antidepressant, and pain reliever. Suggested dose is one cup of infusion, three times a day. Do not take this herb with any other antidepressants.

Valerian root (Valeriana officinalis)
Since pain-related anxiety and tension are so often a component of RSD, you can use valerian to calm your nervous system. Herbalists suggest that you drink two to three cups of infusion a day.

Passionflower (Passiflora incarnata)
The intense, unremitting pain of RSD can cause great anxiety. This herbal tranquilizer will calm you down and ease nerve pain. The recommended dose is 1 to 4 ml of tincture or one cup of infusion, twice a day. An interesting note: This herb has been patented for use in a chewing gum in Romania.

Herbal Creams and Ointments

Traumeel ointment (See page 158)

Arnica cream
The German Commission E has approved arnica as a topical agent. It reduces pain, numbness, and tingling.

Do-It-Yourself

Contrast baths
Inflammation and swelling decrease blood supply to the affected area. Because contrast baths boost circulation, they increase the supply of nutrients from the blood, help to eliminate waste, and reduce pain. Immerse the limb in hot water for three minutes, then in cold water for thirty seconds. Repeat this process three to five times.

Homeopathy (use dosage on the package)
 • Sulfur, a mineral found in rocks around hot springs and volcanoes, can soothe red, hot, burning skin.

Aromatherapy
- Mix a few drops each of lavender oil, sandalwood oil, and calendula oil into a neutral lotion or oil, and massage the area.
- Add one cup of vinegar to a hot bath to help balance your skin.
- Apply a compress soaked in verbena or thyme tea to soothe and cool the area.
- To relax, take a bath with valerian. Mix 100 mg of herb in 2 liters of hot water and add it to your bathwater.

Mind/Body

Yoga

PASCHIMOTTANASANA (POSTERIOR-STRETCH POSTURE)
This helps relieve skin diseases. (See pages 344–351 for postures.)

Qi Gong
This ancient Chinese exercise combines deep breathing with movement, and helps to circulate internal *chi*, or vital energy. In some studies, it has helped people with RSD by reducing pain and anxiety.

Imagery (See page 341 for technique)
Using imagery is an effective way to control pain.

Seeking Help from Complementary Practitioners

Acupuncture
I've found that this therapy provides relief for some patients.

Biofeedback (See page 341 for technique)

Red Flags

Call your doctor if you have:

- Persisting pain
- Fever
- Elevated white count
- Inflammation
- Redness that gets worse

PERIPHERAL NEUROPATHY

Description

The peripheral nerves are part of a network that connects the central nervous system (brain and spinal cord) to the muscles, skin, and internal organs. Peripheral neuropathy is a malfunction of these nerves. When it affects a single nerve, it is called a mononeuropathy. In contrast, a polyneuropathy affects many different nerves simultaneously.

Symptoms of peripheral neuropathy include pain, numbness, tingling, muscle wasting, and loss of strength. Also, loss of sensation may cause ulcers, cuts, small burns, and other injuries to go unnoticed, raising the risk of infection or other damage.

Since many peripheral nerves lie close to the surface of the body, they are particularly vulnerable to compression. Entrapment neuropathy, a common type of peripheral neuropathy, can occur because of physical injury to a nerve, or compression of a nerve by neighboring structures. Some types of entrapment neuropathy are:

- Median nerve peripheral nerve injury and entrapment. Better known as carpal tunnel syndrome, this is the result of repeated compression of the median nerve in the narrow carpal tunnel at the wrist (see page 175). Women are especially prone to this condition.
- Ulnar nerve peripheral nerve injury and entrapment. The ulnar nerve lies close to the surface of the elbow, so it is easily damaged. Symptoms range from numbness and tingling to muscle weakness in the hand and a claw-hand deformity (see cubital tunnel syndrome, page 180).
- Radial nerve peripheral nerve injury and entrapment, also known as Saturday-night palsy. This condition results in a wrist drop, where the wrist assumes a bent position with the fingers flexed.
- Peroneal nerve peripheral nerve injury and entrapment. This causes weakening of the muscles that lift the foot.

Peripheral neuropathy is especially common among people over the age of fifty-five, afflicting as many as 3 to 4 percent of those in this age group. It usually strikes the nerves of the limbs, especially the feet. Women, especially during pregnancy, postpartum, and breast-feeding, may be more vulnerable to some types of peripheral neuropathy:

- Bell's palsy, which affects the facial nerve and causes paralysis and weakness of the forehead and lower face, is three times more frequent in women during pregnancy. It usually occurs in the third trimester or during the first two weeks after birth.

· Meralgia paraesthetica is one-sided or bilateral entrapment of the lateral femoral cutaneous nerve of the thigh, when it passes under the inguinal ligament. While it's sometimes the result of trauma, this painful condition is also associated with obesity and/or the weight gain of pregnancy. It usually occurs during the third trimester and improves within three months after birth.

· Carpal tunnel syndrome, involving entrapment of a nerve in the wrist, occurs in 20 to 40 percent of pregnant women because of fluid retention (see above).

· Breast-feeding-related neuropathies
  · Pressure on the nerves under the arm (axilla) may occur when the breasts get engorged with milk. You may feel numbness and tingling in your forearm, especially on the outer, or ulnar, side. The symptoms may improve as the baby suckles.
  · If you use a hand-operated breast pump, you may experience pain and tingling when you bend your elbow.

· Postpartum foot drop can happen when the fetal head presses against the lumbosacral spine, or if there is compression of the peroneal nerve by leg braces during delivery. What happens is that you are unable to extend your ankle upward, so your foot slaps down when you walk. This injury is common in small women who deliver large infants.

Causes

Peripheral polyneuropathy may be associated with a number of factors, including infection, autoimmune disease, toxic agents, cancer, and nutritional deficiency. Here are the major causes:

· Illnesses, including: AIDS, diabetes (a very common cause), kidney failure, and syphilis.
· Nutritional deficiencies, such as low levels of vitamin B12 and folate.
· Medications, including: AIDS drugs, antibiotics (metronidazole, an antibiotic used for Crohn's disease, and isoniazid, a tuberculosis treatment), chemotherapy drugs (such as vincristine), and gold compounds (used for rheumatoid arthritis).
· Exposure to chemicals, including: arsenic, lead, mercury, and pesticides made from organophosphates.

Signs and Symptoms

You may feel any or all of the following in your affected limb(s):

- Decreased feeling or sensation distributed like a "glove and stocking"
- Weakness
- Loss of reflexes
- Numbness or insensitivity to pain or temperature
- Tingling, burning, or prickling
- Sharp pains or cramps
- Extreme sensitivity to touch, even light touch (wearing clothes, walking, or other activity may feel unbearable)
- Loss of balance and coordination
- Symptoms may get worse at night

Conventional Treatments

The pain of peripheral neuropathy is often a challenging problem. Both analgesics and neuropathic pain agents (drugs that act on nerves) are used as a first line of attack. Tricyclic antidepressant drugs, like amitriptyline and nortriptyline, are also sometimes prescribed for pain and depression. Their side effects include urinary retention and low blood pressure. Trazodone is another drug that can be substituted if you cannot tolerate them. A second tier of drugs sometimes used for pain include anticonvulsants, such as gabapentin (Neurontin), carbamazapine (Tegretol), and phenytoin (Dilantin).

There is also a topical pain medication. Lidocaine, a short-acting anesthetic, is now available in patch form (Lidoderm).

Preventive treatment for peripheral neuropathy often depends largely on the cause. For example, if your problem is caused by diabetes, your physician will focus on controlling your blood sugar; vitamin therapies will be used if you're found to have a nutritional deficiency.

Dietary Strategies (See Chapter 14 for food sources of specified nutrients)

Fats

Not all fat is unhealthy. Substitute good oils for bad. Called "essential fatty acids" (EFAs), omega-3 and omega-6 oils are used by the body to make EPA and DHA, which are critical for healthy cell membranes. This is true for every cell in the body, and it's especially important in the nervous system and brain. Tragically, the American diet has traditionally relied on saturated fats or oils lacking the correct balance of omega-3 and omega-6 fatty acids.

Make sure that you avoid saturated and trans fats and consume foods and oils that have plenty of omega-6 and omega-3 fatty acids.

In general, don't burn oil and don't allow it to get rancid. Keep it in the refrigerator.

- Drink plenty of water. Season it with lemon or citrus.
- Vitamin B6 is involved in producing neurotransmitters. If you are lacking in this nutrient, muscle twitches and weakness, numbness, and tingling may be the result.
- Vitamin B5 (pantothenic acid) is important for cellular metabolism.
- Vitamin E is an antioxidant that can prevent nerve damage.
- Vitamin B1 (thiamine) occupies a site on the nerve cell membranes and improves their functioning.
- Zinc protects the body from chemical damage.
- Chromium is a trace mineral that acts as a helper to insulin. It unlocks the cell membrane door, allowing glucose to enter. Considerable research exists on its ability to help diabetics, even women with pregnancy-induced diabetes, control blood sugar. Since peripheral neuropathy is associated with diabetes, anything that helps you manage your glucose level is worth doing.

Supplements

Vitamin B6
A deficiency of B6 can cause muscle twitching, muscle weakness, numbness, and tingling. The accepted dose range is 2 to 100 mg a day.

Vitamin E
The accepted dose range is 15 to 1,000 mg a day.

Vitamin B1
Enhances nerve cell functions. The accepted dose range is 1.4 to 50 mg a day.

Zinc
The accepted dose range is 8 to 40 mg a day.

Chromium

As described above, this important trace mineral helps maintain the body's blood glucose level. The lower limit for chromium is 25 mcg; no safe upper limit has been established.

Gamma-linolenic acids (GLAs)

Found in black currant seed oil, borage oil, and evening primrose oil, GLAs have been shown to help the symptoms of some types of neuropathy, including diabetic neuropathy. I prefer that you use it in its natural form (i.e., in food); however, if you want to take supplements, the dose is 1,500 mg a day.

Lipoic acid

This supplement is used extensively in Germany to treat diabetic complications like peripheral neuropathy as well as diabetic autonomic neuropathy (neuropathy affecting the nerves that supply the digestive tract and the heart). Although there isn't a huge body of literature yet, there is some evidence that supports its use, especially when combined with GLA. Doses used for treating diabetic complications are usually 300 to 600 mg daily; people in a recent study used 800 mg. Up to 1,800 mg daily of lipoic acid appears to be safe, but more is not necessarily better.

Herbal Creams and Ointments

Capsaicin cream (0.025–0.075 percent) (See page 96)

This is a "hot" botanical remedy harvested from red peppers, or cayenne. It can be a potent analgesic for peripheral neuropathy. A 1992 study of 277 diabetics with peripheral neuropathy demonstrated a significant improvement in pain when they applied capsaicin to their extremities.

Do-It-Yourself

- Examine your ailing limb(s) every day. Injuries must be treated early to prevent infection. Lacking sensation, you are especially prone to breaks in the skin, so vigilance is the watchword.
- Eat a nutritious diet.
- If your neuropathy is diabetes-related, strict control of your sugar is helpful.
- Exercise regularly.
- Abstain from excessive alcohol consumption.

Exercise

If you can, keep up your aerobic exercise. Swimming is particularly beneficial. Without any pain from impact, it strengthens the muscles and tones the body.

Seeking Help from Complementary Practitioners

Acupuncture
Some of my patients benefit from this therapy.

Biofeedback (See page 341 for technique)

Red Flags

Call your doctor if you experience:

- Numbness or tingling in your extremities
- Chronic weakness or heaviness in your muscles, which may be accompanied by cramping
- Prickling, burning, stabbing or any other uncomfortable and spontaneous sensation on your skin

TRIGEMINAL NEURALGIA

Description

This excruciating condition leads to brief, recurrent bursts of severe, knife-like pain in the face that follows the distribution of the trigeminal nerve. There are two trigeminal nerves, one on each side of the face. Often, the pain happens instantaneously and without provocation. It can also be triggered by chewing, speaking, or swallowing or by stimulation as mild as a touch to the area or a breeze. Typically, the pain is felt in the cheek near the nose, or in the mouth or jaw.

Trigeminal neuralgia affects twice as many women as men. It does not usually strike people under age fifty, although it may be associated with multiple sclerosis in younger individuals.

Causes

We don't know what causes this ailment. It usually occurs spontaneously, with no precipitating event or disease, although it does occasionally happen after a dental procedure.

Symptoms

- Blinding facial pain, lasting from a few seconds to one to two minutes.
- Tic douloureux—A facial muscle tic caused by repeated wincing after each paroxysm of pain.

Conventional Treatments

With facial pain, a dental evaluation is usually in order. If you do indeed have trigeminal neuralgia, your physician will probably prescribe seizure medications, such as carbamazepine (Tegretol), and antidepressants. She may also prescribe baclofen, a drug that acts on the central nervous system to help relax muscles and relieve spasms.

Dietary Strategies

Celery (Apium graveolans)

In ancient times, Hippocrates believed that celery was able to calm nerves. Today we also know that celery has anti-inflammatory properties. You can drink celery juice or celery tea. In addition, you can make a celery tonic by steeping 2 tablespoons of bruised celery seeds in a pint of brandy. Then, two or three times a day, drink 2 tablespoons of water mixed with 1 tablespoon of infused brandy.

Supplements

Vitamin B2

To help growth and repair of the skin, the accepted daily dose range is 1.6 to 50 mg a day.

Vitamin E

An antioxidant that may prevent nerve damage. The accepted daily dose range is 15 to 1,000 mg a day.

Do-It Yourself

- Apply warm compresses steeped in cider vinegar or chamomile tea to the painful area.
- Using organic fruit, cut a lemon in half and rub it on the painful spot.
- Rub peppermint onto the affected area.

Seeking Help from Complementary Practitioners

Acupuncture or deep tissue massage may be helpful.

Red Flags

Call your doctor if you experience:

- Persisting pain
- Fever
- Generalized aches and pain

HERPES ZOSTER (SHINGLES)

Shingles is an infection characterized by intensely painful blisters that follow the path of a nerve. It begins with a feeling of weakness, fever, tingling, or pain on one side of the body. In a few days, along a line that follows the affected nerve, a rash appears. As the rash develops, it turns into small, fluid-filled blisters that are initially highly tender and painful. It may even hurt when your clothing touches the lesions. After a couple of weeks, the blisters begin to heal, becoming itchy scabs. Herpes zoster usually occurs on the chest, abdomen, back, face, or neck.

After the initial infection subsides, some people develop deep pain, known as postherpetic neuralgia.

Causes

Shingles is a reactivation of the herpes zoster virus, which also causes chickenpox. The virus can remain dormant in the body for many years. We don't know what brings about the recurrence of infection; it may be triggered by stress.

Conventional Treatments

In addition to pain relievers (analgesics), your doctor may prescribe antiviral medications, such as valacyclovir (Valtrex) or acyclovir (Zovirax). Check with your doctor before taking these drugs if you may become pregnant. You may also be given corticosteroids. For longer-lasting pain, she may prescribe tricyclic antidepressants. And if any of the blisters become infected, antibiotics may be in order.

Supplements

- Vitamin E prevents damage to tissue. The accepted daily dose range is 15 to 1,000 mg a day.
- Vitamin C speeds healing. The accepted daily dose range is 90 to 2,000 mg a day.

Herbal Creams and Ointments

Capsaicin cream (0.025–0.075 percent) (See page 96)

Do-It-Yourself

Aloe vera
The best way to use aloe is to buy a plant, break off a leaf, and apply directly to the rash the sticky gel that oozes out.

Calamine lotion
It may be an old standby, but it still works.

Cold
Ice relieves pain and reduces inflammation. To protect your skin from direct contact with the ice, I recommend putting it in a plastic sandwich bag, covering it with a cloth, and applying it to the inflamed area.

Aromatherapy
Make a compress using essential oil of lemon balm (*Melissa officinalis*) mixed with water and apply it to the lesions.

Colloidal oatmeal powder (Aveeno)
Add a few drops of water to the powder, make a paste, then apply it to your rash.

Red Flags

Call your doctor if you have:

- Persisting pain
- Fever
- Your lesions appear infected (signs include redness, warmth, swelling, and tenderness)

9

When It Really *Is* All in Your Head

Headache is one of the top ten reasons for visits to the doctor. While there are many types, migraine or tension headaches are the most common. Although the pain they cause can be frighteningly severe, headaches are rarely the sign of a serious disorder. Nonetheless, you should take them seriously.

Depending on the type of headache you have, you may feel the pain all over your head or in only one spot—your forehead or the side or back of your head. Sometimes the pain moves from one place to another during the course of your headache. It may be dull and throbbing, or excruciatingly sharp and piercing.

With the exception of cluster headaches, which occur less frequently than migraines or tension headaches, women are more likely than men to experience most recurrent headache disorders. In surveys of the general population, women also suffer more headache-related emotional distress and disability, such as anxiety and depression.

It's not always possible to identify the culprit causing your headache, but the most common triggers are psychological stress, sleep difficulties, irregular eating habits or responses to specific foods, and hormonal shifts. Working in a noisy or stuffy office, exposure to chemicals, cigarette smoke, or fluorescent lights, and other environmental factors may also play a role.

MIGRAINE HEADACHES

Description

Migraines, from the Greek word *hemikrania*, which means "half the head," affect more than 25 million Americans. Whether it comes on suddenly or with a warning aura, the intense throbbing or pounding of a migraine may last for hours or even days. You may also experience nausea, vomiting, and sensitivity to light and sound. Migraines can be so debilitating that 35 percent of people polled say they have wished they were dead during an attack! In addition, new research has revealed that people with migraines report lower levels of mental, physical, and social well-being than people who do not experience headaches, and they are also more likely to suffer from depression.

Almost one in five women—three times as many as men—suffer from migraine headaches. They are most common between the ages of twenty-five and forty-five. Not only do women experience migraines more frequently, they are also more severely disabled by them. Nearly 52 percent of women, compared to 38 percent of men, miss at least six workdays per year because of this painful disorder. Women also cancel normal activities and report disruptions in their family or social relationships more often.

Because there is no cure for migraines, you'll need to focus on preventing the attacks and treating their symptoms.

Causes

Migraines used to be considered an emotional problem. Thankfully, that idea has now been dismissed. Still, we don't really know what causes them. They do run in families; if both of your parents suffer from migraines, your chance of developing them is a whopping 75 percent. We now believe that some sequence of events causes blood vessels in the brain to tighten and then relax, a process that irritates the nerves surrounding those blood vessels. The nerve endings then transmit sensations of pain, resulting in the throbbing misery of a migraine. This sickening process is caused by certain migraine triggers, which activate parts of the brain and cause the release of neurotransmitters, or brain chemicals, such as serotonin and dopamine, which carry nerve impulses between brain cells. Triggers include:

- Foods and/or alcohol
- Emotional stress
- Environmental factors—perfume or other odors, loud noises, cigarette smoke, household cleaners and chemicals, insufficient ventilation, bright lights or glare, or changes in humidity or temperature
- Lifestyle—sleeping too little or too much, missed meals, lack of exercise or an irregular exercise routine, getting too much sun, or air travel
- Certain types of medications

Hormones, especially estrogen, have a powerful, though as yet unexplained, impact on migraines. The headaches often begin during puberty, when hormone levels are fluctuating. Do your migraines occur just before or during your menstrual period? This may be due to sustained high levels of estrogen, followed by a sudden drop, that comes about during the normal course of your menstrual cycle. Migraines frequently diminish with menopause, although in some cases they worsen. Pregnant women usually report an improvement in migraines, probably because they have consistently high levels of estrogen. But about 4 to 8 percent of women experience worse headaches during pregnancy. And estrogen-containing medications, such as birth control pills and hormone replacement therapy, are also associated with increased headaches.

Signs and Symptoms

Prodrome
You may notice symptoms such as hunger, water retention, mood changes, and irritability many hours before your migraine begins.

Aura
Most migraines occur without any warning. But about 20 percent of women experience an aura, which is a visual, motor, or sensory occurrence that goes on for about ten to thirty minutes before the actual headache starts. This is different from the aura of a seizure, which lasts only a couple of seconds before the seizure. Symptoms of an aura may include flashing lights, dancing spots or blindness, auditory hallucinations, as well as dizziness or numbness.

Pain
You may feel pounding, tapping, or severe throbbing on one or both sides of the head. Noise, light, and movement—especially bending over—intensify the pain.

Nausea and vomiting

Weakness or numbness in parts of your body

Cold, blue feet and hands

Women tend to report more severe, more frequent, and longer-lasting headaches than men. They also suffer more nausea, vomiting, numbness, and tingling. But they experience visual auras far less frequently than men.

Conventional Treatments

Conventional pain relief includes both prescription and over-the-counter medications. Nonprescription analgesics (pain relievers) include Tylenol, aspirin, and nonsteroidal anti-inflammatory drugs (NSAIDS), such as ibuprofen. Your doctor may prescribe a Cox-2 inhibitor, a drug in the new category of NSAIDS. There are also some pain medications available in oral, nasal spray and injection form (Zomig, Maxalt, Imitrex).

Other conventional techniques for pain relief include cold compresses for your forehead and eyes, complete rest, and minimizing light, noise, and smells.

Standard prevention strategies for migraines include avoiding food (see below) and other triggers. Wearing polarized sunglasses whenever you are outside in the sun can help tame a common trigger—bright light or intense glare. If you suffer frequent or particularly severe migraines, or if pain relief medicines don't help, your doctor may prescribe any of a wide range of preventive medications. These include beta-blockers, calcium channel blockers, serotonin antagonists or agonists, tricyclic antidepressants, serotonin reuptake inhibitors, anticonvulsants, or alpha-adrenergic blockers. Like any powerful medications, these all have significant side effects (see Chapter 13 for details).

Keeping a Headache Diary

Do a little detective work to find out what triggers your migraines by keeping the headache diary on page 205. Pay close attention to recurring trends. Do your headaches come at a particular point in your menstrual cycle? Do they occur after eating particular foods or when you haven't had enough sleep? Note when you start nutritional supplements or other treatments, and see if your pattern improves.

Dietary Strategies (See Chapter 14 for food sources of specified nutrients)

Food triggers
One of your most important strategies for managing migraine headaches is avoiding food triggers. Check your headache diary to see if your headaches occur after eating certain foods. If you notice a connection between your headaches and a particular food, try avoiding it for two weeks and then

Sample Migraine Diary

Date	Possible Triggers	Point in Menstrual Cycle	Warning Signs	Time Headache Began and Ended	Other Symptoms	Location and Type of Pain (throbbing, dull; left, right, both sides)	Pain Intensity (mild, moderate, severe)	Treatments Used

reintroduce it, noting your response. This is called an elimination/challenge. If the reintroduced food does trigger a headache, remove it from your diet for at least six months.

Common food triggers and allergens include:

- Frankfurters and other processed meats containing nitrates
- Foods containing MSG, aspartame, preservatives, colorings, and other additives
- Chocolate
- Cheese, especially those that are aged or strongly flavored
- Shellfish
- Alcohol, especially red wine
- Citrus
- Wheat
- Eggs
- Fermented, cured, pickled, or marinated foods
- Cow's milk and milk products
- Caffeine
- Nuts

Riboflavin (vitamin B2), omega-3 oils, and magnesium

These have been shown to decrease the intensity and frequency of migraines. Aim to include more of these nutrients in your diet.

Water

Be sure to drink enough water. Insufficient consumption can lead to dehydration and exacerbate headaches. Aim for at least six 12-ounce glasses a day. Substituting water for soda or coffee is especially effective; not only will you feel refreshed, but you'll eliminate any caffeine-related headaches. I tell my patients to make regular water drinking more pleasurable by using filtered water or bottled water "seasoned" with a few drops of freshly squeezed organic lemon.

Caffeine

If caffeine does not trigger your headaches, you can try it as a treatment— caffeine constricts blood vessels in the head. Drink one or two cups of strong coffee at the start of an attack and lie down in a dark, quiet room.

Salt

Eliminating salt may be helpful.

Protein

You may have success in reducing migraine attacks with a low-protein diet. This is because protein-rich foods are high in tryptophan, an amino acid that the body converts to serotonin, and serotonin may worsen some migraines.

Migraine Meals

These recipes include many of the key nutrients that prevent and treat migraines — omega-3 fatty acids (fish oil), calcium, magnesium, and riboflavin. They are also rich in zinc, folic acid and other B vitamins, and vitamins A and E — nutrients that are essential for a strong immune system, good circulation, proper cellular functioning, and a healthy nervous system. My recipe for treating a migraine is to start with one of these migraine meals, follow it with a therapeutic lavender oil bath and contrast compresses, and finish your day or evening with a soothing herbal tea to help you get to sleep.

R E C I P E

BAKED SALMON WITH CHICKPEA SALAD

SALMON
1 pound of salmon fillet
½ fresh lemon
Dill
Onion powder
Garlic powder

CHICKPEA SALAD
1 can chickpeas, rinsed and drained
1 red onion, chopped
4 Roma tomatoes, chopped
1 red pepper, chopped
1 cucumber, diced
4 ounces green lettuce, leaves separated
1 teaspoon coriander
1 teaspoon garlic powder, or one clove fresh garlic crushed
½ teaspoon black pepper

1. *To prepare fish*: Heat oven to 400 degrees. Place fish in ovenproof baking dish and squeeze lemon over fish. Sprinkle dill, onion powder, and garlic powder over fish and bake in oven for 40 minutes.
2. *While the fish is baking, prepare the chickpea salad*: Place all the ingredients for the chickpea salad into a bowl and toss well.

3. *To serve*: Cut the baked salmon into cubes. Place chickpea salad on individual plates and arrange salmon cubes on top of the salad.

SERVES 2–3

Supplements

Riboflavin (vitamin B2)
In a study published in *Neurology* in February 1998, patients taking riboflavin reported 37 percent fewer migraines than those taking a placebo; their headaches went away faster, too. The dose used in the study was 400 mg, which is more than the RDA. If you want to try this dose, you will need a doctor's prescription. It may take about a month before the vitamin's protective benefits kick in.

Essential fatty acids (EFAs)
Essential fatty acids play a role as precursors to prostaglandins, hormonelike substances that are part of the body's anti-inflammatory responses. They may also affect the widening and narrowing of blood vessels that cause migraines. You can try supplementing with refrigerated flaxseed, 1,500 to 3,000 mg a day.

SAMe (S-adenosyl methionine)
SAMe is an important biological agent that is involved in more than forty different biochemical reactions in the body. It functions as a neurotransmitter and an antioxidant. It's widely used in Europe to treat depression and inflammatory and pain syndromes, such as osteoarthritis. There's preliminary evidence that SAMe also relieves migraines. Recommended daily dosage is 800 mg. Be aware, however, that in large doses it can upset the stomach. Do not take SAMe if you take levodopa for Parkinson's disease. This nutrient may trigger manic episodes in people with bipolar disease.

Magnesium
Magnesium relaxes the muscles and calms excited nerves. Although we don't yet understand the role it plays in migraines, it's clearly important: Decreased blood levels of magnesium have been reported in patients with migraines, and intravenous injection of magnesium can stop a migraine within minutes. More important, though, two double-blind studies suggest that daily supplements of magnesium may reduce the frequency of headaches. The acceptable daily dose range is 320 to 350 mg. Excess magnesium may cause diarrhea; it goes away when you stop taking the supplement.

Calcium and vitamin D

Daily supplements of calcium and vitamin D may reduce the frequency and duration of headaches. The acceptable range for calcium is 1,300 to 2,500 mg a day; for vitamin D, it's 15 to 50 mcg. (You may want to try taking vitamins and minerals in effervescent form, in which you mix the vitamin into water. That way, you're also helping to keep yourself hydrated.)

Herbs

Feverfew (Tanacetum parthenium)

This is the herb of choice for migraines. Its active ingredient is parthenolide, a spasm-reducing chemical that relaxes blood vessels in the head by making the smooth muscle inside them less reactive to possible constrictors. It also helps prevent migraines or makes them less severe by neutralizing vasoconstrictors such as serotonin, prostaglandins, and norepinephrine.

Feverfew has been used for centuries in European folk medicine for the treatment and prevention of migraines. But its worth has also been substantiated by a wealth of scientific studies. In one, patients using feverfew had fewer migraines as well as a significant reduction in nausea and vomiting. In an article published in 1998 in *Cephalgia*, a prestigious headache journal, the authors systematically examined the evidence for and against feverfew. Their conclusion? The majority of studies examined favored feverfew use over placebo.

Feverfew is best used preventively, so you need to take it every day. It may take a month or two to take effect. This herb comes in many formulations, so you can harness its potent ability to reduce inflammation and relieve pain by using it as a tea, a decoction, or in tablet form. Simply follow directions on the package. Be sure that any feverfew product you buy is standardized to contain at least 0.4 percent parthenolide.

Do not take feverfew if you are pregnant or breast-feeding. If you take blood-thinning drugs such as aspirin or warfarin, use feverfew with the supervision of your physician.

Ginger (Zingiber officinale)

Ginger is particularly useful in treating nausea. The usual dose is 250 mg to 1 gram several times a day. My preference is that you get as much as you can from your diet.

Teas

Both chamomile (*Chamaemelum nobile* or *Matricaria recutita*) and elderberry (*Sambucus nigra*) teas have a calming, sedating effect. If your headaches are related to stress, these infusions may help relieve anxiety. You may use commercially available tea bags or, if you prefer, steep 1 teaspoon of dried herb in a cup of hot water.

Herbal Creams and Ointments

Nature's Chemist

This product contains menthol and a copaiba extract, harvested from the Amazon. It's a counterirritant—that is, a chemical that promotes the release of the body's natural pain relievers. Use it during your headache by rubbing small amounts onto your neck muscles and forehead.

Do-It-Yourself

Acupressure massage (See page 353 for technique)

Because it is unobtrusive, you can use acupressure on the subway, during a meeting, or whenever you feel a headache coming on. It is also an effective technique to use while in the throes of a migraine. Press one or more of the points listed here, depending on where your headache is, for two to five minutes each. Repeat the process for at least twenty to forty minutes.

- LI4 (Large Intestine-4) is the point on the back of the hand in the web between the thumb and index finger. Press here for general pain in the front of the head.
- GB20 (Gallbladder-20) is found in the hollow between the front and back neck muscles, behind the bony prominence behind the ears (there are two GB-20 points). Use this spot if you have general pain at the side and back of your head.
- For headache, toothache, and earache, try TH23 (Triple Heater-23), the "Silk Bamboo Hole," located at the outer edge of the eyebrow where the brow departs from the bone.

Scented bath

Lavender oil is traditionally used to relieve anxiety and nervousness. Since migraines may be associated with stress, soaking in a bath to which you've added several drops of lavender oil is a good strategy when you feel a headache coming on.

Contrast compresses
Alternate cool and warm compresses for five minutes each, with a two-minute break in between. Apply the compresses to your forehead or, if the back of your head aches, to your neck.

Peppermint oil (Mentha piperita) *compress*
Peppermint is an effective tension-reliever. Soothe your headache by applying to your forehead a washcloth saturated with cool water to which you've added two drops of peppermint oil.

Try a commercial compress, like the ones sold by Johnson and Johnson. The effectiveness of these convenient heated compresses is supported by clinical studies.

Mind/Body

Biofeedback (See page 341 for technique)

Relaxation and imagery (See pages 340–341)

Exercise

Aerobic exercise promotes the release of the body's natural painkillers or endorphins (sometimes called a "runner's high"). But this fact is often neglected when it comes to migraines. Still, exercise can help prevent *and* treat headache-related pain.

Regular aerobic exercise at least three times a week can reduce both the frequency and intensity of your migraines. And if you can bear it, try exercising when you feel a headache coming on. Avoid isometric or other exercises that produce abrupt variations in blood pressure. Instead, aim for activity that uses the large muscle groups, such as bike riding or swimming.

Seeking Help from Complementary Practitioners

Acupuncture
In a 1997 report, the National Institutes of Health approved acupuncture as an effective treatment for headaches. It reduces headache frequency and severity with no side effects. In some cases, patients receiving acupuncture can reduce their medications by as much as 50 percent.

Massage

Classical Swedish massage affects the interaction between the muscles and the nervous system. The muscles are stimulated by nerve cells to contract and relax. The stroking and deep kneading of a Swedish massage softens "knots" in the muscles and relieves migraines by releasing chronic neck and shoulder tension, and maintaining an even blood flow to the head. In addition, as the muscles relax, the body releases endorphins, which relieve pain and enhance feelings of well-being.

Red Flags: When to Call Your Doctor

Call your doctor if:

· Your migraine persists longer than usual, or after several days.
· You experience prolonged visual changes or neurological symptoms, such as motor loss, numbness, weakness, or tingling; slurred speech, a change in balance; or memory loss.
· The headache started after you injured your head or were knocked out.
· Along with the headache, you have fever, vomiting, and a stiff neck.

TENSION (MUSCLE CONTRACTION) HEADACHE

SARAH'S SAGA

Sarah's woes began shortly after she and her boyfriend of seven years decided to split up because she was moving to another city. Young, enthusiastic, and eager to make it professionally after graduating college with a degree in education, Sarah had decided to take a job as a "big city" schoolteacher. She soon learned that the pressure of her job was intense. Each day she faced twenty screaming, unruly children. For hours, she sat scrunched at a small desk. At lunchtime, she often grabbed a candy bar and a cup of coffee rather than a square meal; she preferred to use her time to prepare her afternoon lessons. Unfortunately, her stressed-out colleagues and supervisors offered little support or camaraderie.

Sarah came to me for help while she was in Baltimore during her holiday break. She was hurting, and extremely anxious about it. Although she had always experienced headaches, her pain had been getting progressively more ferocious since she started the new job. "It begins every morning and worsens as the day goes on. By late afternoon, I feel like I've been hit by a Mack Truck," she sighed. After a comprehensive examination and workup, I concluded that she was suffering from tension headaches.

Recognizing the value of a multipronged approach toward this problem, I sat down with Sarah and reviewed her lifestyle, especially diet and exercise. Then we talked about medications, relaxation, and other treatments.

That day I started Sarah on an acupuncture regimen. Since she was going back home after her break, I taught her some simple reflexology and acupressure techniques she could do on her own. She could even do some of them while in class, without attracting the attention of her students. Because I could sense her anxiety and tension, I provided her with several self-hypnosis tapes and strategies for meditating.

I suggested that she exercise before work and make some changes in her diet. Especially important were cutting back caffeine and drinking more water. I recommended that she continue to use Tylenol or other nonprescription pain relievers, but also told her that once her lifestyle changes and self-help "tools" kicked in, she might no longer need medication.

A couple of weeks later, Sarah called with the kind of news I love to get from patients—she was feeling better.

Description

Nearly 90 percent of headaches are tension headaches, which occur when muscle spasms irritate the nerves and cause tension or tightness in the head, face, and neck. When tension headaches occur more than fifteen times a month, they are considered chronic. Episodic tension headaches happen less than once or twice a week, but still often enough to make you miserable.

Although no one has yet figured out why, disabling chronic tension headaches occur in 5 percent of women compared to only 2 percent of men. And when women get tension headaches, they report higher levels of tenderness in all the muscles surrounding the skull. Among women, the frequency of this debilitating disorder rises at around age forty-five and peaks between the ages of fifty and fifty-nine. Although the gender disparity isn't as large, women also have more episodic tension headaches.

Causes

The most common triggers of tension headaches are:

- Stress
- Unbalanced diet
- Inadequate sleep
- Hormone changes
- Depression
- Poor posture that causes tension in neck, scalp, or facial muscles

Signs and Symptoms

Tension headaches may last for as little as thirty minutes or for as long as several days. They may occur once or twice a month or nearly daily, and they may be mild or severe. With a tension headache, you're likely to experience:

- A gradual onset of steady, dull aching
- Pressure on your head (sometimes described as feeling as if your head is in a vise)
- Tightness and discomfort in your back, shoulders, face, or neck
- Tenderness in the muscles surrounding your skull

Conventional Treatments

If you avoid your known triggers, such as staying up too late or skipping meals, you may be able to prevent tension headaches. If stress is the trigger, try to figure out what is causing it and either remove the problem or deal with it more effectively by learning relaxation or other stress management techniques.

Once your headache begins, the usual treatment includes painkillers, such as aspirin, ibuprofen, or acetaminophen. For severe cases, muscle relaxants or prescription pain relievers may be necessary.

Dietary Strategies

- Aim for at least six 12-ounce glasses of water a day. Not drinking enough fluids can leave you dehydrated and will worsen your headaches. I tell my patients to make regular water drinking more pleasurable by using filtered water or bottled water "seasoned" with a few drops of freshly squeezed organic lemon.
- Curb your caffeine consumption.
- Don't skip meals; eat regularly.

- Cut down on sugary, sweet foods; these cause a sudden surge and then a dip in blood glucose levels, which can lead to a headache.
- Drink invigorating carrot juice.

Supplements

Melatonin

Melatonin is a hormone manufactured by the pineal gland, an organ that controls your wake/sleep cycle. Taken as a supplement, it can help improve your sleep patterns. Follow dosing on the bottle.

Herbs

Valerian root (Valeriana officinalis)

Herbalists suggest this herb to relieve anxiety and stress. Follow package instructions for dosing.

Chamomile (Chamaemelum nobile or Matricaria recutita)

This sweet-smelling herb fights anxiety and helps you relax. To help you sleep, make a double-strength tea before bedtime by steeping two tea bags or 2 teaspoons of dried flowers in one cup of boiling water. Avoid contact with your eyes; it may cause irritation. Chamomile may cause an allergic reaction.

Stress reducer tea

Mix three parts chamomile, two parts sage, and one part basil with one cup of boiling water. Drink it twice a day. Or look for Tension Tamer, a commercially available herbal tea.

Do-It-Yourself

Every day

- Keep your neck muscles relaxed when working or exercising and try to maintain good posture, paying special attention to slumping shoulders.
- Try to identify and avoid situations that cause tension or stress.
- When you feel a headache coming on, rest in a quiet, dark room.
- For simple but effective pain relief, apply a cold pack to your forehead, eyes, and neck or take a hot shower.
- To relax your muscles and relieve dull, steady pain, make a ginger compress. Cut and peel one fresh gingerroot; boil it in three cups of

water until the water turns cloudy. Soak a washcloth in the mixture and apply it to the back of your neck.

Aromatherapy

Try aromatherapy for pain relief. Soak for twenty to thirty minutes in a bath to which has been added two or three drops of lavender (reduces nervousness; useful for all types of headaches) or peppermint (its calming, cooling scent relieves headache pain). Do not use these oils for long periods of time or during pregnancy.

Massage

Give yourself a massage in one of these tension-laden areas:

For the neck: Sit in a chair and tip your head back slightly to relax your muscles. Grab the back of your neck lightly and squeeze. Start at the bottom of your skull and work down. After five squeezes, increase the pressure and repeat.

For the shoulder: Use your right hand to grasp your left shoulder. Knead toward your neck, using increasing pressure. Repeat on the other side using your left hand to grasp your right shoulder. Find the most sensitive places and press up to one minute or until the pain eases.

Acupressure

Try these acupressure points (see page 353 for technique).

- GV-16 (Governing Vessel 16), on the back of the head at the base of the skull. This relieves a stiff neck and pain in the eyes, ears, and nose.
- GB-20 (Gallbladder 20), on the back of the head at the base of the skull, on either side of the large vertical muscle that helps control movement of the head. Use this if you have a stiff neck.
- Bl-2 (Bladder 2), in the upper hollows of the eye sockets, where the eyebrow meets the bridge of the nose. Try this for frontal headaches, eyestrain, and tension.
- GB-41 (Gallbladder 41), on the top of the foot, one inch up from the web connection between the fourth and fifth toes. Use this point for tension and muscle pain.
- To improve blood circulation in the head, brush your hair and scalp using firm, downward strokes. Then, starting at your left temple, make tiny circles over your ear and down the back of your head to your neck; repeat on the right side.

Mind/Body

If you suffer from frequent tension headaches, one of the best things you can do is learn how to manage stress. Try the relaxation and meditation techniques described in Chapter 18.

Yoga
Try Siddhasan (Perfect Posture), on page 349.

Exercise

Regular exercise helps to relieve tension. Particularly useful in this regard is aerobic exercise. I recommend twenty to thirty minutes of biking, swimming, walking, dancing, tennis, or aerobics at least three times a week.

Seeking Help from Complementary Practitioners

Hypnotherapy
If you can discover what they are, hypnotic suggestion may help to eliminate your headache triggers.

Chiropractic treatments
These may help tension headaches.

Red Flags

Call your doctor if:

- Self-help strategies don't work after three days.
- You experience prolonged visual changes or neurological symptoms, such as motor loss, numbness, weakness, or tingling; slurred speech; a change in balance; or memory loss.
- The headache started after you injured your head or were knocked out.
- Along with the headache, you have fever, vomiting, and a stiff neck.
- Your headaches are unusually severe or recur frequently.

TEMPOROMANDIBULAR DISORDERS

Description

Temporomandibular disorder (TMD) is the name for a collection of medical and dental conditions that affect the hingelike joint that attaches the lower jaw to the skull, as well as its surrounding muscles and tissues. Pain and dysfunction in this joint can be frightening, since you use it for speaking, chewing, and swallowing.

For a long time, many authorities doubted the existence of TMD because it involved such a broad array of symptoms, ranging from mild to very severe. Perhaps the fact that it predominantly affects women—as many as seven times more women than men—also had something to do with their dismissive attitude. Today, however, TMD is recognized as a legitimate ailment, although there is still controversy over its causes and proper treatment. This is unfortunate because TMD is very common; about one in four young women suffer from this painful problem.

If you have TMD, you may get frequent headaches. They occur when muscles around the joint go into spasm, causing facial pain, primarily in the jaw, mouth, and around the ear. As pressure builds on other parts of the skull, you may also get pain that is similar to a tension headache.

Causes

There is no one clearly identifiable cause for TMD. But we do know that these factors can lead to problems:

- Jaw misalignment
- Clenching or grinding your teeth
- Dental problems (tooth decay, impacted wisdom teeth, gum disease, infection, crooked teeth)
- Degenerative arthritis or trauma to the jaw
- Poor posture
- There is some evidence that TMD is linked to fibromyalgia, another predominantly female ailment (see Chapter 12)

I'm intrigued by evidence that reproductive hormones play a role in this ailment. I've already mentioned how much more common TMD is in women. In addition, using oral contraceptives or estrogen replacement therapy raises your risk for TMD. And pain from TMD ebbs and flows across the menstrual cycle. You may notice that your pain is worse just before or during your period. Finally, there seems to be a link between premenstrual syndrome (PMS) and TMD. Women with PMS are more likely to report TMD; likewise, a recent study suggests that women with TMD have more PMS symptoms.

Signs and Symptoms

The range of aches and pains associated with TMD can be bewildering. Your symptoms may be so mild that they have little impact on your daily life. Or they may be persistent and seriously debilitating. You may experience:

- Headaches, similar to tension headaches (see page 212)
- Pressure on top of your head
- A clicking or popping sound from your jaw
- A tendency to chew on one side
- Earache
- Neck, head, face, and shoulder pain
- Tenderness around your jaw
- Dizziness
- Difficulty opening or closing your mouth
- Pain when you chew, yawn, or open your mouth wide
- Disturbances in sleep or mood

Conventional Treatments

Conventional treatments for TMD range from simple stretching exercises to surgery, depending on the severity of the problem. Nonsteroidal anti-inflammatory drugs are used for pain; if muscle spasms are involved, your doctor may prescribe muscle relaxants. Physical therapy, electrical stimulation, moist heat, and ultrasound are all possible therapies. Spray and stretch, a technique where the muscles around the jaw are sprayed with a coolant spray and then stretched, may be recommended. You may also be referred for laser treatments, which can increase blood flow to the affected area, or for a mouth guard, a device that keeps your upper and lower teeth apart and helps your jaw muscles relax. If your joint is seriously deteriorated, your doctor may suggest arthroscopic surgery or joint replacement.

Supplements

Melatonin
Melatonin is a hormone manufactured by the pineal gland, an organ that controls your wake/sleep/wake cycle. Taken as a supplement, it can help improve your sleep patterns. Follow dosing on the bottle.

Herbs

Valerian root (Valeriana officinalis)
This herb may relieve anxiety and stress. Follow package instructions for dosing.

Do-It-Yourself

Visit your dentist
Correcting crooked or misaligned teeth and fixing any damaged fillings or crowns may alleviate your headaches.

Stress
Avoid activities that put stress on your teeth and jaw:

- Excessive yawning
- Chewing gum, candy, ice, and hard candies
- Resting your chin on your hand
- Cradling the telephone between your jaw and shoulder
- Clenching your teeth
- Nail biting
- Eating hard foods

Massage
Try some of these:

- Use your fingers to locate sore spots around your eyes. Press these spots with your finger and hold for ten seconds.
- Grab your ears and gently pull them down and away from your head.
- Rub your ears between your forefinger and thumb.
- Press the areas where your neck and skull meet and hold 10 seconds.
- Finally, using your thumb, find tender points along your jaw and apply pressure for 10 seconds.

Acupressure (see page 353 for technique)
- GB-14 (Gallbladder 14), one finger width above each eyebrow, for jaw pain.
- LI-4 (Large Intestine-4) is the point on the back of the hand in the web between the thumb and index finger. Press here for general pain in the front of the head.

- ST-7 (Stomach 7), place your middle finger one thumb width in front of your ear. Find the indentation on your upper jaw and press for one minute.

Ice

If your jaw is swollen, apply ice for twenty to thirty minutes. You can do this frequently, but take one-half hour breaks in between treatments.

Warmth

To reduce pain, apply a warm compress or a hot-water bottle to your jaw for twenty minutes.

Exercise

Here's a simple jaw exercise:
1. Open your mouth 1 inch wide.
2. Make a fist and put it in front of your chin.
3. Using your lower jaw, push your chin into your fist.
4. Then, put your fist on one side of your jaw and push your jaw toward it.
5. Repeat on the other side
6. Repeat 6 times. Do this exercise twice a day.

Seeking Help from Complementary Practitioners

Hypnotherapy and biofeedback may give some symptomatic relief.

Red Flags

Call your doctor if you have persistent pain or swelling, or if your jaw is misaligned.

SINUS HEADACHE

Description

The sinuses are hollow areas under the bones of the face that connect the nose and throat. When they get irritated or inflamed, they cause a throbbing headache that is centered in the face. True sinus headaches are rare; they account for only 2 percent of all headaches. Instead, most "sinus headaches" are actually tension or cluster headaches, mild migraines, or headaches due to allergies.

Causes

Most sinus headaches are caused by an inflammation or infection of the sinuses. They may be aggravated if you have noncancerous growths, called nasal polyps, or anatomic abnormalities, such as a deviated septum or deformities in the sinus ducts that inhibit normal drainage.

Signs and Symptoms

- Dull, aching pain in your face, especially your forehead, cheeks, across your nose and behind your eyes
- Pressure between your eyebrows and above or below your eyes
- A runny or stuffed nose
- Postnasal drip
- Watery eyes
- Feeling worse as the day progresses
- More pain when you bend your head forward

Conventional Treatments

Treatment depends on the cause. If you have a sinus infection, your doctor may prescribe antibiotics to clear it up. (Because antibiotics may cause yeast infection, be sure to take an acidophilus supplement or eat yogurt that contains live cultures every day.)

Likewise, if allergies are the culprit, antihistamines may provide some relief. You may also use nasal sprays or decongestants to unclog your sinuses; I find that sprays usually work better than pills. Carefully follow the directions and warnings on the labels of over-the-counter products.

The usual treatments for temporary pain relief include aspirin, ibuprofen, or acetaminophen.

Herbs

Echinacea (Echinacea angustifolia, Echinacea purpurea)
This popular remedy, made from purple coneflowers, has been proven in well-constructed, double-blind, placebo-controlled research to reduce the symptoms, frequency, and duration of colds. Laboratory studies have proven

that it can increase antibody production and bolster cellular immune function. The recommended dose is 1 cup of tea or 1 teaspoon of tincture three times a day.

Do-It-Yourself

Every day
- Stop smoking and avoid other people's smoke, as well as other airborne irritants.
- Use oral or nasal decongestants before flying, travel to high altitudes, or swimming in deep water, especially if you have a cold.
- Use a humidifier if the air in your home is dry.
- When you have a sinus headache, avoid leaning over. In bed, keep your head elevated to relieve pressure.
- Try these treatments to relieve congestion and pain:

Salt water nasal douche: Salt water shrinks swollen tissues and blood vessels. Add 1 tablespoon of sea salt to 1 cup of warm water; lean your head back and apply one eyedropper-full into each nostril. Repeat two to three times a day until the swelling is gone.

Warm herbal compress: Boil 3 cups of water and pour it over 1 tablespoon of dried lavender and 1 tablespoon of dried chamomile. Steep for twenty minutes. Soak a cloth in this mixture, wring it out and apply it to the back of your neck or your forehead.

Acupressure
Try these acupressure points (see page 353 for technique).

- GV-26 (Governing Vessel 26), located directly under the middle of the nose, is a useful point for anything to do with the head or sinuses.
- LI-20 (Large Intestine 20) helps many nasal problems, including sinusitis and allergic rhinitis. To find these points, smile. They are in the creases in the face, near the nose.

Aromatherapy
Lavender reduces pain and is an anti-inflammatory. Add two to three drops to a hot bath and soak for twenty to thirty minutes.

Sinus massage
Using a circular motion, massage the bridge of your nose with your index finger and thumb for thirty seconds. Then press your thumb into your brow-

line—the spot where your nose meets your forehead, between your eyebrows. Apply pressure there for thirty seconds. Move up your forehead, halfway between your browline and the middle of your forehead and massage in a circular motion for thirty seconds.

Exercise

Perform these cranial stretch exercises at least twice a week.

FRONTAL SINUS RELEASE
1. Hold your nose with one hand and your hair above your forehead with the other.
2. Pull your nose down and your hair up.
3. Hold 15 to 60 seconds.

MAXILLA SINUS RELEASE
1. Place your right thumb on the roof of your mouth on the left side and your left thumb on the roof of your mouth on the right side.
2. At the same time, hold your hands out in front of your face in a prayer position.
3. Press your thumbs into the roof of your mouth.
4. Hold 15 to 60 seconds.

Red Flags

Call your doctor if:

- Your symptoms don't go away in three to five days.
- Your temperature is higher than 102 degrees.
- You experience nosebleeds, blurred or double vision, or balance problems.

EYESTRAIN HEADACHE

Description

Steady pain and pressure behind the eyes and on the forehead and face is often a sign of eyestrain. When you overwork your eye muscles by squinting, straining, prolonged close work, or blinking this type of headache may be the result.

Causes

- Reading or staring at a computer monitor for long periods of time
- Reading or working with insufficient lighting
- Incorrect eyeglass or contact lens prescription
- Wearing contact lenses for too long, or wearing ill-fitting contact lenses
- Trouble seeing things close-up (presbyopia)
- Blurred vision or an inability to see objects clearly (refractive disorders)
- Irregular curvature of the eye, resulting in blurred vision (astigmatism)

Signs and Symptoms

If your headaches are caused by eyestrain, you're likely to experience:

- Steady frontal pain, often behind your eyes
- Pain in your forehead and face, and sometimes in the back of your head and neck
- Pressure around or on top of your head
- Symptoms that often occur when your read or focus on objects that are close to you

Conventional Treatments

In addition to pain relievers, the usual treatments for headaches caused by eyestrain include getting glasses (or new glasses) and eye exercises. Your doctor will also remind you to rest your eyes and avoid excessive computer use.

Dietary Strategies (See Chapter 14 for food source of specified nutrients)

Vitamin A
Improves vision and helps relieve chronic eyestrain.

Vitamin B12
This, too, helps relieve eyestrain.

Supplements

Vitamin A
To improve vision and relieve eyestrain, take between 900 and 3,000 mcg a day. Do not take vitamin A supplements if you are pregnant; they may cause birth defects.

Do-It-Yourself

Every day
- Get regular eye exams with an optometrist or ophthalmologist.
- Clean your contact lenses daily. Use an enzymatic or heat cleaner once a week to remove protein buildup.
- Look up from close work and change your focus every fifteen minutes.
- Make sure your work and reading areas are well-lit.
- Wear sunglasses and a hat when you're out in bright sunlight.
- To reduce inflammation, roast an apple. Lie down for half an hour and put slices of the pulp on your eyes. You can do the same with slices of cucumber.

Acupressure
Use this acupressure point for eyestrain headaches:

- Bl-2 (Bladder 2), in the upper hollows of the eye sockets, where the eyebrows meet the bridge of the nose, relieves frontal headache, eyestrain, and tension.

Aromatherapy
- Add a few drops of fennel, chamomile, rosemary, or parsley oil to cool water. Soak a cloth in the mixture and wring it out. Lie in a dark room and apply the compress to puffy, swollen eyes.
- Mix 1 drop of lemon or rose oil and 2 tablespoons of a neutral carrier oil, such as wheat germ, almond oil, or sunflower oil, and massage it into your temples and the bony areas around the eyes.

Palming
This will relax your eyes. Try it!
1. If you wear contact lenses, take them out.
2. Turn down the lights and sit or lie down.
3. Place your hands over your eyes, palms down to block out light.
4. Keep your eyes open and stare into the darkness for 30 to 60 seconds.
5. Close your eyes and remove your hands.
6. Slowly open your eyes.

Exercise

To relieve eyestrain, relax your mind, strengthen your eyes, and prevent future vision problems, do this eyeball stretch:

EYEBALL STRETCH
1. Sit comfortably in a chair.
2. Without moving your head, move your eyes up toward the ceiling and down toward the floor.
3. Move your eyes from left to right.
4. Move your eyes diagonally from the upper left to the lower right, and then from the lower left to the upper right.
5. Rotate your eyes clockwise, then counterclockwise.
6. Repeat these steps 10 times.
7. Rub your hands together until they feel warm. Cup them over your eyes; do not press. Allow the warmth to relax your eyes.

Mind/Body

To relax and relieve your eyes, try relaxation, imagery, or meditation (see Chapter 18).

Red Flags

Call your doctor if:

- Self-help strategies don't work.
- You experience prolonged visual changes or neurological symptoms, such as motor loss, numbness, weakness, or tingling; slurred speech; a change in balance; or memory loss.
- The headache started after you injured your head or were knocked out.
- Along with the headache, you have fever, vomiting, and a stiff neck.
- Your headaches are unusually severe or recur frequently.

CLUSTER HEADACHES

Description

With pain so intense they are sometimes described as "suicide" headaches, cluster headaches are a daunting ailment. Cluster headaches rarely affect women; 90 percent of them occur in men.

The excruciating pain is caused by abnormal contraction and expansion of blood vessels. Why are they called "cluster" headaches? Unfortunately it's because they occur in a series that can last for weeks or even months, followed by a remission for some period of time. Episodic cluster headaches strike from one to six times a day for several weeks; the chronic form brings almost daily headaches with no relief for six months or more. Thankfully, they usually last only about an hour.

Causes

We don't yet know why cluster headaches occur. Some of the likely causes are:

- Problems with the hypothalamus gland, which controls normal body cycles such as sleep, appetite, and hormone secretion.
- Hormones or hormone imbalance are always a possible suspect whenever an ailment strikes one sex more than the other. One study found that men's testosterone levels were lower during an active cluster cycle than during a remission.
- Digestive disorders, such as peptic ulcers, constipation, hypoglycemia (low blood sugar), and food allergies increase your risk for cluster headaches. It may be that your body is thrown off balance if you don't absorb nutrients normally.
- Swelling and inflammation of the nerves behind your eye may play a role.
- Alcohol consumption can trigger a cluster headache; it also increases your risk of developing this disorder to begin with.
- Smoking tends to increase your chances of having cluster headaches; it also worsens attacks.
- Bright or glaring lights.
- Lack of sleep.

Signs and Symptoms

Cluster headaches often occur early in the morning and may wake you from sleep. Symptoms include:

- Localized, intense pain, usually on one side of your head or around or behind one eye. The throbbing, knifelike pain comes in frequent, stabbing bursts.
- Pain may also occur in your forehead, cheek, nose, ear, or chin and jaw area
- Sweating on your forehead and abdomen
- Watery eyes
- Flushed face

Conventional Treatments

The best treatment for cluster headaches is prevention; in other words, avoid any triggers you're aware of.

Aspirin, ibuprofen, and acetaminophen don't usually work because the headache disappears before they take effect. Prescription medications, such as quick-acting inhalants or sprays, are a better choice for pain relief.

Dietary Strategies

Raw honey may help prevent a cluster headache. Take 1 tablespoon at the first sign of a headache, followed by another tablespoon in half an hour if symptoms develop.

Do-It-Yourself

Breathing exercises
These techniques bring more oxygen into your blood and may help prevent cluster headaches.

DEEP INHALATION
1. Lie flat on the floor, a couch, or your bed. Inhale deeply, dividing your breath into three parts: First raise your stomach, then fill your lungs, and finally fill your chest.
2. Hold your breath for 3 seconds.
3. Slowly exhale.
4. Repeat 5 times.

WU BREATHING
This is a Chinese breathing technique for headache relief.
1. Lie down with your arms by your sides, and your feet hip width apart.
2. Put the tip of your tongue on the roof of your mouth, behind your teeth.
3. Breathe in through your nose.
4. Imagine your breath coming through the nose, to the top of the head, and down to your belly.
5. Continue breathing in this way for 20 to 30 minutes.
6. Do every day, in the morning and at night.

Seeking Help from Complementary Practitioners

Acupuncture is sometimes effective for cluster headaches.

Red Flags

See your doctor if you have pain around your eyes. This may be an indication of glaucoma.

TREATMENTS USEFUL FOR
ALL TYPES OF HEADACHES

Dietary Strategies

Coriander (*Coriandrum sativum*), an herb known as cilantro in its fresh form, provides pain relief for headaches. Try sprinkling it on your food or using it in salsa.

Do-It-Yourself

Acupressure (See page 353 for technique)
For headache pain, in general:

- SI-1 (Small Intestine 1), on the outside of the pinky finger, next to the nail.
- LI-4 (Large Intestine 4), in the web between the thumb and forefinger.

For face and head pain:

- BL-1 (Bladder 1), in the inner corners of the eyes.

For eye pain:

- ST-1 (Stomach 1), on the cheekbones, directly below the pupils.
- BL-1 (Bladder 1), in the depression above the inner corner of the eye.
- GB-1 (Gallbladder 1), at the outer corner of the eye.

For toothache:

- SI-19 (Small Intestine 19), in the depression next to the ears when your mouth is open.

Aromatherapy

A combination of eucalyptus (*Eucalyptus globulus*) and peppermint (*Mentha piperita*) relieves headache pain. Use it in a diffuser or sprinkle a few drops into your bath.

Seeking Help from Complementary Practitioners

Acupuncture

A recent review of the use of acupuncture for headaches asked this question: Does acupuncture have any value in the management of patients with headaches? After reviewing twenty-seven studies over the last twenty years, the authors answered yes: Acupuncture has clear potential, and should be one of the first approaches to consider when dealing with headaches.

10

—

Are You a Good Sport?

It's enormously gratifying when my women patients tell me how good they feel after they exercise or participate in sports or fitness programs. There is no doubt in my mind that physical activity helps you stay trim and fit and keeps your pain in check. It boosts your spirits and can leave you downright exhilarated. My patients' anecdotes are bolstered by the scientific literature, which again and again substantiates the many benefits of regular exercise. Unfortunately, exercise also has a down side—the risk of musculoskeletal injury—and that's the subject of this chapter.

One question I frequently hear is: Are women more prone to sports injury and pain? Although this issue is still debated in scientific journals, we do know that women are at greater risk for getting hurt from certain activities and sports. Women playing sports that involve pivoting, such as soccer, volleyball, and basketball, have the highest injury rates—higher than men who play these sports and higher than women in other sports. Women are especially prone to certain types of problems, particularly knee injuries, which they suffer between two and eight times as frequently as men, and stress fractures.

You may be more susceptible to pain and injury in certain parts of your body because of innate sex-linked differences in anatomy, hormonal makeup, and the elasticity of your ligaments. During pregnancy, as well as other times during your menstrual cycle when your hormones are fluctuating, joint dislocations are more common, and they may be exacerbated by sporting activity.

Some of the anatomical factors that predispose you to suffer more sports injuries than your male partner or friends include:

- Leg alignment, or how the femur (the thigh bone) and the tibia and fibula (lower leg bones) are connected to one another.

- Increased knee valgus — the knees point out to a greater degree. Combined with the wider pelvis, this means that the stresses and strains placed on certain structures, especially the knee, are different. Women's knees are more unstable, and because they bear such high forces, they are particularly susceptible to injury.
- More joint laxity, leading to a greater risk of sprain, strain, and dislocation.
- The hormonal cycle may also cause greater laxity of the ligaments, soft tissue, and support structures.

Fitness level also influences whether you are likely to be injured. Are women less fit than men? A recent study of 861 army recruits enrolled in an eight-week basic training course found that woman were *twice* as likely as men to experience exercise-related injury because they had a general lower level of fitness. This distressing finding is consistent with the U.S. Surgeon General's recent report that 60 percent of adult women in our country don't get enough physical activity. In fact, according to both the Centers for Disease Control and the Surgeon General, women are consistently less physically active than men.

These appalling statistics persist, despite landmark legislation that encourages female participation in sports. For example, as a result of Title IX, which prohibits sex discrimination in schools, women's involvement in high school athletics jumped from 300,000 when the law was passed in 1972, to 2.7 million in 1999. And today, women are actively involved in the U.S. Olympic Team; 37 percent of American Olympians are women.

But we can't all be Olympians. Whatever you do, I can't emphasize too strongly how important it is to get out there and move.

In this chapter, I'll start by providing general how-to advice for all types of sports injuries. Many of the dietary strategies and home remedies listed here will enhance your sports performance and fitness, as well as minimize pain should you suffer an injury. In later sections, you'll find more particulars about specific problems.

Prevention

- Get a medical check-up before you start any exercise program.
- Choose an activity that is appropriate for you. For example, if you have bad knees, swimming or cycling is more appropriate than running.
- Start slowly, especially if you are not used to strenuous exercise. Injuries frequently occur when you push your body too fast or too hard. You

can add more activities, or increase the intensity or duration of your workout, as your body becomes accustomed to more activity.

· Use proper form. Any exercise can be unsafe if you don't do it correctly. Get advice from a certified exercise leader or personal trainer.

· Warm up for five to ten minutes before exercising. For instance, if you are a jogger, walk for the first five minutes of your run.

· Cool down for five to ten minutes after your activity and then stretch. This will help loosen muscles that have become tight and contracted while you exercised.

· The key to staying injury-free is daily activity. An estimated 20 million "weekend warriors" suffer sports-related injuries leading to permanent or temporary disabilities. I recommend that you do *at least* thirty minutes of moderate exercise *at least* three times a week. You don't have to join a gym. Moderate exercise includes vacuuming and cleaning your house, washing your car by hand, going for a 2-mile walk, gardening, or taking a couple of brisk laps around the mall. I also suggest doing strength training (with weights) once or twice a week.

· "No pain, no gain" is a damaging myth. Exercise may be tiring, but it should not be painful. If it hurts, stop! Remember, pain is a warning; along with swelling, tenderness, or redness of your skin it is often the first sign of injury.

· Old, worn-out shoes can lead to hip, knee, ankle, and foot injuries. These areas of the lower body account for 90 percent of all sports injuries. Wear supportive, cushioned footwear appropriate for your activity. There are shoes designed for aerobics, running, and tennis, as well as cross trainers if you do several different sports.

· Wear appropriate clothing. Lightweight, breathable clothes are important in hot weather; when it's cold, wear warm, protective clothing. Clothes that are too tight restrict movement and circulation.

· Use safety equipment designed for the type of exercise you do—a bicycle helmet if you bike, a safety helmet and guards for wrists, elbows, and knees if you Rollerblade.

· In one study, 71 percent of women complained of breast discomfort after exercise. This led to the development of ergonomically designed sports bras that provide comfortable support and limit movement of the breasts during exercise. The American Council on Exercise (ACE) suggests that you consider these pointers when you buy a sports bra:

    · Sports bras work in one of two ways, through compression or encapsulation. Compression bras, which are better if you are small-breasted, push your breasts against your chest. Harness-type sports bras, appropriate if you have larger breasts, encapsulate and provide support for each breast.

- Select a bra based on comfort, not on size.
- Bras that provide adequate ventilation prevent chaffing and minimize friction caused by sweating.
- Pay attention to the clasps or straps on the bra and make sure they don't dig into your skin.
- Before making the purchase, try the bra on and mimic the movements of your activities to ensure that it fits comfortably.

Conventional Treatments

Sports injuries happen, even if you are super careful. Don't ignore them. Some injuries can take a long time to heal.

The standard treatment for sports injuries is known by the acronym R.I.C.E, which stands for:

Rest
Avoid activities that cause pain or swelling. Don't resume until your exercise is pain free. Exercising before your injury has healed may make it worse; it can also increase your chance of reinjury.

Ice
Ice is a pain reliever, slows blood flow to the injury, and reduces swelling. It also limits tissue damage and speeds repair. Apply it as soon as possible and continue for ten to thirty minutes at a time, intermittently for two to three days. Do not apply ice for more than thirty minutes. To protect your skin from direct contact with the ice, I recommend putting it in a plastic sandwich bag, covering it with a cloth, and applying it to the inflamed area.

Compression
Apply a compression bandage, such as an ACE wrap, to reduce swelling and limit motion. Do not make the bandage too tight—you don't want to impair blood flow to the injured area.

Elevation
To reduce swelling, elevate the injured limb above the level of your heart using pillows, a sofa back, or a chair.

For relief of pain and inflammation, take ibuprofen or aspirin.

Dietary Strategies (See Chapter 14 for food sources of specified nutrients)

Calcium

Since more than 99 percent of the calcium in the body is warehoused in the bones, you can imagine how important calcium is for sports competition. It's also critical for preventing osteoporosis. Calcium is most effective when combined with vitamin D, which helps ensure its adequate absorption.

Vitamin E

A potent antioxidant, this vitamin can increase your immune response and may offer protection against the formation of free radicals during heavy exercise. Because free radicals can cause tissue damage leading to muscle soreness, vitamin E can help curb pain. It may also be helpful during weight training, since lifting weights also induces muscle fiber damage.

Vitamin C

This vitamin helps your body make collagen, which is an important protein found in cartilage, tendon, and connective tissue. These structures "play overtime" when you exercise. Researchers have studied vitamin C and sports injuries for decades. In one study, done in 1960, vitamin C and bioflavonoids decreased athletic injury potential in football players. There's also evidence that vitamin C relieves muscle soreness, reduces the frequency of cold and upper respiratory symptoms in marathon runners, and limits bruising tendencies for people who play contact sports. And a recent study, published in the journal *Pain*, showed that vitamin C intake reduced exercise-related soreness. Unlike animals, humans cannot manufacture ascorbic acid, so you must get it from food or supplements.

Other antioxidants

Your muscles may hurt if you overexert yourself during heavy-duty exercise. Since muscle soreness and pain may be caused or exacerbated when free radicals damage tissue, it is helpful to use antioxidants, which quench or neutralize them. Besides vitamins C and E, other helpful nutrients are selenium and beta-carotene.

OPCs (Oligomeric Proanthcyanidins)

This is a tongue-twisting fancy name for a class of compounds originally discovered in a French maritime pine tree. Most commercially available supplements are made from grapeseed or pine bark.

Few studies have directly examined the effects of OPCs on women's sports injuries; however, in some research they've been shown to decrease swelling, strengthen tissue, and fortify blood vessels. I'm impressed by scientific evidence showing that OPCs strengthen and protect elastin and collagen, some of the building blocks for muscles, tendons, and cartilage.

OPCs are present in a wide variety of everyday foods, such as blueberries, bilberries, red wine, onions, green and black tea, legumes, and parsley. If you're a normal, healthy woman, I believe that eating OPC-laden foods is sufficient. You can beef up your consumption of OPCs by cooking with grapeseed oil. Unlike flaxseed or other healthy oils, grapeseed oil has an extremely high boiling point, making it ideal for cooking.

B complex vitamins

These serve a multitude of purposes. I'd emphasize these:

- B1, or thiamine, is important for the processing of carbohydrates, fats, and proteins. Your cells need this vitamin to manufacture ATP (adenosine triphosphate), a critical energy-transporting chemical, which is obviously valuable for athletics.
- B2, or riboflavin, is also needed for the production of ATP. It aids processing of fats and amino acids and helps to activate folate and vitamin B6.
- B3, or niacin, enables more than fifty of the body's enzyme reactions. It helps to manufacture energy and fat from carbohydrates and sex hormones. There are several forms of vitamin B3, including nicotinic acid, niacinamide, and inositol hexaniacinate. The latter improves walking distance in people with intermittent claudication. (This painful condition is a result of hardening of the arteries in the leg; it can be a real problem for older people who want to exercise.)
- B6, or pyridoxine, is an extremely versatile vitamin that helps manufacture neurotransmitters, hormones, and proteins. Although deficiencies of this vitamin are scarce, certain drugs can accelerate its depletion. These include penicillamine (used for arthritis), hydralazine (blood pressure), isoniazid (TB), and MAO inhibitors (depression).
- B12, or cobalamine, helps your body produce SAMe, a potent pain reliever. B12 is also needed for nerve cell activity and to prevent anemia. Since adequate stomach acidity is needed to absorb B12, if you are on acid-reducing drugs like Prilosec (omeprazole), Zantac (ranitidine), or one of the others, you are likely to need supplemental B12. This vitamin is a perfect illustration of one of my mottos: "for every force, there is a counterforce." Acid-reducing drugs are frequently pre-

scribed for people who take nonsteroidal anti-inflammatory drugs for pain. The irony is that one of their side effects is to diminish production of SAMe, a natural pain reliever. Other drugs that hinder B12 absorption are AZT (for AIDS), phenformin and Metformin (for diabetes), nitrous oxide, and colchinine (for gout).

· Get plenty of water. Be sure to drink an 8-ounce glass before you start and after you finish exercising. If you're out there for a long time, especially in hot weather, take frequent water breaks. To get all that water to go down the hatch more easily, you can spice it up with a few drops of orange, lemon, or grapefruit juice.

RECIPE

WILD RICE SALAD WITH CITRUS DRESSING

This delicious dish contains B vitamins, vitamins C and E, and OPCs.

4 cups cooked wild and brown rice
1 red pepper, chopped
1 small red onion, chopped
2 bok choy stalks including leaves, chopped
1 carrot, diced or thinly sliced
½ cup cashews or pecans

DRESSING
¼ cup orange juice
¼ cup lemon juice
1 clove garlic, minced
¼ cup olive oil
1 tablespoon rice syrup

1. In a large bowl combine the rice, red pepper, onion, bok choy, carrots, and nuts.
2. In a separate small bowl, whisk together the dressing ingredients, and then mix it into the rice mixture.
3. May be served warm or cold.

SERVES 6

Supplements

Coenzyme Q10

Since muscle soreness and pain after exercise may be caused or exacerbated when free radicals damage tissue, it's helpful to use antioxidants, which quench or neutralize them. CoQ 10 is a powerful antioxidant, but it's hard to get a therapeutic dose from food. I recommend supplements. The U.S. Dietary Reference Intake has not been established for CoQ 10. The typical dose range suggested in the literature ranges from 30 to 300 mg divided into three doses daily.

Minerals

Minerals, including magnesium, zinc, chromium, and copper, are important for many of the body's enzymatic functions. You can get them from a daily multivitamin and mineral supplement.

Sports drinks

Another source of minerals is a good sports beverage, containing water, minerals, electrolytes (potassium, sodium, chloride), and carbohydrates. The water prevents dehydration during or after an intense sports workout. The carbohydrates give the body fuel for energy production, preventing the breakdown of muscular stores of glycogen.

Vitamin B

As discussed earlier, you need B vitamins. Take a B-complex vitamin that includes vitamins B1, B2, B3, B6, and B12. It's best to take a complex rather than individual B vitamins because they work as a team and you want to get the correct ratio.

Creatine

Found naturally in the body, creatine is converted to phosphocreatine, which helps produce energy. As a nutritional supplement, it's been touted as a great way to enhance athletic performance. It's been shown to help in high-intensity, short-duration exercises like swimming, soccer, and volleyball. Men may benefit more from creatine than women, possibly because women's muscles contain more creatine to begin with. I'm waiting for more scientific proof before I wholeheartedly endorse this supplement for all sporting activity. If you want to try it, follow dosing instructions on the package.

HMB (Beta-hydroxy-beta-methylbutyric acid)

This is another chemical that occurs naturally in the body; it is related to leucine, an amino acid. Based on two small but well-designed studies of women, it looks like HMB supplements have no effect on body mass and strength if you are sedentary. But if you do weight training, it may improve your response. It might also keep you from developing muscle damage during a heavy workout. In addition, HMB may prevent muscle damage and pain during exercise. I'm waiting for more research before I recommend it conclusively.

Ergogenic aids

You may hear about these products or see them in your health food store. They are said to build muscle or enhance athletic performance (and as a consequence may reduce pain), but there is insufficient evidence for me to recommend them. As far as I'm concerned, their value still needs to be scientifically proven. They include:

- Conjugated linoleic acid
- Amino acids
- Phosphatedidylserine
- Branched chain amino acids (leucine, isoleucine, valine)
- Carnitine
- Phosphate
- Pyruvate
- Stimulants, such as ephedra (Ma Huang)
- Caffeine (tea, coffee, guarana)
- Ribose
- NADH (Nicotinamide Adenine Dinucleotide)

Herbs

Ginseng

Ginseng is sometimes used as a sports supplement, and there is some evidence that it can significantly improve aerobic capacity. There are three species: American ginseng (*Panax quinquefolius*), Asian ginseng, Korean ginseng (*Panax ginseng*), and Siberian ginseng (*Eleutherococcus senticosus*).

Most of the positive research that I have seen utilized *Panax ginseng*. The usual dose is 200 mg of an extract. Ginseng can interfere with drug metabolism, so check with your doctor if you regularly take any medications. It can also cause breast tenderness, menstrual abnormalities, insomnia, and tachycardia (rapid heartbeat).

White willow bark (Salix alba)

The bark of willow trees contains an anti-inflammatory compound similar to aspirin. It's appropriate for exercise-related musculoskeletal pain. Unlike other anti-inflammatory drugs, willow is less likely to upset your stomach because it is converted into its active ingredient (salicylic acid) after it is absorbed by your gut. The recommended dose is one cup of infusion, three to five times a day. Do not use willow if you are allergic to aspirin or other NSAIDS, or when pregnant or breast-feeding. Use caution if you take blood-thinning medications.

Meadowsweet (Filipendula ulmaria)

This flowering plant of the meadows acts as an anti-inflammatory because it contains salicylates, the active ingredient in aspirin. It is helpful for exercise-related musculoskeletal pain. Use 1 to 2 teaspoons of dried herb per cup of hot water for a tea. The recommended dose is up to three cups a day. Avoid meadowsweet if you are allergic to aspirin.

Herbal Creams and Ointments

Aloe vera

A common house plant, aloe cools, soothes, and relieves inflammation. Creams are readily available. Be sure to buy one with a high aloe content; it should appear as one of the first listed ingredients.

Joint-Ritis (See page 96)

Sports Gel

Made from *Bellis perennis* (daisy), *Hypericum perforatum* (St. John's wort), *Rhus toxicodendron* (poison ivy), and *Ruta graveolens* (rue), you can rub this homeopathic gel into sore, aching muscles, tendons, or joints up to four times a day.

Do-It-Yourself

Every day

- Apply a vinegar compress to reduce inflammation.
- Wrap a wet plantain leaf around the affected area to reduce swelling and stiffness and encourage healing.
- Give yourself an herbal massage to ease muscle pain and stiffness. Make a muscle rub by combining 2 drops of coriander oil, 4 drops of juniper

oil, 4 drops of black pepper oil, and 4 teaspoons of grapeseed oil. Use the oil to massage the painful spot.

Aromatherapy
  · Rosemary (*Rosmarinus officinalis*): To fight inflammation and relieve pain, add a few drops of rosemary oil to water for a compress. You can also add it to a neutral oil or lotion and use it to massage the sore area.
  · After-Sport Shower Formula: You might also enjoy this. Add two drops of rosemary oil, two drops of pine oil, and four drops of lemon oil to a small dollop of unscented shower gel. Work it into a lather with a sponge or washcloth and use it in the shower. Avoid rosemary during pregnancy or if you have epilepsy or high blood pressure.

Mind/Body

Yoga
Try Tree Pose, Chair Pose, and Standing Yoga Mudra. (See pages 344–351 for postures.)

Red Flags

Call your doctor if you have:

  · Any injury that doesn't improve after ten days of home care and rest.
  · Pain that lasts for more than an hour or wakes you at night.
  · Any injury where a joint "pops" and immediately becomes difficult to use.

SPRAINS AND STRAINS

Description

Sprains and strains are the most common sports-related injuries. A sprain is an injury to the ligaments around a joint that results in an excessive stretch or a tear. Ligaments are bands of tissue that bind joints together; they also support many internal organs.

Sprains may occur around any joint, but they usually affect the back, fingers, knees, wrists, and, especially when it comes to sports injuries, the ankles. Day in and day out, the ankles support the body's entire weight. Making matters worse, when you run or jump they absorb forces three times your body weight. Small wonder, then, that the ankle is your most vulnerable joint.

The ankles are prone to many sports-related injuries, including fractures and dislocations, but sprains are the most common. They may be more of an issue for women than men — in at least one study, women suffered mild ankle sprains 25 percent more frequently. If you play basketball or tennis, or do aerobics or other activities that involve jumping, quick starting, and stopping, watch out.

Sprains may be mild, moderate, or severe. Depending on their severity, they are graded from I to III:

- Grade I (mild): The ligament stretches but does not tear and there is no looseness of the joint. You still have full range of motion with only mild pain. Treatment includes ice with physical therapy, and the prognosis for recovery is excellent.
- Grade II (moderate): The ligament is partially torn and there may be some looseness of the joint. You have pain, bruising, and swelling and it may hurt to walk. Treatment includes ice, bracing, and/or a cast. The prognosis is good.
- Grade III (severe): The ligament is completely torn and the joint is loose and unstable. Your pain is severe and you also have swelling, bruising, and occasional bleeding under the skin. In addition to ice and a splint, treatment involves surgery. The prognosis for recovery is variable.

A strain is an injury, without a tear, of a muscle. Muscle strains are also called pulled muscles.

Causes

Strains are caused by overuse, overstretching, or overloading the muscles in a particular area. This causes inflammation and fluid buildup.

Sudden or unexpected twisting is the most frequent cause of sprains. Improper footwear or poor athletic form can also cause problems.

Signs and Symptoms
- Swelling
- Immediate pain, mild to severe
- Burning or popping

- Because there may be bleeding into the injured area, it may appear swollen or bruised
- In the case of a sprained ankle, it hurts when you move the ankle or try to put weight on it

Conventional Treatments

Your doctor will do a physical exam and may order an MRI (magnetic resonance imaging) to evaluate the damage. R.I.C.E. and anti-inflammatory medications are standard treatments for strains and sprains. Physical therapy is sometimes recommended, too. Depending on how severe the sprain is, your other options include braces, crutches, and surgery.

Supplements

In addition to the dietary strategies mentioned at the beginning of this chapter, I recommend these nutrients to hasten healing:

Vitamin C
The acceptable daily dose range is 90 to 2,500 mg. Try to spread your intake over the course of the day. Large amounts of vitamin C may cause kidney stones or gout, or cramps and diarrhea.

Vitamin E
The acceptable dose range is 15 to 1,000 mg a day.

Vitamin A
The acceptable dose range is 900 to 3,000 mcg a day.

Zinc
The acceptable dose range is 8 to 40 mg a day.

Selenium
The acceptable dose range is 60 to 400 mcg a day.

Herbs

Ginger (Zingibar officinale)
Ginger is a natural anti-inflammatory. Herbalists suggest adding five to twenty drops of tincture to your favorite herbal tea once a day. Use caution if you take blood-thinning medication.

Chamomile (Chamaemelum nobile *or* Matricaria recutita)
This sweet-smelling herb helps fight inflammation, promotes relaxation, and decreases spasms. To help you sleep, make a double-strength tea by using two tea bags or steeping 2 teaspoons of dried flowers in a cup of boiling water. Avoid contact with your eyes; it may cause irritation. Chamomile may cause an allergic reaction.

Herbal Creams and Ointments

Arnica (Arnica montana)
Also called leopard's bane, mountain tobacco, and sneezewort, arnica is helpful for sprains, strains, and bruising. Use an arnica cream, or add several drops of a tincture to a cold compress and apply hourly for the first eight hours to reduce swelling. Do not use on open wounds.

Capsaicin cream (0.025–0.075 percent) (See page 96)

Traumeel ointment (See page 158)

Triflora Arthritis Gel
You can use this homeopathic ointment to relieve minor muscle aches and stiffness that result from overexercising or sports injuries.

Do-It-Yourself

Prevent ankle injuries
- Wear quality athletic shoes with good ankle support. Be sure they are specific for your activity.
- Consider high-top shoes, which provide extra ankle support.
- If your ankle is weak, tape it or wear a brace.

Injuries
When you get a strain or a sprain, elevate the area and apply a cold compress as soon as possible. Continue with the cold compresses until you've reduced the swelling. While a compress using plain old cold water is fine, here are some options that will promote quicker healing:

- Add cider vinegar to your compress to relieve pain and swelling.
- Mix ½ teaspoon of ginger powder and 1 cup of boiling water; let it cool and use it on your compress.
- Pour boiling water into a bowl containing a handful of chamomile

flowers and stir until it turns into paste. Let it cool, spread it on a cotton wrap, and apply it to the affected area for at least fifteen minutes.

Aromatherapy
- Lavender: This herb calms and soothes your spirits as it reduces pain. Add 3 drops of lavender oil to a foot bath or cold compress. Or try adding 3 drops of lavender oil, 3 drops of chamomile oil, and 2 drops of neroli (made from bitter orange blossoms) to a warm bath. You can also add this mixture to 3 teaspoons of grapeseed or sweet almond oil and use it for a massage. Be careful with lavender if you have hay fever or asthma since it may cause an allergic reaction.
- Rub in a small amount of peppermint oil onto the injured area to numb it.
- Add a few drops of sweet marjoram oil and rosemary oil to a compress to encourage healing and reduce inflammation.

Homeopathy
Use these remedies one at a time, following the dosages listed on the package labels:

- Arnica (*Arnica montana*, leopard's bane, mountain tobacco, sneezewort) stimulates healing of damaged tissue.
- *Ruta graveolens* (rue, bitter herb, herb of grace) is used primarily for bruising and ligament strains.

Acupressure (see Chapter 19 for instructions)
To cut pain, use ST 44 (Stomach-44), on the top of the foot, in the web space between the second and third toe.

Exercise

If you have a sprained ankle, it's important to stop exercising until the pain and swelling resolves and your ankle has healed. Still, it's important to do gentle stretches and range-of-motion exercises to preserve movement in the joint.

First phase
- Ankle pumping: With your knee fully extended, bring your toes and foot up and then down, repetitively in sequence. Repeat five times.
- Sit comfortably and write the alphabet in the air with your big toe. Move only the foot and ankle, not the leg.

- Stretch the gastrocnemius-soleus, a major muscle in the calf, by standing 30 inches from a wall, placing your palms on the wall and leaning into the wall until you feel a stretch in the back of your leg.

Second phase
When you are able to bear weight on your ankle, you can balance on your leg for twenty to sixty seconds. If it hurts, put a foam cushion under your foot.

Third phase
You can strengthen the major muscles of your foot and ankle by using elastic tubing to move your foot up, down, in and out.

Seeking Help from Complementary Practitioners

A massage may be helpful.

Red Flags

Call your doctor if you experience:

- Pain, stiffness, or swelling that lasts longer than two to three days
- Inability to bear weight on or move the joint
- Popping when you move a sprained joint
- Poor alignment or crooked bones

COMMON SPORTS-RELATED KNEE INJURIES

Your knee is a critically important joint that flexes and extends the leg. The collateral ligaments, one on each side, connect the upper bone, or femur, to the bones of the lower leg, the tibia and fibula. These ligaments also prevent the knee from moving from side to side. Within the knee itself are the anterior cruciate and posterior cruciate ligaments. They provide stability and serve as guide wires, stopping the knee from overextending or rotating too much.

Whether you're a young runner who leads an active lifestyle or an older woman suffering from arthritis, your knees are particularly vulnerable to pain and injury. Far more than men, women are prone to get runner's knee and other knee ailments. Women have a relative risk of injuring the anterior cruciate ligament, the patellofemoral (knee cap) joint, and the meniscal cartilage (the knee's shock absorber) that is respectively 3.5, 2.3, and 2.1 times higher than in men.

RUNNER'S KNEE

Description

Also called chondromalacia patella, patellofemoral disorder, or patellar mal-alignment, runner's knee is an overuse injury. Besides running, it's associated with walking, jumping, or bicycling and can also occur if you ski, play soccer, or do high-impact aerobics. Sometimes, when you repeatedly bend and straighten the knee, you irritate the inside surface of the kneecap, which then grinds against the thigh bone, or femur. This causes the cartilage behind the knee, which usually helps absorb shock, to break down. The result is pain.

Causes

- Imbalanced muscle strength or flexibility
- Unequal leg lengths
- Alignment problems—turned-in thighbones, wide hips, underdeveloped thigh muscles, or knock-knees
- Flat feet (overpronation), where the feet roll inward, the arches collapse, and the mid-feet flatten out more than normal when you walk or run

Signs and Symptoms

- Dull, aching pain under, behind, or around the kneecap
- Snapping, popping, or grinding in the knee
- Swelling
- Pain when you walk, run, or sit for a long time
- Going down stairs or hills is particularly painful

Conventional Treatments

Standard care for this and many other sports injuries includes R.I.C.E. (see page 235) and anti-inflammatory medication. To take pressure off the knee, switch to a nonweight-bearing exercise, such as swimming or rowing, until you are better. You may need a knee sleeve or brace to support the knee.

It's wise to have your muscle strength, gait pattern, and flexibility assessed by a physiatrist, orthopedist, or sports medicine physician. You can be fitted for semirigid orthotics if it turns out that you overpronate. In addition, your doctor or a physical therapist may recommend exercises, specifically a quadriceps strengthening program.

Do-It-Yourself

To prevent runner's knee, I recommend these tips:

- Avoid running straight down a hill; instead, walk down or run in a zigzag fashion
- Don't do deep knee bends
- Stay away from shoes with cleats or high heels
- Buy shoes made for running with arch support and cushioning (see page 262 for details about how to choose proper shoes)
- Replace your running shoes every three hundred to five hundred miles

Exercise

Try the Hamstring Stretch, Quadriceps Set, and Straight Leg Raises to gently strengthen and stretch your injured knee. (See pages 331–338 for exercises.)

Red Flags

Call your doctor if you have:

- Pain, stiffness, or swelling that lasts more than two to three days
- Inability to bear weight on or move the joint
- Popping sounds
- Poor alignment or crooked bones

COLLATERAL LIGAMENT INJURY

Description

The collateral ligaments are found on both sides of the knee. They connect the femur, or thigh bone, with the bones of the lower leg, the tibia and fibula. Collateral ligaments prevent the knee from moving from side to side.

Bending or twisting can sprain or tear them (also see "Sprains and Strains," page 242).

Causes

Collateral ligament injuries are common in activities such as running, jumping, and contact sports. Like other knee injuries, they are also more likely to happen if you are overweight.

Signs and Symptoms

- Poor alignment of the knee joint
- Pain on the outer side of the knee
- Swelling and tenderness
- The knee feels as if it's going to give way
- An audible pop or snap at the time of injury

Conventional Treatments

Standard care for this and many other sports injuries includes R.I.C.E. (see page 235) and anti-inflammatory medication. Until you get better, switch to a nonweight-bearing exercise such as swimming or rowing. If the damage is severe, you may need to use crutches, a knee immobilizer, or a knee brace to prevent further injury.

To prevent further problems, have your muscle strength, gait pattern, and flexibility assessed by a physiatrist, orthopedist, or sports medicine doctor. If you overpronate, you can be fitted for semirigid orthotics. Also, your doctor or a physical therapist may recommend a quadriceps strengthening program or other exercises.

Do-It-Yourself

To prevent collateral ligament injuries, I recommend these steps:

- Be sure to warm up before exercising
- Wear proper shoes and use appropriate knee protection for the sport
- Learn weight-lifting techniques to build the muscles that support and strengthen the knee

Exercise

Do not return to sports until you are fully recovered and have been cleared by your doctor. I suggest that you meet these conditions before you start exercising again:

- You can bend and straighten the injured knee without pain.
- The swelling has improved.
- You have regained normal strength in the knee and leg.
- You can bear weight enough to resume.

In the meantime, do these rehabilitation exercises for your knee: Heel Slide, Prone Knee Flexion, Straight Leg Raise, and Wall Squat. However, do the Wall Squat only after your pain has lessened. (See pages 331–338 for exercises.)

Red Flags

Call your doctor if you have:

- Pain, stiffness, or swelling that lasts more than two or three days
- Inability to bear weight on or move the joint
- Popping noises when you move your knee
- Poor alignment or crooked bones

PATELLAR TENDONITIS (JUMPER'S KNEE)

Description

If you exercise too much or train too hard, you may develop pain in the patellar tendon. This strip of fibrous, cordlike tissue connects the kneecap to the shin. Patellar tendinitis is a risk if you run, walk, bike, or do sports that involve jumping. (*Note:* There is more information on treatments for tendinitis in Chapter 7.)

Causes

In addition to overuse, several kinds of movements can damage the patellar tendon. These include twisting with your feet in a fixed position, rapid squatting, or sharply extending your knee. In severe instances, you can tear the tendon.

Signs and Symptoms

- Pain, swelling, and tenderness around the patellar tendon
- Swelling of the knee joint
- Pain with jumping, running, or walking
- Pain when you bend or straighten the knee
- Tenderness behind the knee

Conventional Treatments

It's likely that your physician will simply recommend ice and compression, along with anti-inflammatory medication for the pain. She may also suggest that you use a knee brace or immobilizer to support the knee. Sometimes, shoe orthotics can be helpful.

Do-It-Yourself

- To prevent injury, add shock-absorbing insoles to your shoes to reduce the impact of activity on your knee.
- Try an ice massage for the pain.
  1. Freeze water in a Styrofoam cup.
  2. Peel the top of the cup away to expose the ice and hold on to the bottom of the cup.
  3. Rub the ice into your leg for five to ten minutes.

Exercise

Until you are fully recovered, switch to a sport that is less stressful for your knee, such as swimming. Meanwhile, you can do the Hamstring Stretch and Patellar Mobility Exercise to promote strengthening and healing. (See pages 331–338 for exercises.)

Once the pain in your knee has lessened, try Quadricep Sets, Quadriceps Stretches, and Straight Leg Raises, which strengthen the muscles that support and stabilize your knee. (See pages 331–338.)

Red Flags

Call your doctor if you have:

- Pain, stiffness, or swelling that lasts more than two or three days
- Inability to bear weight on or move the joint
- Popping when you move the joint
- Poor alignment or crooked bones

ANTERIOR CRUCIATE LIGAMENT (ACL) TEARS

This ailment has begun to receive national attention, thanks in part to the terrible spectacle of women NCAA basketball players in agony after tearing their ACLs on live television. It's estimated that a female athlete will tear this ligament once out of every three hundred times she participates in practice or games.

We don't know why women are so vulnerable to ACL injuries, but apparently certain female anatomical characteristics tend to put you more at risk. As a woman, you have a wider pelvis and more flexible hips so the ACL, located inside the knee, is under more strain than a man's. Over the past couple of years, medical researchers have found that women's knee muscles don't provide as much protection as do their male counterparts, even when they use the same strengthening and conditioning programs. They suggest that innovative strengthening exercises, designed especially for women, may need to be developed.

The bottom line is that women suffer more injuries from noncontact sports, including basketball, soccer, gymnastics, snow skiing, and handball. If you participate in sports where you pivot or jump and land on one foot, you are particularly susceptible to ACL tears. These injuries can be very painful. What's more, because the ACL gives your knee most of its ability to rotate, you lose stability when you make lateral and twisting motions.

ACL tears are usually diagnosed by MRI (magnetic resonance imaging). Immobilization of the knee and, depending on the severity of the ACL tear, surgery to reconstruct the knee is often required.

Signs and Symptoms

- Loud audible pop, signifying a tear
- Difficulty standing on the injured leg

- Swelling of the leg and knee (hemorrhage)
- Intense pain

Red Flags

Pain, swelling, and loss of motion in the knee are signals for you to call your doctor.

OTHER SPORT-RELATED INJURIES

ANDREA'S STORY

Andrea, a thirty-four-year-old caterer, appeared to be in great shape. This was not surprising, given her exercise habits. "Twice a week I take aerobic dance at the local community center and I run two to three miles a day," she told me.

Andrea had come to see me shortly after a midwinter vacation. She had decided to surprise her husband and their seven-year-old son and four-year-old daughter with a weeklong stay at a Miami Beach resort. While enjoying the sun, the sand, the surf, and the "early-bird specials," she made it a point to keep up her exercise. "I did my daily run on the beach, finishing up on the boardwalk," she explained.

Unfortunately she was now in exquisite pain. "It started toward the end of my vacation—this awful pain and discomfort in my shins," she said. I already had an inkling of what her problem was; then, she mentioned the kicker: "I keep thinking it's getting better; then, when I start to run, it starts up again."

Andrea had shin splints, a common condition that is sometimes caused by running on an uneven surface. Those otherwise-glorious runs on the beach in Miami were the reason for her misery.

I told her to ease off on high-impact sports, like running and aerobics, and substitute swimming, in-line skating, or biking until her sore, damaged muscles felt better. To speed up the process, I suggested a diet loaded in antioxidants, such as vitamins C and E, selenium and beta-carotene, which encourage healing. In addition to the Arnica cream she was already using on her legs, I suggested that she whirlpool her legs twice a day and gave her instructions for an easy-to-make herbal rub she could use to massage away muscle pain and stiffness. Finally, I gave her a series of stretches to do every day.

As she was getting ready to leave, I asked Andrea when she had last bought running shoes. "Gosh, I can't even remember," she replied. Because worn-out running shoes can cause or aggravate shin splints, new shoes were added to her list of "prescriptions."

A month later, I ran into Andrea at our local sporting goods store. She was buying new running shoes, which I took as a good sign. She flashed me a big smile and a thumbs-up. "Cured!" she said.

SHIN SPLINTS (SHIN PAIN)

Description

If you're a runner, shin splints can stop you dead in your tracks. This ailment comes in two varieties: anterolateral and posteromedial. The anterolateral, as its name implies, affects the muscles and causes pain in the front and outer part of the lower leg. You're prone to this type of shin splints because of the normal imbalance between the muscles in the front of the shin (tibialis anterior, whose job is to raise the foot up), and the overpowering calf muscle (gastrocnemius muscle) in the back. When the calf muscle is significantly stronger, it can cause damage to the front shin muscles.

Posteromedial shin splints affect the muscles in the back, inner part of the leg. It hurts along the inner leg above the ankle, and gets worse when you lift up on your toes or move your ankle inward. Often, these shin splints are provoked by running on uneven roads or a banked track, or if your feet deviate inward without the support of a good pair of running shoes.

Although runners are especially susceptible to shin splints, other athletes get them, too. You can develop inflammation of the shin bone (tibia), or the muscles and tendons that attach to it, if you run or jump on hard surfaces or exercise too much, too fast, or too soon. The tibia is where the muscles that raise the arch of the foot are attached, so shin pain can also occur if you have tight calf muscles or wear worn-out shoes.

Causes

Overuse is the usual cause of shin splints. They often occur when you increase your mileage or pick up your pace. If you participate in aerobics, basketball, volleyball, or other activities that involve repetitive pounding, you may also develop this problem. And your shins may object if you switch your exercise routine to a hard surface, like asphalt or the hard wooden floor of a gym.

If your arches collapse when you walk or run—your foot flattens out more than normal—you are at greater risk for shin splints. This condition, called overpronation, puts more stress on the leg muscles.

Signs and Symptoms

- Pain is in the front, outer part or the back, inner part of your lower leg. Your shin bone or the muscles on either side of it may hurt.
- Tender and/or swollen shins.
- Generally, it hurts most during exercise and feels better when you rest. You may, however, have pain at rest.
- Usually, but not always, shin splints affect both legs.

Conventional Treatments

R.I.C.E. (see page 235) and rehabilitation exercises are standard treatments for shin splints. You may use ibuprofen or aspirin for pain relief and inflammation. You can get prescription, custom-made arch supports (orthotics) to correct overpronation, if that's part of the problem.

Do-It-Yourself

To prevent shin splints
- Wear well-cushioned, stable running shoes.
- Run on soft surfaces (grass or dirt) and do aerobics on an exercise mat.
- Increase the intensity of your workout gradually.
- Include calf stretches in your warm-up and cooldown (see exercise section below).
- Check with a podiatrist about getting orthotic inserts for your shoes.
- If you are a runner who's had recurrent shin splints, examine your running style and correct improper form. Get help from a trainer if necessary.

Ice massage for pain
1. Freeze water in a Styrofoam cup.
2. Peel the top of the cup away to expose the ice and hold on to the bottom of the cup.
3. Rub the ice into your leg for five to ten minutes.

Hydrotherapy
Submerging your legs in a whirlpool can be helpful.

Exercise

My patients with shin splints often ask me when they can return to their activity. Although I know it's frustrating to hear this, my answer is: "It depends." My general rule of thumb is that the longer you have symptoms before you start treatment, the longer it will take to get better. Still, everyone recovers from injury at a different rate. Remember though, if you start too soon you may worsen your problem or even cause permanent damage. You can return to your normal activity when you have complete range of motion and full strength in both legs, you can jog or sprint straight ahead without pain or limping, and you can jump on either or both legs without pain. Until then, to tide you over and help you stay in shape, substitute swimming or another low-impact activity.

When it's time to go back to your regular routine, start slowly. If it hurts, stop and resume your treatment.

In the meantime, you can do therapeutic exercises, including Calf Stretch with Towel, Standing Calf Stretch, Active Range-of-Motion of the Ankle, Heel Raises, and Sitting and Standing Toe Raises. (See pages 331–338 for exercises.)

Seeking Help from Complementary Practitioners

Massage
Deep massage of sore muscles can help relieve soreness and pain.

Acupuncture
I've found this therapy to be very helpful for my patients with shin splints.

Red Flags

If you develop tightness, numbness, or tingling in the lower leg while you work out, or shin pain that doesn't subside with rest, see your doctor. You may have *compartment syndrome*. Your lower leg muscles are separated into compartments by membrane walls. When you overindulge in your favorite sport, your muscles may get too big for their compartments, putting pressure on nearby nerves and blood vessels. Symptoms may clear up when you stop exercising; however, it may take several hours to a few days for them to clear up. Compartment syndrome is a serious problem that may require surgery. Left untreated, it can become a surgical emergency.

STRESS FRACTURE

Description

Stress fractures are hairline cracks in bone that can cause severe pain. They are serious injuries; if left untreated, stress fractures may get worse, or even lead to complete fractures. The most common sites for them are the bones of the mid-foot (metatarsals), shin bone (tibia), outer lower leg bone (fibula), thigh bone (femur), and back bones (vertebrae).

Causes

Stress fractures are the result of repeated or prolonged activity, which is why they're common in long-distance runners and ballet dancers. Suddenly increasing your workout time or intensity can also cause a stress fracture. They occur more often in women, especially women with thinner bones, so if you're a postmenopausal woman with osteoporosis, watch out and be sure to take calcium.

Discrepancy in leg length, high arches, and using shoes with poor shock absorption may also predispose you to stress fractures.

Signs and Symptoms

- Pain at the site of the fracture, triggered by a workout. Unlike shin splints (see page 255), this is not muscle pain. The fractured bone is what hurts.
- Site is tender and sore to touch.
- Activity makes the pain worse.
- Pain gradually becomes more intense over time.

An X ray doesn't always reveal a stress fracture during the early stage. When the bone heals and callus tissue develops around it, an X ray is more helpful. A bone scan can pick up a stress fracture earlier than an X ray.

Conventional Treatments

If you have shin pain, apply ice packs for twenty to thirty minutes every three to four hours for two or three days until the pain subsides. You can also take anti-inflammatory drugs. If the pain doesn't diminish, you will need an X ray or bone scan to see if you have a stress fracture. If you do, the most important treatment is rest; you'll have to stop exercising for a while. In addition, you may need to wear a cast for three to six weeks while the bone heals.

Seeking Help from Complementary Practitioners

Hypnosis
One interesting study suggests that hypnosis that focuses on the healing process, including the stages of fracture healing, and on speeding up the process, may reduce your recovery time and promote faster healing.

Red Flags

Call your doctor if you experience pain, swelling, or immobility around a bone.

TENNIS ELBOW

Description

Tendons attach the muscles to the bones. Tennis elbow, also known as lateral epicondylitis, is a type of tendinitis, or inflammation of the tendons. Tennis elbow affects not only the tendons but also the epicondyle, the bony point where they are anchored. (For more information on conventional and complementary treatments for tendinitis, see Chapter 7.)

Causes

Tendons are strong and fibrous but not especially flexible, so overuse or sudden, abrupt movement may irritate or inflame them. Tennis elbow is frequently the result of improper form. For example, if you turn your wrist during a serve or hit a stroke poorly, you may be jarring or putting extra stress on your muscles and tendons. Obviously, this ailment affects tennis players, but it can also be a problem if you play golf or do other activities where you repeatedly bend your wrist up against resistance.

Signs and Symptoms

Pain and tenderness on the outside of your elbow and sharp pain when you grip something or twist your hand and forearm are the hallmarks of tennis elbow. Simple actions that involve bending your wrist up may make the pain worse; it may hurt just to carry your briefcase or shake hands with a friend.

Exercises

Try Wrist Range-of-Motion, Forearm Range-of-Motion, and Elbow Range-of-Motion. (See pages 331–338 for exercises.)

Red Flags

Call your doctor if you:

- Have excessive pain
- Can't fully move your elbow
- Have swelling, numbness, or tingling around your elbow

GOLFER'S ELBOW

Description

Tendons attach muscles to bones. Golfer's elbow, also known as medial epicondylitis, is an inflammation of the tendons, known as tendinitis. It causes pain and tenderness on the bony bump located on the inner side of the elbow. (For more information on conventional and complementary treatments for tendinitis, see Chapter 7.)

Causes

Overuse may irritate and inflame the tendons because they are strong and fibrous but not especially flexible. Repeated bending of the wrist and fingers is the usual suspect in golfer's elbow. Besides golf, you can get this injury if you play baseball or racquet sports, as well as from carpentry, typing, and other occupations.

Signs and Symptoms

- Pain in your elbow, at the side closest to your body
- Bending your wrist causes pain along the inner side of your forearm
- It hurts to make a fist
- Pain worsens when you flex your wrist (bend it down) against resistance

Exercises

Try Wrist Range-of-Motion, Forearm Range-of-Motion, and Elbow Range-of-Motion. In addition, wrist strengthening exercises include Wrist Flexion, Wrist Extension, Wrist Radial Deviation Strengthening, and Pronation and Supination Strengthening. (See pages 331–338.)

Red Flags

Call your doctor if you:

- Have excessive pain
- Can't fully move your elbow
- Have swelling, numbness or tingling around your elbow

ACHILLES TENDINITIS

Description

This ailment, common among runners, is an inflammation of the thick tendon that attaches the calf muscles to the heel. If you love basketball or other sports that involve jumping, or if you play racquetball and other activities that use frequent stop-and-go movements, you are putting considerable stress on your Achilles tendon. You can prevent Achilles tendinitis with good shoes, proper training, and stretching. (For more information on conventional and complementary treatments for tendinitis, see Chapter 7.)

Causes

There are many causes of Achilles tendinitis:

- Poor conditioning
- Frequent uphill running
- Running on your toes
- Doing too much too soon or increasing your activity too quickly
- Tight calf muscles
- Wearing worn-out shoes
- Insufficient stretching
- Anatomical factors, such as bowlegs, having one leg shorter than the other, or high arches

Signs and Symptoms

You'll feel pain and tenderness along the cordlike tendon at the back of your heel and calf.

Exercises

Start out with the Calf Stretch with Towel and then move on to the Standing Calf Stretch and the Stair Stretch. When the pain has let up, you can try Toe and Heel Raises and the One-Leg Balance.

(See pages 331–338 for exercises.)

Low Back Pain (See Chapter 6)

HOW TO BUY ATHLETIC SHOES

I find it perplexing that people continue exercising in poor-fitting, worn-out shoes. It's relatively inexpensive to keep yourself well-shod, athletically speaking. And it can help prevent so many injuries. Here are some tips for getting the right shoes for you:

- Determine your correct shoe width by placing your bare foot on a white piece of paper and tracing it. Compare the width of this tracing with the width of your shoe. If your shoe is less than one-quarter of an inch of the maximum tracing width it is too narrow. Shoes that are too narrow can aggravate bunions and toe deformities.
- Feet normally swell as the day goes on. To get the right size, shop for shoes late in the day when your feet are their largest.
- When you buy shoes, wear the same socks you use when you exercise.
- If your feet are wide, look for shoes with a wide toe box; be sure you can easily wiggle your toes.
- You probably have one foot that is larger than the other; most people do. Always size your shoe to your bigger foot.
- Do not buy snug-fitting shoes assuming they'll be okay after you break them in. They should be comfortable as soon as you try them on.
- Don't be surprised if your feet get longer and wider as you age and after pregnancies.

THE FEMALE ATHLETE TRIAD

Certain sports ailments are related specifically to the menstrual cycle. Amenorrhea, or lack of periods, occurs in nearly 20 percent of vigorously exercising women. Some girl and female athletes suffer from a complex interplay of menstrual irregularity, eating disorders, and premature osteo-porosis—a syndrome called the Female Athlete Triad. The pressure many young women feel to achieve or maintain unrealistically low body weight only makes the problem worse.

Not only does this syndrome diminish your physical performance, it is a serious risk to your long-term health. If you have any component of the Triad, you are at risk and should be screened for the others. Keep accurate records of your menstrual cycle; if it begins to diverge from its normal pattern, take note and follow it carefully. Mention it to your physician. She may want to evaluate your bone mass and make recommendations for pre-venting osteoporosis. It may be necessary for you to train less intensely and increase your total calories and calcium intake. It may also be wise to begin a program of resistance training to increase your muscle strength and mass (see Chapter 6 for more information about osteoporosis).

11

Oh, My Aching Feet

At some point in their lives, three-quarters of Americans have foot problems. When you think about it, that's not surprising. Just by standing, we put a force on our feet that is 50 percent greater than our body weight. Nor did Mother Nature have concrete sidewalks or high-heeled shoes in mind when our feet and upright stance evolved. Our long life spans don't help either; as we age, our feet widen and get flatter, and the protective padding of fat on the soles wears down.

Women are at higher risk than men for most kinds of severe foot pain. This has a lot to do with high-heeled shoes, which are responsible for most women's foot deformities and problems. Think about it: Are you, like Cinderella's sisters, forcing your feet into shoes that are too tight? In a 1992 survey done by the American Podiatric Medical Association, 44 percent of women said they wear shoes that look good but don't fit well.

Ironically, the same design features that make your shoes fashionable — narrow width, pointed toes, and high heels — are deadly for your feet. Two-inch heels increase the pressure on the front half of your foot by 57 percent; in 3-inch heels, that pressure rises to an astounding 76 percent. And because high heels cause your feet to slide forward in your shoes, your toes are also under duress. In fact, most foot problems can be prevented or successfully treated by wearing proper footwear.

Pregnancy may also make your feet more vulnerable to foot trouble. Enlargement of the belly, breasts, and thighs, along with swelling of the feet and ankles, leads to changes in posture, movement, joint stability, and weight distribution. This has a dramatic effect on your feet and the way you walk. Also, you widen your base of support — the amount of distance between your feet — to compensate as your center of gravity migrates up and forward, and to give yourself greater stability. The net effect is greater pressure on different parts of your feet. In addition, you release hormones that relax ligaments, further weakening your feet and ankles.

Other risk factors for foot problems include:

- Being overweight
- High-impact sports, such as tennis, jogging, or racquetball
- Heavy lifting
- Extensive walking
- Diabetes

In this chapter, I'll start by providing several all-purpose, do-it-yourself treatments for painful foot ailments, such as heel spurs, diabetic feet, ingrown toenails, athlete's foot, and warts. Following that, you'll find more particulars about other specific problems. One note: For information about Achilles tendinitis and ankle injuries, please go to Chapter 10.

Prevention

You can prevent many foot ailments simply by wearing well-fitting, comfortable shoes. The ideal shoe is roomy and has low heels, a thick sole, and arch support. Here are some tips for buying shoes:

- Your feet swell as the day goes on; they also change shape and size, depending on whether you are walking, sitting, or standing. Shop for shoes in the evening, when your shoe size is biggest. Be sure the shoe fits the widest part of your foot.
- Foot size changes with age and after pregnancy, so have your feet checked every few years and after each baby.
- Soft glove leather allows breathing room and stretches to accommodate your feet. Avoid synthetics and patent leather.
- Get shoes with enough room for you to wiggle your toes. Avoid pointy-toed styles and allow one-half inch between the end of your longest toe and the shoe.
- Be sure that the heel fits snugly and doesn't slip. Shoes with laces, straps, or buckles can be helpful.
- Avoid shoes with stitching around bunions or other sensitive areas.
- Wear high-quality athletic shoes that have good ankle support and are made specifically for your activity (for tips on buying athletic shoes, see Chapter 10).

Do-It-Yourself

Self-massage for your feet

WATER MASSAGE
1. Fill a bathtub or basin ankle deep with cool water.
2. In tandem, rhythmically move your feet back and forth, allowing the water to gently caress them, for 2 minutes.
3. Raise your feet completely out of the water after each stroke.

For added pleasure, you can add a few drops of a pleasant-scented herbal essential oil, like lavender or rosemary. If athlete's foot is a concern, try adding several drops of tea tree oil, which has documented antibacterial and antifungal effects.

BALL ROLL
1. Sit on a chair and place a tennis ball or another small rubber ball under the arch of your foot.
2. Roll your foot backward and forward for 1 minute.
3. Repeat with the other foot.

Reflexology
1. Use your thumb and index finger to rotate your toes in a circular motion.
2. Then, make a fist and rotate it around the bottom of your foot.
3. Finally, twist your foot as if you're wringing wet clothes, moving the top and bottom in opposite directions.

Contrast baths to ease aching feet
Soak your feet in cool water, then in warm water, alternating every few minutes for about fifteen minutes.

Exercises

Try Sitting and Standing Toe Raises and Head and Foot Bounces. (See pages 331–338 for exercises.)

Mind/Body

Yoga for your feet
Try Guptasana (Concealed Posture), Utkatasana (Squatting Posture), and Kneeling Foot Stretch. (See pages 344–351.)

METATARSALGIA

GILDA'S STORY

Gilda is a seventy-year-old woman who works as a candy striper in our local hospital, where she delivers newspapers and magazines to the patients. She is on her feet a great deal.

I've known Gilda a long time, ever since she came to me for rehabilitation after suffering a stroke about seven years ago. When I ran into her one day in the elevator, she told me she had developed a sore, aching pain in the balls of her feet. "It gets worse when my husband and I go out on the town, and I wear my high heels," she explained. Gilda and her husband loved ballroom dancing, and this pain was putting a cramp in their style. "I'm afraid I may have to give it up," she said, wistfully. I watched the way she walked down the hall, and noticed that she tended to shift her weight abnormally.

The next time I saw her, I offered to take a quick look at her feet. When she stopped by my office, I noted that the skin over her metatarsal bones was thinned out, which is common in women of her age. But I also noticed that the shoes she was wearing looked "tired" and lacked cushioning. "I know they're worn," she confessed. "But I just love these shoes. I won them in a dance contest a couple of summers ago, when I was vacationing at a bungalow colony."

Gilda had metatarsalgia, a painful condition that is common among middle-aged and older women. I suggested that she try herbal foot soaks, as well as a new pair of cushioned sneakers for everyday use. I also gave her the name of a podiatrist colleague who could fashion a metatarsal bar, or some other form of metatarsal support for her feet. Finally, I gave her some exercises that she could do while she watched TV at night. With these tips, Gilda's pain improved. The next time I saw her, she said: "My feet hurt so much less. In fact, we're going out dancing tonight."

Description

Metatarsalgia, or pain in the metatarsal bones, is probably the most common cause of foot pain among middle-aged women. The metatarsal bones are the long bones of the foot; they lie in the mid-foot area. These bones connect with the tarsal bones and heel bones (calcaneus) in the rear, and the phalanges (toe bones) in the front. The agonizing pain of metatarsalgia feels like a bruise, or a dull aching pain in the ball of the foot (on the underside of the forefoot, underneath the metatarsal heads). Occasionally, the pain radiates to other areas. Metatarsalgia generally occurs because you abnormally distribute weight on your forefoot when you walk, and this leads to inflammation. You can sometimes get relief by walking or standing on the outside of your foot, since this removes pressure from the ball of the foot.

Causes

You can develop metatarsalgia for many reasons. The aging process causes thinning of the fat pad in the foot, making you more vulnerable to metatarsal forces. Other common causes include:

· Wearing narrow pointy shoes, with high heels and a narrow toe box
· Being overweight or obese
· Repeated, forceful pounding of your foot when walking or running or doing too much of a weight-bearing activity, such as jumping
· High arches or foot abnormalities that flatten the front of your foot
· Arthritis
· Trauma

Signs and Symptoms

· Pain on the bottom of the middle of the foot, made worse when you stand or bear weight.
· Tenderness over the bony surfaces of your feet.

Conventional Treatments

Treatments for metatarsalgia focus on relieving pressure on the bottom of the foot. More comfortable shoes are certainly in order. If you are currently using shoes that give you pain in your metatarsal area, it may be time for a shoe "checkup":

· Make sure your shoes are not worn out—that the tread on the bottom is intact and the wear pattern is even.
· If your foot has a tendency to pronate, or migrate inward, you might benefit from a shoe that provides greater restraint.
· Look for a shoe with forefoot cushioning.

If you are a do-it-yourselfer, you can create your own padded shoe inserts simply by fabricating a circular shoe insert, made of moleskin, that you can place under your metatarsals. This will provide some cushioning and give you some relief.

If that doesn't help, a podiatrist can fit you for custom-made arch supports (orthotics), or work with you to devise other mechanical methods to relieve the pain in the mid-foot. These include redistributing weight-bearing pressure and force behind the metatarsal head.

- Internal: An orthotic, known as a "cookie" or metatarsal pad, can be conveniently placed inside your shoe, right in back of metatarsal heads 2, 3, and 4. The orthotics should fit snugly between the inner border of the big toe and the outer side of the small toe.
- External: A metatarsal bar is a ¼-inch piece of tapered durable plastic that is placed on the sole of the shoe.

You may need to take anti-inflammatory medications for pain or change your choice of athletic activity, if that's what's causing the problem.

Do-It-Yourself

Every day
- Put your feet up to get relief, whenever possible.
- Watch your weight, staying at the appropriate level for your height and build.
- Avoid high-heeled shoes or narrow, pointy footwear. Instead, wear comfortable shoes with a small heel and plenty of room for your feet.
- Soak your feet in Epsom salts nightly for twenty minutes.
- Use ice. You can make a convenient ice applicator by freezing water in a 12-ounce paper cup. Then, remove the icicle and place it in a plastic bag before applying it to your foot.
- Massage your feet:
    1. While sitting comfortably in a chair, cross your right foot over your left leg.
    2. Sprinkle several drops of massage oil (or lavender oil) on your left hand.
    3. Using your thumb, gently stroke the bottom of your foot in a circular fashion, beginning with the outer circumference and working your way toward the center.
    4. Do this for three minutes. Then, switch to your other foot. CAUTION: Never massage cracked, blistered, or broken skin, especially if you are diabetic.

Herbal foot bath
Add five to eight drops of lavender, rosemary, or juniper oil to a basin of warm water and allow your feet to soak for thirty minutes. Allow them to air dry.

Exercise

To condition the small muscles of your feet and keep them in good shape, try the following exercise:
1. Obtain a set of marbles.
2. Set them out on the floor.
3. One by one, pick up the marbles with your toes and deposit them into a 16-inch Styrofoam cup.

Seeking Help from Complementary Practitioners

Acupuncture
Your acupuncturist can help relieve the pain of metatarsalgia.

Massage
A professional foot massage can work wonders.

Red Flags

Call your doctor if:

· Your pain significantly limits how far you can walk
· You have a fever or your foot looks red (you may have an infection)
· The pain lasts more than seven days

MORTON'S NEUROMA

Description

A neuroma is a benign (noncancerous) tumor of nerve tissue. But benign is a strange word to use for this ailment, which can cause horrible, shooting pain, as well as numbness and tingling. Often confused with metatarsalgia, because the pain is found in the metatarsalgia area, Morton's neuroma is not, technically speaking, a true neuroma. It is actually a fibrosis, or tissue thickening, around the nerves that supply the toes. It strikes the nerve that passes between the base of two toes, most commonly between the bones of your third and fourth toes, or those of your second and third toes. This ailment causes the nerve to thicken and become inflamed and very painful. Usually, it's a result of repetitive irritation that occurs when the bones of your toes rub together. Like so many of the foot ailments I've described in this chapter, it's often connected to constrictive shoes—the sure giveaway being that it affects five times as many women as men.

Causes

Although it may develop for no reason, Morton's neuroma is commonly caused by:

- Wearing shoes that are too tight
- Running or walking too much
- Running on hard surfaces

Signs and Symptoms

- Burning pain, often worse when your toes are pointed up or when your toes are squeezed together
- Numbness or tingling
- Tenderness and pain on the bottom of the foot, between the bones of the third and fourth toes, or the second and third toes
- Pain travels from the outer side of one toe to the inner side of the adjoining toe
- Tight and/or high-heeled shoes make the pain worse
- Walking barefoot relieves the pain

Conventional Treatments

To ease the sharp pain of a neuroma, the best thing you can do is to allow your toes plenty of room by wearing properly fitting shoes with a wide toe box. A metatarsal pad worn in the shoes will help spread your toes and take pressure off the inflamed nerve. Custom-made arch supports (orthotics) sometimes serve the same purpose.

If the pain is bothering you and ibuprofen and aspirin don't provide relief, your doctor may suggest using a whirlpool with cold water, or ultrasound. Or she may recommend Xylocaine or cortisone injections. Should all else fail, surgery may be required.

Herbs

Ginger (Zingibar officinale)
Ginger is a natural anti-inflammatory. Herbalists suggest adding five to twenty drops of tincture to your favorite herbal tea once a day. Use caution if you take blood-thinning medication.

Herbal Creams and Ointments

Triflora cream
This is a homeopathic gel; its ingredients include comfrey (*Symphytum officinale*), poison ivy (*Rhus toxicodendron*), and marsh tea (*Ledum palustre*).

Do-It-Yourself

- Herbal foot bath: Add five to eight drops of lavender or rosemary oil to a basin of warm water. Soak your feet for thirty minutes. Allow them to air dry.
- Regularly treat yourself to a barefoot walk on the beach. Walking on hard surfaces provokes pain, so the beach can be quite a relief. CAUTION: If you are diabetic, do not walk barefooted.
- Stop any activity that makes the condition worse.
- Use ice to massage the top of your foot. Cold can physiologically slow down the trapped nerve transmission, relieving the tingling, burning pain. Fill a 12-ounce paper cup with water and freeze. Then, remove the icicle and put it in a plastic bag before applying it to your foot.
- Avoid high-heeled shoes or narrow, pointy footwear. Instead, wear comfortable shoes with a low heel and plenty of room for your toes.
- In your shoe, use a foam rubber pad under the sole of your foot to keep your toes spread apart and decrease pressure on the nerve.
- Remove your shoes frequently and massage your feet.

Exercise

To condition the small muscles of your feet and keep them in good shape, try this exercise: Stand with your feet parallel. Bend your toes up into the air. Hold for a couple of seconds, then release.

Red Flags

Call your doctor if:

- You develop loss of sensation or worsening tingling
- Your pain significantly limits how far you can walk
- Your pain gets progressively worse
- The pain lasts more than seven days

BUNIONS

Description

Also known as hallux valgus, a bunion is a painful, bony lump that forms on the joint at the base of the big toe (the metatarsophalangeal, or MTP joint). This occurs when the bone or tissue that make up the big toe migrates out of place, usually because the toe is squeezed inward. In addition to the bump, the joint swells and the toe turns in. Because this part of the foot bears much of the weight when you walk, bunions can really hurt. A "mini bunion," or a bunionette is a similar deformity that develops beside your little toe.

Bunions are common only in shoe-wearing societies. What's more, they occur ten times more frequently in women than in men. It's likely that their major cause is—you guessed it—women's high-heeled shoes.

Causes

Bunions form when the big toe is forced inward, putting pressure on the joint at its base. This is usually the result of a lifetime of abnormal forces and pressure on the joints and tendons during normal walking. It happens for a variety of reasons:

- Genetic predisposition—you may be born with a foot type whose mechanics, or distribution of forces, is vulnerable to bunion formation
- Flat feet or low arches—a normal arch is one inch or more above the ground
- Frequently wearing high-heeled shoes, especially those that squeeze the toes together
- Foot injuries
- Tight Achilles tendon

- Arthritis
- Inflammatory joint disease
- Neuromuscular disorders
- Congenital deformities
- Being a ballet dancer or having another occupation that stresses the feet

Signs and Symptoms

- A bony bump at the base of the big toe, which may be accentuated when you put weight on your foot
- Swelling, redness, and soreness of the big toe joint
- Thickening, irritation, or blistering of the skin on the bunion
- Restricted movement of the big toe
- Pain, especially caused by pressure when wearing shoes

Conventional Treatments

Bunions don't go away unless you have them surgically removed. But non-surgical treatments can reduce pain and stop them from getting worse. To relieve pressure on the bunion, wear shoes with flat heels and a wide toe box. Avoid any shoes with heels more than 2 inches high.

You can cover the bunion with commercially available pads to prevent irritation and shield the bone from external pressure. There are also special inserts you can wear between your first and second toes to correct their alignment. A podiatrist can apply padding and taping to further reduce stress and pain.

If the bunion is swollen, apply ice packs several times a day. Anti-inflammatory medications can relieve pain. Traction or corticosteroids can also relieve severe pain.

For severe pain, hydrotherapy and ultrasound can offer an additional measure of relief.

I believe surgery to correct bunions should be a last resort, to be used only when the deformity has advanced, more conservative measures have failed, and you still have significant pain. Any surgery is risky, but in the case of bunions it may result in a decrease in the range of motion of your great toe, a particular problem if you are a dancer or an athlete.

Herbal Creams and Ointments

Marshmallow (Althaea officinalis)

You can use a paste made from this wild, light pink–flowered plant to relieve inflammation and swelling. Use enough root powder to cover the affected area and add cold water to make a paste. Apply a thick layer to your bunion and let it dry. Reapply as often as necessary, every two to three hours if needed. Do not apply to any open areas.

Comfrey (Symphytum officinale)

If you have an open abrasion on the skin overlying your bunion, you can apply a comfrey compress to help heal the wound. Comfrey contains an oil that forms a protective, soothing film over the area that will help speed healing. Please note that you should never take comfrey for internal use.

Do-It-Yourself

- Give your feet a rest and go barefoot every now and then.
- Switch shoes frequently.
- Switch to a flat-heeled shoe instead of high heels. High heels put extra pressure on your toes and joints. Also, be sure your shoes have plenty of room for your toes.
- Soak your feet in warm water and massage them.
- Aromatherapy: Add a drop of the essential oil of lemon balm (*Melissa officinalis*) or chamomile to a massage oil and rub it into the area.

Exercise

Because bunions may be caused by tight Achilles tendons, try the Stair Stretch. (See pages 331–338.)

Red Flags

- Worsening deformity that prevents walking
- Excessive pain

CORNS

Description

Corns are tough, thickened skin on your feet, caused by pressure or friction. They are harder than calluses and may be quite painful.

Causes

Anything that causes prolonged pressure or rubs on the skin of your foot, especially in an area covering a bony prominence, can result in a corn. Common culprits are:

- New, tight, or poor-fitting shoes
- Wearing sandals or shoes without socks
- High-heeled shoes
- High arches, which may put added pressure on your toes when you walk
- Any physical deformity that distributes your weight unevenly when you walk
- Protruding bones or not enough flesh to cushion the bones of your feet.

Signs and Symptoms

- A hard, tough area of thickened skin. It is usually yellow, but it may become red when irritated or inflamed.
- Tenderness or pain under the skin
- Sensitivity to pressure

Conventional Treatments

Standard care for a corn involves removing the source of friction or pressure on the area. Change to more comfortable, foot-friendly shoes and use a special shoe insole for added cushioning. You can also apply a special sock or protective sheath over the corn.

Corns are made of keratin, thickened skin that forms as a protective padding in response to outside pressure. You can dissolve the keratin layer by covering it with salicylic acid paste and applying a foam pad to protect it from friction. You can also use a pumice stone after bathing to debride it. If you prefer, a podiatrist can shave the corn down with a scalpel.

Dietary Strategies (See Chapter 14 for food sources of specified nutrients)

Vitamins A and E
These vitamins encourage healthy skin.

Vitamin C
This vitamin encourages healing.

Supplements

To encourage healing you can take:

- Vitamin A—the acceptable daily dose range is 900 to 3,000 mcg.
- Vitamin E—the acceptable daily dose range is 15 to 1,000 mg.

Herbal Creams and Ointments

Tea tree (Maleluca alternifolia) *mix*
Mix 4 drops of tea tree oil, 3 drops bergamot oil, 3 drops lavender oil, and 2 teaspoons of jojoba oil. Dab onto the affected area. This helps provide pain relief while softening up your corn and preventing infection.

Goldenseal (Hydrastis canadensis) *cream*
This herb has astringent, anti-inflammatory properties. Used topically, it can prevent infection and speed healing.

Do-It-Yourself

- Always wear loose comfortable shoes with a wide toe box.
- Use a file or pumice stone to rub down a corn. This works best if you first take a bath or soak your foot in water. You can also use fresh lemon juice or vinegar to soften the skin. Repeat this process daily until the corn disappears. Use a pad or a piece of moleskin, available at any drugstore, to cover the area and prevent another corn from forming.

Red Flags

Call your doctor if you see any signs of infection, including:

· Redness
· Swelling
· Fever
· Discharge

HAMMERTOE

Description

Hammertoe usually involves the second toe, which bends under, and takes on a cramped, hammer, or clawlike appearance. As the toe bends, it may rub against the top of your shoe, causing painful, hard corns to develop.

Causes

Hammertoe is often a congenital condition, but other contributing factors include:

· Wearing shoes that are too tight or too narrow. This causes the second toe to buckle
· A flat front arch
· A bunion, which may cause the big toe to slide under the second toe
· Muscle and nerve damage from diabetes or other diseases

Signs and Symptoms

· A toe that bends under
· A callus or hard corn on top of the toe
· Redness and inflammation
· Pain at the tip of the toe, where it hits your shoe

Conventional Treatments

It's especially important to wear shoes that don't cramp your toes. You can also tape the affected toe to an adjacent toe to maintain their proper alignment. A lambswool insert or a splint can also keep your toes in position.

Hammertoe is not especially painful, but you can take ibuprofen, acetaminophen, or aspirin to relieve pain or inflammation, if necessary. Available in pharmacies are small, doughnut-shaped pads you can wear on top of the toe to reduce friction and irritation.

In extreme cases, surgery may be needed to straighten the toe or remove any bony prominence that develops on top of it.

Do-It-Yourself

- Be sure your shoes are roomy, with a wide toe box
- Take an evening foot bath
- Stretch out your toe
- Try taping the affected toe to an adjacent toe
- Consider wearing sneakers or running shoes as often as possible

Exercise

Exercises that stretch your toes may provide some relief. For example:

PICK UP MARBLES
1. Obtain a set of marbles and set them out on the floor.
2. One by one, pick up the marbles with your toes and deposit them into a 16-inch Styrofoam cup.

TOWEL PICKUP
Lay a towel flat on the floor and, keeping your heel in the air, use just your toes to move it toward you and crumple it up. When it becomes too easy, put a book or some other weight on the towel.

Red Flags

- Worsening deformity
- A wound or open abrasion from pressure on the toe
- Difficulty walking

PLANTAR FASCIITIS AND ARCH PAIN

Description

The plantar fascia is a broad band of connective tissue that runs along the bottom of the foot, from the ball to the heel. It helps to maintain the arch of the foot. If you overstretch it, small painful tears and inflammation may develop.

Runners and other athletes are particularly prone to plantar fasciitis, which is one of the most common causes of painful feet I see in my practice. It frequently strikes people over fifty, developing twice as often in women as in men.

Sometimes, plantar fasciitis becomes chronic and severe, even disabling. About half the time, bone spurs develop near the front of the heel, causing a related ailment known as heel spur syndrome.

Plantar fasciitis is also the most common cause of arch pain (sometimes called arch strain). What happens is the tissue pulls away from the heel, causing pain, inflammation, and a burning sensation at the arch of the foot. Arch pain may also develop if you have a structural abnormality such as flat feet.

Causes

While overuse is the usual cause of plantar fasciitis, there are others:

- Flat feet or overpronation
- Suddenly increasing how much you run, especially up and down hills
- High arches
- Bowlegs
- Knock-knees
- Differences in leg length
- Poor running shoes

Signs and Symptoms

- Pain and tenderness, especially in the front of your heel and your arch
- Local swelling in the affected area
- More pain in the morning, just after you get up, or after periods of rest
- Pain increases when you walk, run, or do anything else that puts pressure on your feet

Conventional Treatments

You can take anti-inflammatory medications, such as aspirin or ibuprofen, for the pain and swelling. Acetaminophen relieves pain but not inflammation. If you get no relief, your doctor may recommend a steroid injection, which will provide immediate relief. But there are side effects, including local trauma, bleeding, or black-and-blue marks. I discourage repeated (more than three times a year) injections with steroids.

Your doctor may also recommend that you be fitted for arch supports or orthotics to treat flat feet.

If this ailment becomes severe or chronic, you may require surgery.

Do-It-Yourself

- Wear comfortable shoes with thick soles.
- Put cushioned heel lifts or heel cups in your shoes; this shifts your weight forward and cushions the sore spot; a shoe with a *slightly* elevated heel — ½ to 1 inch — will do the same thing.
- Use arch supports, which will limit the movement of your plantar fascia and allow it to heal.
- Roll an old-fashioned glass soda bottle, a rolling pin, or a foot roller back and forth with the sole of your bare foot.

Exercise

- Take a break from any activity that involves pounding. Switch to swimming, biking, or another sport that is kind to your feet.
- Once pain has subsided, resume your regular exercise slowly. If you feel any pain, stop.
- Meanwhile, to speed healing, try these exercises: Plantar Fascia Stretch, Gastroc Stretch, Soleus Stretch, and Bicycle Stretch. (See pages 331–338.)

Red Flags

- Worsening pain
- Inability to walk

MISCELLANEOUS FOOT AILMENTS AND HELPFUL REMEDIES

- Horsechestnut (*Aesculus hippocastanum*), used both externally and internally, helps leg swelling and circulatory disorders. Used as a lotion, it helps to heal leg ulcers. The seed coating can be toxic, so peel them if you are making remedies yourself.
- Tea tree oil, oil of bitter orange, peppermint oil, and garlic are useful treatments for athlete's foot.

12
—

Unending Pain

Pain is aptly labeled the most vicious of all evils. I was intimately acquainted with the terrific torment of chronic pain when, several years ago, my mother was stricken with terminal cancer during the prime of her life. Like many advanced cancer patients, Mom endured the torture and indignity of excruciating pain with a delicate blend of stoicism, melancholy, cautious optimism, and a strong will to overcome.

As each day brought her a fresh onslaught of demonic pain, I came to realize the power of complementary medical approaches. My mother received world-class care from her doctors. Yet, when I reflect back, I see that their conventional approaches to managing her pain included little creativity or innovation. Notwithstanding their stalwart and compassionate pleas to us to rely exclusively on narcotic painkillers to do the trick, I knew better. Traditional painkillers were okay in small measure, but they were by no means a sole solution.

My philosophy was shaped by my conviction that chronic pain, especially cancer pain, demands a holistic approach incorporating the best in nutrition, mind-body techniques, acupuncture, and other complementary strategies. These therapies fortify your spirit and give you the strength and resolve to endure.

Recognizing the critical yet intangible link between environment and healing, my wife, Marlene, insisted that we move my mom to our house. A budding clinical nutritionist and biologist with a flare for creative, healthful cooking, Marlene developed several customized therapeutic recipes, based on a thorough review of the literature. Motivated by the work of the acclaimed scientist Dr. Judah Folkman, the father of the angiogenesis theory of cancer—which posits that starving cancer cells of their blood supply helps wage the war against cancer—my wife used many soy products in her prescriptives. Soy products contain genistein, which may act by inhibiting

endothelial growth (the inner cell lining) of capillarie
velopment of blood vessels to aid tumor tissue.

We found music therapy to be a wonderful way
mother's spirits during the painful and dark days she
going chemotherapy and radiation. Although she was
ually diminished in intensity, and her days became m
used exercise, acupuncture, and "grandchildren therapy." I observed first-
hand the power of mind over body: snug in our family's nest, my mother
kept herself alive for several months so she could welcome the birth of her
youngest grandchild.

Cancer pain is but one of many types of unending pain. Although it's
often impossible to cure chronic pain, there's a lot you can do to ease your
misery, discouragement, and frustration. Taking something positive from a
very challenging time in the life of my family, I now use complementary
therapies as an adjunct to conventional modes of treatment to help em-
power my chronic pain patients. And I should add that many patients are
well ahead of their doctors on this issue; more than 50 percent of cancer
patients use complementary therapies, and a U.S telephone survey found
that cancer was one of the top five reasons for using alternative medicine.

CANCER PAIN

Cancer is a chronic illness that can occur anywhere in the body. Up until
ten or twenty years ago, a cancer cell was a black box. Today, scientists
know a great deal about carcinogenesis—the development of cancer. Still,
the antidote to cancer pain remains a mystery.

Today's researchers, using the techniques of cellular and molecular biology, look at the fundamental mechanisms that underlie cancer. The target
of research is DNA, which makes up the genetic material, or building
blocks, of the body's cells. In each cell, genes encode the proteins necessary
to perform all body functions. For some reason—spontaneously, as a result
of environmental damage, or even because of viral infection—genetic
changes, or mutations, occur in a normal cell. There may be many varieties
of cancer, but in all cases, something that is supposed to limit a cell's growth
has broken down. Instead of growing and replicating normally, the cell
becomes malignant. Your body has "fail-safe" mechanisms to destroy these
abnormal cells, but they don't always work. So malignant cells may begin
to accumulate. At some point, they reach a critical mass that is identified
clinically as a tumor growth. Finally, the cancerous cells become invasive,
entering the bloodstream to metastasize at other sites in the body. Pain is

ᴐehind. The pain associated with cancer can be ravaging, and if left
ᴐated, can become all-consuming.

Despite three decades and billions of dollars spent on research, the war
on cancer has not produced a "cure." That's because cancer has many
forms; it is not a single virus, like polio. Yet, many types are curable, if
detected and treated early.

Causes

When you consider cancer pain, it's important to recall the old adage: an
ounce of prevention is worth a pound of cure. Preventing cancer by con-
sidering its causes and modifying your risk factors is an ideal way to avert
the disaster of cancer pain. There is no one cause of cancer, or the pain
that derives from it.

Signs and Symptoms

Although these depend largely on where the cancer is located, common
symptoms include:

- A lump or thickening
- A wound that doesn't heal
- Unexplained weight loss
- Night sweats or unremitting fevers
- Pain that is present at night and when at rest

Conventional Treatments

There are three major conventional treatments for cancer. These invasive
and difficult-to-endure approaches are intended to shrink tumor bulk,
thereby decreasing pain and minimizing functional impairment. They may
be used on their own or in combination:

Surgery to remove abnormal cells

In addition to traditional surgery, your doctor may use cryosurgery, where
liquid nitrogen is applied to freeze tumors. This technique is used especially
for skin cancer. With laser surgery, the doctor uses a high-intensity light
beam to destroy cancer cells.

Radiation to shrink and destroy tumors

Radiation may be used by itself or in addition to surgery. Treatment involves
regular exposure, every day or every couple of days, for several weeks. You

may be treated with a machine that emits radiation or with an internal radiation source that is implanted in the body. Often, shrinkage of a tumor leads to a considerable reduction in pain, especially if the tumor is pressing on the spinal cord and neighboring roots.

Chemotherapy, or drugs that kill cancer cells
You may undergo chemotherapy by taking pills or injections, or having the chemicals infused intravenously. Chemotherapy usually goes on for two to twelve months. Then your body is given time to recover from the often-severe side effects, the most common of which are nausea and hair loss.

The following complementary approaches are meant to be used in conjunction with conventional treatments, not instead of them. Whenever you use complementary treatments, it's important to keep your doctor informed.

Dietary Strategies (See Chapter 14 for food sources of specified nutrients)

It's been estimated by some experts that diet alone accounts for 60 percent of cancers in American women. To help prevent cancer:

- Eat at least five servings of fruits and vegetables every day, especially those with antioxidants, such as beta-carotene and vitamin C. Antioxidants help to counter the effects of free radicals, by-products of normal bodily processes that cause cell damage.
- The cruciferous (cabbage family) vegetables, including broccoli, cauliflower, cabbage, and brussels sprouts, also contain anticancer substances called indoles.
- A high-fiber diet speeds food through the intestines and contributes to regular bowel movements, thereby allowing the body to get rid of cancer-causing substances more rapidly. Fiber also appears to lower blood estrogen levels.
- Consuming flaxseeds or flaxseed oil is helpful, since it may have an antiestrogenlike effect.
- Cut back on animal fat from meat and dairy, which has been linked to higher rates of colorectal cancer. Instead, emphasize foods of plant origin. In addition to high levels of vitamins, minerals, and fibers, these foods contain phytonutrients that play a protective role in many cancers.
- You can also substitute fish for meat. A growing body of evidence shows that fish oils slow tumor growth.
- Eat foods containing vitamin E, which is an antioxidant that boosts your immune system and may prevent some cancers.

- Lycopene, found in tomatoes and pink grapefruits, may reduce your risk of cancer.
- Landmark research at the Johns Hopkins Hospital has shown the benefit of broccoli as an anticancer food.
- Soy can reduce the risk of hormone-related cancers. Soybeans contain estrogenlike compounds, called isoflavones (genistein and daidzein), which bind to estrogen sites and prevent your body's natural estrogen from attaching to these sites. In so doing, they may prevent stimulation and growth of cancer cells.
- Tart cherries have potential value in fighting cancer and cancer-associated pain because of their high concentrations of anthocyanins and bioflavonoids. These two potent antioxidants inhibit cyclooxygenase 1 and 2 in a way that is similar to aspirin, Naprosyn, and other NSAIDS. So promising is the potential therapeutic value of tart cherries that the National Institutes of Health (NIH) has awarded an $8 million grant to Johns Hopkins University to study the effects of tart cherries and soy on cancer pain.
- Eat berries — blueberries, blackberries, strawberries, and cherries are full of flavonoids and antioxidants.
- Eat pomegranate. This fruit is very rich in antioxidants and it appears to have enormous medicinal properties. Several universities are conducting clinical trials to evaluate its cancer-fighting potential. Interestingly, the healing power of the pomegranate is thought to be related to its stature as a sacred fruit in several major religions, including Judaism, Christianity, Buddhism, and Islam. In Judaism, the number of commandments — 613 — corresponds to the number of seeds in a pomegranate. And the ancient Greeks hailed it as a form of life and regeneration.

RECIPES

BERRY SMOOTHIE

Use organic fruits if possible.

1 cup frozen blueberries
1 cup frozen strawberries
1 banana
1 mango, peeled and pitted

1 *cup orange juice*
1 *cup tangerine juice*

Place all ingredients in a blender and mix thoroughly.

SERVES 6

POMEGRANATE-TANGERINE JUICE

Peel 4 pomegranates. Peel and pit 5 tangerines. Press the fruit in a citrus press.

SERVES 2

BRAN MUFFINS

3 *cups raisin bran cereal*
1 *cup sugar*
2½ *cups unbleached white flour*
2½ *teaspoons baking soda*
1 *teaspoon salt*
4 *egg whites*
⅓ *cup orange juice*
⅓ *cup olive oil*
1¾ *cup soy milk*
¼ *cup rolled oats*

1. Preheat oven to 375 degrees.
2. Lightly grease a muffin pan or line it with paper baking cups.
3. In a large mixing bowl combine cereal, sugar, flour, baking soda, and salt.
4. In a separate bowl, slightly beat the egg whites. Beat in the orange juice, oil, and soy milk. Stir in the dry ingredients and mix well.
5. Fill muffin pans ¾ full, and sprinkle the tops with rolled oats.
6. Bake at 375 degrees for 25 minutes.

MAKES ABOUT 12 MUFFINS

Dietary Supplements

To help prevent and fight cancer, try these supplements:

Selenium

In a double-blind study, half of the patients were given 200 mcg of selenium and followed for six years. They had a 50 percent reduction in overall cancer mortality, including significantly less lung, colon, and prostate cancer. The acceptable daily dose range is 60 to 400 mcg.

Vitamin C

Vitamin C (ascorbic acid), a powerful antioxidant, boosts your immune system and helps you fight cancer. In addition, a deficiency in vitamin C has been linked to certain types of tumors. The acceptable dose range is 90 to 2,000 mg a day. Spread it out over the course of the day for best results. This vitamin may cause diarrhea or cramps at high doses.

Zinc

Zinc facilitates more than three hundred enzymatic reactions in the body. A deficiency may lead to decreased immunity and impaired healing. The acceptable dose range is 8 to 40 mg a day.

Vitamin E

Another antioxidant that boosts your immune system, reduces fatigue, and accelerates healing, we also think vitamin E may prevent certain types of cancer. The acceptable daily dose range is 15 to 1,000 mg.

Folate

Research has shown that this nutrient, also known as folic acid, helps to prevent certain types of cancer. The acceptable dose ranges from 400 to 1,000 mcg a day.

Herbs

Garlic (Allium sativum)

Garlic has shown promising ability to inhibit or reverse growth of certain tumor cells. For example, one large observational study of nurses found that garlic consumption led to a 30 percent reduction in colon cancer. Garlic also reduces blood pressure and lowers cholesterol. Take garlic tablets, following the dose on the package. Or you can chop garlic and mix it with an equal amount of honey and take 1 teaspoon, three to six times a day.

Green tea (Camellia sinensis)

Polyphenols, the active ingredient in green tea, may detoxify carcinogens, so drinking this beverage can protect you against stomach, breast, lung, esophageal, pancreatic, colon, and duodenal cancers. Drink three cups a day.

Do-It-Yourself

Health habits

Prevent cancer with healthy habits:

- Quit smoking and/or avoid secondhand smoke
- Abstain from alcohol, or use it only in moderation
- Avoid overexposure to the sun; wear sunscreen
- Do monthly breast self-exams and regular mammograms
- Have regular gynecologic exams
- Drink plenty of water

Aromatherapy

Do not use essential oils as a massage immediately before or after chemotherapy because this can encourage the spread of cancer cells through the body. In the early stages of cancer, use oils only in a bath or diffuser.

- Rosemary (*Rosmarinus officinalis*) — for fatigue: Avoid this oil during pregnancy or if you have epilepsy or high blood pressure.
- Fennel (*Foeniculum vulgare*) — for nausea: Do not use fennel during pregnancy or if you have epilepsy.
- Geranium (*Pelargonium graveolens*) — for depression: Do not use during the first three months of pregnancy; if you have a history of miscarriage, do not use at all.

TENS (transcutaneous electrical nerve stimulation)

This therapy helps you manage pain by applying brief pulses of electricity that block pain messages to the brain. I've found it very helpful for my patients; studies show that it provides relief for 30 to 50 percent of people with chronic pain. Although this is often a conventional treatment, performed in a physician's or physical therapist's office, home units are available.

Seek support

I always refer my cancer patients to support groups. Those who go feel less overwhelmed by depression and hopelessness. Studies show that people in support groups experience psychological improvement, and tend to live longer than those who try to deal with cancer on their own. I believe that the positive change in outlook and mood helps bolster the immune system. Other forms of support include psychotherapy and creative arts therapy, especially music and painting.

Mind/Body

Meditation (See page 340)

Imagery (See page 341)

Yoga
Siddhasan (Perfect Posture), Kagasana (Crow Posture), and Shavasana (Corpse Posture) can ease muscles that may be tense from pain. They will also calm you, helping you fight depression, restlessness, and insomnia. (See pages 344–351 for postures.)

Autogenic training (see page 341)

Music therapy
My colleague Professor Mathew Lee, chairman of physical medicine and rehabilitation at New York University's prestigious Rusk Institute, has co-authored a book called *On Music for Health*. Dr. Lee, himself a cancer survivor, states that "Music is a joyful expression of life. We have witnessed the power of music. We have watched how music can lift our fallen spirits, enrich our busy minds and heal our battered bodies." I saw this in a direct and powerful way, as I watched my mother benefit from the beauty of Brahms during the painful throes of her struggle with terminal illness. My recommendation is that you listen to music that you love; music that penetrates your soul, whether it's songs from your childhood, Sondheim, or Schubert. If you're a musician, making music counts, too.

Exercise

My esteemed colleague and mentor, the late professor emeritus Heinz Lippman of the Albert Einstein College of Medicine in New York, used to joke that exercise allowed his old age to outlive his cancer. There is no doubt about the power and vitality of exercise. Even in the face of life-threatening illness, exercise helps you feel good. For example, in a ten-week randomized study of twenty-four breast cancer survivors, the women who did aerobic exercise four days a week had significantly less depression and anxiety over time compared to women in a control group.

You may not feel up to such a rigorous regimen. But I still recommend that you do as much light aerobic exercise as you can tolerate. For physical and spiritual healing, many of my patients enjoy light gardening or taking time to walk around, appreciate nature, and smell the roses.

Seeking Help from Complementary Practitioners

Hypnotherapy
In studies of breast and other cancers, self-hypnosis reduced pain and suffering more effectively than therapy groups and other supportive treatments. Once you learn how, you can use this technique on your own.

Acupuncture
Acupuncture is a scientifically validated method for relieving the nausea of chemotherapy.

Red Flags

See your doctor if you have:

- Persisting fevers
- Weakness
- Malaise
- Intractable nausea and vomiting

CHRONIC FATIGUE SYNDROME (CFS)

Description

The subject of controversy for a long time, chronic fatigue syndrome used to be dismissed as "psychosomatic" or imaginary. Since the late 1980s, when the Centers for Disease Control first acknowledged it, CFS has gained acceptance as a legitimate diagnosis. Women with CFS outnumber men by two to one, and it is especially common among women between the ages of eighteen and thirty-five.

CFS is a collection of many clinical features. Symptoms linger for months and sometimes never go away completely. Instead, they periodically come and go with no apparent reason. One of the most salient hallmarks of CFS is pain. This is a miserable illness that causes unexplained, persistent, or relapsing pain. It is not due to overexertion; nor is it relieved by rest. But it is usually so bad that it forces you to reduce your activity level.

According to a small, recently published study, if you have chronic fatigue syndrome, you may be at higher risk of developing other health problems, including fibromyalgia (CFS shares some features with fibromyalgia; see page 296), irritable bowel syndrome, chronic pelvic pain, and temporomandibular disorder (see Chapter 9). CFS sufferers bear other costs as well—high unemployment and disability rates, and large health care expenses.

We make a diagnosis of CFS if someone has at least four of the following:

- Muscle pain
- Pain in many joints, but without inflammation or infection
- Headache
- Sore throat
- Tender lymph nodes in your neck or armpit
- Poor sleep pattern
- Generalized weakness, caused by physical exertion, that lasts more than twenty-four hours
- Problems with memory or concentration

Causes

The roots of CFS are still being debated. It seems, however, to be a complex interaction of biological, psychological, and environmental factors. Researchers are investigating possible viral infections, including herpes, polio, and Epstein-Barr. Some experts think it may stem from damage to the immune system, while others believe it is a psychological or neurological disorder.

Signs and Symptoms

- Extreme fatigue
- Fever
- Headache
- Nausea
- Dizziness
- Muscle and joint pain
- Sleeping problems
- Depression

- Memory loss
- Sore throat
- Tender lymph nodes

Conventional Treatments

Many physicians find CFS baffling and difficult to deal with. Drugs are the usual conventional answer. Your doctor will probably recommend traditional pain medications including NSAIDS, such as ibuprofen or naproxen. If you have allergy-type symptoms, you'll be given antihistamines and decongestants. And to improve your energy and mood, your physician may prescribe Prozac, Zoloft, amitriptyline, or other antidepressants.

Dietary Strategies (See Chapter 14 for food sources of specified nutrients)

Elimination/challenge diet
Sometimes food allergies cause or contribute to CFS. The most common allergies are dairy products and wheat. Try avoiding all dairy products for two weeks and then reintroduce them, noting your response. This is called an elimination/challenge. Keep a diary and see if your symptoms improve while you are off dairy products; then watch what happens when you start eating them again. You can repeat the same process with wheat and/or with any other foods that appear to aggravate your symptoms.

Bromelain (See page 324)

Vitamin B6
This nutrient increases the brain's production of a chemical that helps control pain.

Astragalus (Astragalus membranaceus)
This perennial plant in the pea family strengthens the immune system. To make an immune-enhancing broth that you can use as a stock for vegetable soup or for cooking brown rice, simmer 1 ounce (25 grams) of chopped astragalus root in a pint of water. Drink one cup every day.

Mustard (Synapse arvensis)
As an herb, mustard is useful for relieving depression and melancholy. I prefer you use it in its nutritional form, in recipes or as a condiment.

Olive (Olea europea) and olive oil
These small, evergreen fruits are the source of olive oil. They help fight extreme fatigue and exhaustion.

Supplements

B-complex vitamins
For a healthy nervous system and more energy, take one pill a day.

Evening primrose oil (EPO) (Oenothera biennis)
This is a type of essential fatty acid that is available as capsules or as an oil. Take 500 mg a day.

Acidophilus (Lactobacillus acidophilus)
Because chronic yeast infections may have a connection to CFS, it's a good idea to take these "friendly" bacteria, often found in high-quality yogurt, that help to prevent yeast overgrowth in your body. Acidophilus is also available in tablets, and it's safe and nontoxic. Follow dosage on the package.

NADH (nicotinamide adenine dinucleotide)
This is a natural chemical that helps the cells produce energy. Some research has shown an improvement in symptoms after patients took 10 mg a day for four weeks. However, the research is not yet strong enough for me to endorse its use.

Carnitine
This is another substance that occurs naturally in the body. It converts fatty acids into energy. Some researchers have found that supplements relieve CFS symptoms. I have not seen enough solid research to recommend it.

Herbs

Echinacea (Echinacea angustifolia, Echinacea purpurea)
This popular remedy, made from purple coneflowers, has been proven, in well-constructed, double-blind, placebo-controlled research, to reduce the symptoms, frequency, and duration of colds. Because its effects are attributed to stimulation of the immune system, it has been touted as a treatment for CFS. Laboratory studies have proven that it can increase antibody production and bolster cellular immune function. Recommended dose is 1 cup of tea or 1 teaspoon of tincture three times a day.

Ginseng root (Panax ginseng, Eleutherococcus senticosus)
This tonic herb increases energy and strengthens the immune system. Herbalists suggest 3 cups of tea a day. Do not take ginseng during pregnancy, or if you have high blood pressure.

Gingko (Gingko biloba)
This herb, which is actually leaves from the maidenhair tree, improves blood flow, boosts energy, and acts as an anti-inflammatory. Recommended dose is 3 cups of tea a day. Tablets are also available; follow dosing listed on the package.

Licorice (Glycyrrhiza glabra)
No, it's not just a candy. This healing root stimulates white blood cell formation and helps the body heal itself. It also, however, raises blood pressure, so avoid regular use if you have hypertension. Recommended dose is 3 cups of tea a day if your symptoms are acute; use half that dose for chronic ailments.

Exercise

A study in the *British Medical Journal* found that patients who were put on a program of mild-to-moderate aerobic activity (walking, cycling, or swimming) for thirty minutes, five days a week reported less fatigue. I suggest that you do thirty minutes of brisk walking or bike riding at least three times weekly.

Do-It-Yourself

Aromatherapy
Here are three choices of essential oils, and several methods for using them:

- Neroli (Orange Blossom, *Citrus aurantium var. amara*), a blossom from the bitter orange tree, and bergamot (*Citrus aurantium bergamia*), the oil from the fruit of a bergamot tree, will help to lift your spirits.
- Tea Tree (*Maleluca alternifolia*) works against infection and strengthens the immune system.

Methods:

- Add five to ten drops of the oil to your bath.
- Steam inhalation: add three to four drops of oil to a pot of boiling

water, cover your head with a towel, bend over the pot, and breathe deeply for a few minutes.

· Add six to eight drops of oil to the water in a vaporizer.
· Make a massage blend (for neroli only): Add 3 drops of neroli, 3 drops of celery, and 4 drops of rose to 5 teaspoons of grapeseed or vegetable oil. Use it to massage sore, aching parts of your body.

Mind/Body

Yoga
Siddhasan (Perfect Posture), Vajrasana (Adamantine Posture), and Virasana (Hero's Posture) ease pain, encourage relaxation, and fight depression. (See pages 344–351 for postures.)

Meditation (See Chapter 18)

Red Flags

Call your doctor if you have:

· Fever
· Malaise
· Depression
· Weight loss

FIBROMYALGIA

NATALIE'S STORY

Natalie, a woman in her late thirties, came to see me late one November afternoon. "I have fibromyalgia and I'm in constant pain — in my muscles, in my back, all over," she confessed. I could see the distress in her eyes as she peppered me with questions: "My family doctor told me it's all in my mind. Do you agree? I toss and turn all night — I feel like a rotisserie chicken — and I'm exhausted all the time. Is there anything I can do? Am I just going to feel lousy forever? I'm stressed out. I'm so morose all the time, my friends barely want to see me. Should I take antidepressants?"

It was clear after a few minutes that I was another stop on Natalie's doctor merry-go-round. For months she'd been going from one specialist to another, looking for answers. But she still hadn't found what she wanted—advice on taking charge of her pain.

On examination, it was obvious that Natalie did indeed have pain in multiple tender points—a clear case of fibromyalgia. She was also overweight, which put additional stress on her back. Although she had considerable chronic back and shoulder pain, that didn't mean she needed surgery, as one doctor had suggested. I told her that complementary strategies might be the answer to her problems.

We started by talking about proper nutrition and the role it plays in weight loss. In addition, some research suggests that nutrients like magnesium, 5-HTP (5-hydroxytryptophan), vitamin B1, vitamin E, SAMe, and malic acid might lessen the chronic fatigue, sleep disturbances, and muscle pain of fibromyalgia. Because a healthy diet rich in vegetables, fruits, and other whole foods contains many of these nutrients, a well-planned diet can actually decrease pain.

I also explained to her that vitamins C and E play a healing role by promoting the vitality and longevity of collagen and soft tissues. In addition, calcium, along with vitamin D and the amino acid lysine, improves the durability of bony structures. I reminded Natalie that drinking plenty of water (with a squeeze or two of lemon to enhance taste) helps to fend off dehydration, and promotes important chemical reactions in the body. And I recommended that she try soy foods, since cutting-edge research done at Johns Hopkins suggests that soy protein may promote pain relief.

Next, we discussed body mechanics. "Every step you take places stress on your joints and spine, and the problem is exacerbated if you are overweight," I told her. Natalie might benefit from shoe orthotics, which would act as shock absorbers, protecting her back from repeated strain.

I asked Natalie whether and how much she exercised. "I haven't exercised in months because I'm afraid it will hurt too much," she revealed. I urged her to take up swimming, which would help her lose weight. And far from making things worse, once she got started, the exercise would actually help her feel better. Releasing and mobilizing endorphins through exercise is a time-tested, surefire way to relieve pain.

Exercise also lessens anxiety and relieves depression. As I told Natalie, rock-solid research on the mind-body connection has shown that a more positive outlook reduces pain. Besides, I told her: "Starting and then sticking with an exercise regimen will make you feel better about yourself. When your self-esteem is restored, you'll be surprised how your pain takes less of a toll."

Regular exercise would also help Natalie in another way. Like many women with fibromyalgia, she had trouble sleeping. "I often have to take strong medications to get to sleep, and I hate the way they make me feel in the morning," she confided. I described how she could use meditation and visual imagery to relax, and recommended regular infusions of chamomile tea, an effective and gentle aid to sleep.

After a few months, Natalie came back, looking much better. She had lost 12 pounds. She told me: "I swim every other day and I've been watching my diet. I'm practicing meditation, too. I'm sleeping like a baby again and I can't believe how much better I feel. Best of all, I'm in charge of my own destiny."

Description

This poorly understood and often misdiagnosed disease occurs nine times more often in women than in men. If you have fibromyalgia, you're part of a large sorority—3.4 percent of women suffer from this malady, and the figure rises to 7 percent for women between sixty and seventy-nine.

Fibromyalgia is characterized by widespread, long-term, musculoskeletal pain. Typically, people with fibromyalgia "ache all over." Long dismissed as psychosomatic, it is now accepted as a bona fide disease. The American College of Rheumatology has established criteria for its diagnosis. These include widespread pain on both sides of the body for at least three months in eleven of eighteen "tender points." Tender points are located in the muscles of the upper neck, back, shoulders, and hips. According to these criteria, fibromyalgia is the second most common diagnosis in rheumatology clinics, right after osteoarthritis.

Causes

There are some fascinating clues, but no answer, to the question: What causes fibromyalgia? It does not appear to be an inflammatory disease or a degenerative disorder. Nor has a virus been clearly implicated. Many fibro-myalgia patients have had other ailments, such as chronic fatigue syndrome (see page 291), chronic headaches, irritable bowel syndrome, or depression. They also have intriguing physical abnormalities—some patients have changes in nervous system chemicals, such as substance P or peptides that are related to pain. Others report that they had physical or emotional trauma, or an infection, such as Lyme disease, before they developed fibro-myalgia. Still, the mystery remains.

Signs and Symptoms

Pain is just part of the fibromyalgia picture. The full range of symptoms includes:

- Mild aches to incapacitating pain
- Chronic, stiff, aching muscles
- Chronic headaches
- Depression
- Sleep disturbances
- Fatigue
- Morning stiffness
- Co-existing conditions, including chronic fatigue syndrome (see page 291), irritable bowel syndrome, depression, and other forms of arthritis
- Stress, inappropriate exercise, and weather can worsen the symptoms

Conventional Treatments

Fibromyalgia is a perplexing ailment that conventional physicians treat with medications and, sometimes, psychological counseling. Your doctor will probably recommend traditional pain medications including NSAIDS, such as ibuprofen or naproxen. To improve energy and mood and help you sleep, your physician may also prescribe Prozac, Zoloft, amitriptyline, or other antidepressants. Sleeping pills, antianxiety medications, and muscle relaxants are other possible treatments.

Trigger point injections—injections of a local anesthetic directly into painful spots—may help.

Dietary Strategies (See Chapter 14 for food sources of specified nutrients)

- Eat a healthy diet, emphasizing fruits, vegetables, and whole grains. These foods contain nutrients that can promote healing and reduce pain.
- Eat foods containing vitamins C and E, which boost healing.
- For strong bones, be sure to get enough calcium and vitamin D.
- Limit caffeine and alcohol, which interfere with sleep.
- Eat apples and drink their juice. Apples are high in malic acid, a sub-

stance that has been shown in some preliminary studies to be helpful for fibromyalgia.

· Include soy foods in your diet. Preliminary research has shown that soy protein may help relieve pain.

Supplements

SAMe (S-adenosyl methionine)

SAMe is a natural substance produced from methionine, an amino acid, and adenosine triphosphate (ATP), a metabolic chemical associated with energy production. It can reduce pain and fatigue as well as morning stiffness. SAMe is also an antidepressant. The dose is 400 to 800 mg a day. Be aware, however, that in large doses, it can upset the stomach. Do not take SAMe if you take levodopa for Parkinson's disease. This nutrient may trigger manic episodes in people with bipolar disease.

5-HTP (5-hydroxytryptophan)

This supplement has been shown to decrease the number of tender points and improve sleep patterns, morning stiffness, and fatigue. The dose is 100 to 300 mg a day. Do not take this with antidepressants.

Herbs

St. John's wort (Hypericum perforatum)

For depression and increased tolerance to pain the recommended dose is 300 mg three times a day.

Do-It-Yourself

Aromatherapy (See Chronic Fatigue Syndrome, page 291)

Mind/Body

Yoga

Siddhasan (Perfect Posture) and Virasana (Hero's Posture) ease pain, encourage relaxation, and fight depression. (See pages 344–351 for postures.)

Meditation (See Chapter 18)

Exercise

If you have fibromyalgia, it's easy to get caught in a vicious cycle. You're in pain, so you don't exercise. But not exercising weakens your muscles, and unused muscles are more likely to be vulnerable to pain. It's important to keep your muscles moving, so I recommend low-impact aerobic conditioning exercises, such as swimming or using a stationary bike. Gentle stretching exercises, like the ones below, will improve your general flexibility.

ELBOW CIRCLE
1. With your elbows bent, slowly lift your arms up.
2. On both sides, bring your fingertips up to the tops of your shoulders and point your elbows straight out to the sides.
3. Move your elbows in circles. Begin with small movements and progress to large circles.

HIP ROTISSERIE
1. With feet spread apart, place your hands on your hips, with your thumbs in front.
2. Slowly move your hips from side to side four times.
3. Then, move your hips forward and backward four times.

Seeking Help from Complementary Practitioners

Acupuncture
I've found this therapy to be extremely helpful with my fibromyalgia patients. The massive outpouring of endorphins triggered by needling reduces the pain.

Massage therapy
A good massage can ease stiffness in your muscles and deactivate tender points. In addition, it will help you relax, which will make it easier to get to sleep.

Red Flags

- Persisting pains
- Fever
- Weight loss

MYOFASCIAL PAIN SYNDROME (MPS)

Description

MPS is sometimes confused with fibromyalgia, and indeed, they are similar. Both are characterized by chronic pain in the muscle tissues. But the pain of MPS is localized, not widespread, as it is in fibromyalgia. And MPS affects men and women equally.

Myofascial pain syndrome is a neuromuscular condition that involves inflammation and irritation of the muscles and their supportive tissue, or fascial, lining. The myofascial tissues become thickened and lose elasticity, and you develop trigger points. These sensitive, sore areas in the muscle or the junction of the muscle and fascia are tender and painful to the touch. They also cause referred pain; in other words, when pressure is applied, you feel pain at that point *and* elsewhere in your body. This is in contrast to the "tender points" of fibromyalgia, which cause local discomfort only.

Causes

You may develop or be predisposed to MPS for a variety of reasons:

- Sudden trauma to musculoskeletal tissues (muscles, ligaments, tendons, bursae)
- Injury to an intervertebral disc
- Poor posture that results in muscle overload or spasm
- Generalized fatigue
- Repetitive motions, excessive exercise, or muscle strain due to over-activity
- Systemic conditions, such as gallbladder inflammation, heart attack, appendicitis, or stomach irritation
- Underlying metabolic or endocrine problems, such as thyroid disease
- Inactivity—for example, having a broken arm in a sling
- Nutritional deficiencies, including anemia
- Hormonal changes—you may develop trigger points during PMS or menopause

- Nervous tension or stress
- Getting a chill somewhere on your body—for example, sitting under an air-conditioning duct or sleeping in front of an air conditioner
- Sleep deprivation
- Medications, including narcotics

Signs and Symptoms

The major symptom of MPS is localized and referred pain from trigger points. Here's a look at the differences between MPS and fibromyalgia:

Symptoms	FMS	MPS
Pain	Diffuse	Local
Fatigue	Common	Uncommon
Morning stiffness	Common	Uncommon
Tender points	X	
Trigger points		X
Prognosis	Chronic	Resolves with treatment

Conventional Treatments

You may be given anti-inflammatory medications and/or tricyclic antidepressants, such as amitryptyline, for the pain. Otherwise, physical therapy and other conventional treatments for MPS focus directly on the trigger points. One option is trigger point therapy, also known as myofascial release therapy, myotherapy, or massotherapy, a form of medical massage therapy done by a physiatrist or other medical doctor. A physical therapist or physiatrist may do spray and stretch. She will start by applying a vapocoolant spray to your trigger points to reduce the pain; then she will stretch the affected muscles.

Some treatments mechanically disrupt the trigger point. Trigger point injections involve injecting a local anesthetic, such as lidocaine, directly into the trigger points. Dry needling does the same thing but without injecting any substances. The use of lidocaine is no more effective, but it does reduce the soreness after the injections.

Dietary Strategies (See Chapter 14 for food sources of specific nutrients)

- Vitamin B6 increases the brain's production of a chemical that helps control pain.
- Be sure to eat plenty of fruits and vegetables to prevent nutritional deficiencies.
- Drink at least eight 8-ounce glasses of water a day.

Supplements

5-HTP (5-hydroxytryptophan)

This supplement may decrease trigger point discomfort. The dose is 100 to 300 mg a day. Do not take this with antidepressants or serotonin-acting medications, like Ultram (tramadol) or Ambien (zolpidem tartrate).

SAMe (S-adenosyl methionine)

A natural substance produced from methionine, an amino acid, and adenosine triphosphate (ATP), SAMe is a metabolic chemical associated with energy production. It can reduce pain and fatigue as well as morning stiffness. SAMe is also an antidepressant. The dose is 400 to 800 mg a day. Be aware, however, that in large doses it can upset your stomach. Do not take SAMe if you take levodopa for Parkinson's disease. This nutrient may trigger manic episodes if you have bipolar disease.

Herbs

Gingko (Gingko biloba)

This herb, the leaves of the maidenhair tree, improves blood flow, boosts energy, and has anti-inflammatory properties. The recommended dose is 3 cups of tea a day. Tablets are also available; follow dosing on the package.

Valerian (Valeriana officinalis)

This herb helps calm the nervous system, relieving insomnia and anxiety. Herbalists suggest 2 or 3 cups of tea a day.

St. John's wort (Hypericum perforatum)

For depression and increased tolerance to pain, the recommended dose is 300 mg three times a day.

Do-It-Yourself

Aromatherapy
- Neroli (Orange Blossom, *Citrus aurantium var. amara*), a blossom from the bitter orange tree, and bergamot (*Citrus aurantium bergamia*), the oil from the fruit of a bergamot tree, will help to lift your spirits.

Methods:
- Add five to ten drops of the oil to your bath.
- Steam inhalation: add three to four drops of oil to a pot of boiling water, cover your head with a towel, bend over the pot, and breathe deeply for a few minutes.
- Add six to eight drops of oil to the water in a vaporizer.
- Make a massage blend (for neroli only): Add 3 drops of neroli, 3 drops of celery, and 4 drops of rose to 5 teaspoons of grapeseed or vegetable oil and use it to massage sore, aching parts of your body.

- Rosemary (*Rosmarinus officinalis*) helps prevent fatigue. Use this oil on a compress or to massage tender spots. Avoid during pregnancy, or if you have epilepsy or high blood pressure.
- Geranium (*Pelargonium graveolens*), for depression. Use geranium in a bath or a diffuser. Do not use it during the first three months of pregnancy, and do not use it at all if you are pregnant and have a history of miscarriage.
- Shower rub—To make an invigorating shower rub, add two drops of rosemary oil, two drops of pine oil, and four drops of lemon oil to a small dollop of unscented shower gel. Work it into a lather with a sponge and use on your sore, aching muscles.

Mind/Body

Meditation (See Chapter 18)

Yoga
Try Kagasana (Crow Posture), Boat Pose, and Bow Pose. (See pages 344–351 for postures.)

Seeking Help from Complementary Practitioners

- Massage and chiropractic may help relax muscle tissues and relieve pain
- Acupuncture is also helpful for pain relief

Red Flags

Call your doctor if you experience:

- Persisting sleep disturbances
- Weight loss
- Night sweats
- Fever
- Worsening depression

CHRONIC PAIN

Chronic pain, or pain that continues for six months or more, is more common than you might think. In a recent survey, one in five Americans reported suffering from chronic pain, and seven in ten said the pain interfered with their daily life. Women suffer somewhat more frequently from chronic pain, and they are more likely to become depressed as a result.

Chronic pain ranges from mild to disabling, and it can last from six months to many years. It may be the result of an injury or disease, but it is sometimes difficult to find its cause. Whatever its source, chronic pain often becomes a problem in and of itself, one that overwhelms other symptoms you may have. If you are in constant, long-term pain, you run the risk of falling into what we call the "terrible triad" of suffering, sleeplessness, and sadness. Your appetite falls off and physical activity seems impossible. You may become preoccupied with your pain, depressed, and irritable. Because of your inability to control it, chronic pain can cause low self-esteem and a sense of helplessness. Trouble sleeping aggravates an already miserable situation. And on top of this, you may have side effects from medications, mounting medical expenses, problems getting to work, and strains in your closest personal relationships.

Causes

There are countless reasons why you may develop chronic pain, and sometimes we can't pinpoint any source. Common causes include:

- Improperly treated acute pain
- Chronic diseases or syndromes, such as arthritis, endometriosis, headaches, fibromyalgia, cancer, and interstitial cystitis
- Gastrointestinal diseases and disorders, such as irritable bowel syndrome

- Failed joint or back surgeries
- Back or neck pain from nerve damage, joint problems, muscle loss, osteoporosis, herniated disk, or other sources
- Overuse injuries, often in your hands and wrists, from computer use or other repetitive motions
- Chronic nerve syndromes. These include complex regional pain syndrome, an intense, long-lasting nerve injury with pain, typically in an arm or leg; peripheral neuropathy, which causes tingling, numbness, and pain in your hands and feet; and postherpetic neuralgia, which is nerve damage resulting from a viral infection.
- Dental, nerve, or joint problems may cause mouth, jaw, and facial pain.

Conventional Treatments

Of course, treatment depends on the cause of the pain. A thorough, holistic medical assessment of a chronic pain condition is best performed by a physiatrist (a physical medicine and rehabilitation specialist), who can oversee your comprehensive pain management program.

Analgesics, including aspirin, acetaminophen (Tylenol), and NSAIDS, are a first line of defense. Your doctor may also prescribe other, more potent painkillers. Physical or occupational therapy may be options. TENS, a treatment that uses electrical charges to block pain messages, may also be of some help.

Occasionally, when more conservative measures have failed, your doctor may propose another intervention to temporarily blockade the pain generator. Options include an epidural block, a facet joint block, or a peripheral nerve block. Be aware, though, that loss of all sensation—not just pain—in that part of your body as well as other complications can result.

When all else has failed, your doctor may want you to consider surgery. Yet surgery is risky business, especially when there are no new objective neurologic findings to justify it. Besides the risks attendant with any surgery, there can be additional complications, like scar tissue, infection, or even a worsening of pain. Besides, relief is not always permanent; your pain may return six months or a year later.

Dietary Strategies

Soy foods
Recent studies in Israel and at Johns Hopkins suggest that consuming soy protein may help reduce pain.

Turmeric (Curcuma longa) *and ginger* (Zingibar officinale)

Turmeric is a spice used in Ayurvedic (Indian) and Chinese medicine, both as a seasoning and as a tea, because of its potent anti-inflammatory properties. A study with arthritis patients convincingly demonstrated its effectiveness in helping to relieve pain. And gingerroot has been found to have five known inhibitors of prostaglandin synthesis. In plain English, that means that it's capable of fighting inflammation in a fashion that is similar to aspirin and other anti-inflammatory medications.

Pineapple

Eat pineapple and drink its juice; it contains bromelain. (See page 324.)

Supplements

SAMe

There is mounting scientific evidence for SAMe's ability to relieve osteoarthritis, chronic fatigue syndrome, fibromyalgia, and other forms of chronic, long-term pain. It also has a well-documented antidepressant effect. Take 200 mg twice a day. Do not take SAMe if you take levodopa for Parkinson's disease. This nutrient may trigger manic episodes if you have bipolar disease.

Vitamin E

This nutrient speeds healing, reduces fatigue, and boosts your immune system. The acceptable daily dose range is 15 to 1,000 mg.

Multivitamin with antioxidants

A good daily multivitamin supplement can help counter the effects of free radicals, which have been implicated in the development of many forms of chronic disease. Follow the dosing on the package.

Do-It-Yourself

Alexander technique (See page 310)

Aromatherapy

Aromatherapy is beginning to be recognized as part of an integrated, multidisciplinary approach to chronic pain management. It's thought to encourage deep relaxation, so it changes your perception of pain.

In several clinical studies, lavender oil has significantly reduced pain and discomfort. In one study, patients in a critical care population had a 50 percent reduction in pain perception when they received a lavender oil massage. In another, conducted in a hospice population, researchers hypothesized that this volatile oil reduced pain by limiting the effects of external emotional stimuli on a particular part of the brain, called the amygdala. Other research shows that lavender, applied topically, relieves pain and can enhance the effects of conventional pain medications.

I suggest that you take a warm bath and add several drops of lavender oil (*Lavandula angustifolia*). Other oils that may provide relief are eucalyptus (*Eucalyptus globulus*) and mandarin (*Citrus reticulata*).

Mind/Body

Relaxation techniques and meditation (See Chapter 18)

Imagery (See Chapter 18)
Imagery has proven to be an effective way to control and ease pain.

Biofeedback (See page 341)

Music therapy
In addition to my own personal experiences with patients, there is solid research supporting the effectiveness of music therapy in reducing suffering and the physical sensation of pain. Both listening to music and making music are helpful.

Yoga
Try these postures to relax, ease pain and depression, and help you sleep: Shavasana (Corpse Pose), Vajrasana (Adamantine Posture), and Child's Pose. (See pages 344–351.)

Exercise

If you're in constant pain, you may be afraid to start exercising because you're afraid it will increase your pain. But this is a self-defeating proposition. The body releases pain-killing endorphins during aerobic exercise. And exercise fights depression. By depriving yourself of exercise, you may be making things worse. Instead, make it your goal to maintain as much normal activity as possible, including going to work and your responsibilities around the house. Start your exercise program slowly and increase gradually until you can work out for thirty to forty-five minutes, three to five times a week. Duration is more important than intensity. An ideal way to get started is swimming three times a week, which can make an enormous difference in the way you feel.

Seeking Help from Complementary Practitioners

Acupuncture
I find this treatment very useful as a complement to conventional methods for treating long-term, chronic pain. It is especially helpful for musculoskeletal conditions, fibromyalgia, chronic fatigue syndrome, arthritis, and other forms of long-term pain.

Biofeedback (See page 341)

The Alexander technique
This is a method of reeducating your body with movement patterns. The goal is to learn how to minimize tension in the muscles that support your skeleton. It's an ideal way of improving your posture and battling chronic pain. Once you've learned it, you can do it on your own.

Hypnosis
Studies suggest that hypnosis is an effective way to reduce pain. You'll need some training from a hypnotist, but your ultimate goal is to do it yourself.

Red Flags

Let your doctor know if you experience:

- An abrupt change in the severity or intensity of your pain
- Evidence of weakness in your muscles
- Increasing or worsening fatigue
- Loss of appetite
- Fever

REFLEX SYMPATHETIC DYSTROPHY (RSD) (SEE CHAPTER 8)

PERIPHERAL NEUROPATHY (SEE CHAPTER 8)

YOUR

PAIN

PRESCRIPTIONS

13
—

The Traditional Medicine Cabinet

I consider myself a practitioner of integrative medicine, which combines the best of conventional and complementary care. When we treat something as terrible as pain, we have to use all the tools in the arsenal.

I recognize that conventional treatments can be ineffective, or fraught with side effects or unintended consequences. And because pain is so complex, it doesn't fit as neatly into the "one bug, one drug" model. Despite my emphasis on complementary strategies, however, I still firmly believe that modern medicine and technology can do wonders, and that there is an important place for them in the treatment of pain.

NSAIDS

Nonsteroidal anti-inflammatory drugs, or NSAIDS, are the largest class of pain relievers.

Aspirin

Aspirin, or acetylsalicylic acid, works by inhibiting production of cyclooxygenase (COX), an enzyme in the body, which prevents formation of inflammatory chemicals, known as prostaglandins. Aspirin relieves pain *and* inflammation. However, aspirin may: harm your stomach and gastrointestinal tract; irreversibly affect platelets (blood cells that promote clotting) and cause you to bleed; cause tinnitis, or ringing in your ears and dizziness; worsen asthma and/or cause nasal polyps.

Traditional NSAIDS

There are more than thirty brands of NSAIDS available. Some you can buy over the counter, like ibuprofen (Motrin, Nuprin, or Advil), naproxen (Aleve and Naprosyn), and ketoprofen (Orudis). Prescription NSAIDS are stronger and they may have a longer duration of action. Examples include Mobic (meloxicam), Lodine XL (etodolac), Relafen (nabumetone), Daypro (oxaprozin), Voltaren (diclofenac), Anaprox (naproxen), and Toradol (ketorolac).

A popular NSAID "combo agent" is Arthrotec. It combines diclofenac sodium with misoprostol, a prostaglandin E chemical that protects your gastrointestinal tract. Avoid it if you are of childbearing age because misoprostol can cause abortion or birth defects.

All NSAIDS provide pain relief and reduce redness, swelling, and tenderness. As a result, they can improve your range of motion. Like aspirin, they also reduce fever. NSAIDS don't affect your central nervous system, or cause physical dependence or tolerance, like opioids (narcotics).

However, NSAIDS also have many side effects, including some that are quite serious. Common side effects are stomach pain, nausea, vomiting, and diarrhea. Less frequent side effects include anemia, blood or protein in the urine from kidney damage, hypertension, headache or drowsiness, liver, stomach, and gastrointestinal damage, and abnormal blood platelet function. Prolonged use may cause gastrointestinal ulcers. In some cases, NSAIDS may take weeks or months before there is noticeable improvement in your pain. NSAIDS and other non-narcotic analgesics often have a "ceiling effect." This means that when you increase the dosage above a certain point, it may not improve analgesia.

If you take other medications, or if you are pregnant or breast-feeding, check with your physician or pharmacist.

Cox-2 Inhibitors: The New NSAIDS

Now, a new and exciting generation of NSAIDS has been developed. Rather than inhibiting both Cox-1 (which plays a protective role for your stomach and gastrointestinal tract, kidneys and blood clotting functions), and Cox-2 enzymes, they selectively inhibit only Cox-2 enzymes. Their analgesic effectiveness is comparable to conventional NSAIDS. But because they do not interfere with Cox-1 enzymes, they cause a much lower incidence of ulcers. They result in less than half as many GI complications as the older NSAIDS. In addition, they are better tolerated, causing less nausea and abdominal pain. And preliminary research shows that Cox-2 inhibitors may reduce your risk of colorectal cancer.

There are only two on the market right now—celecoxib (Celebrex) and rofecoxib (Vioxx)—but others are in development. Although Vioxx has been approved by the FDA as a treatment for menstrual pain and other types of acute pain, Celebrex is also often used successfully for these purposes. Vioxx is currently indicated only for osteoarthritis, and studies are in progress to support its use in rheumatoid arthritis. Celebrex is indicated for both rheumatoid arthritis and osteoarthritis. Both of these drugs are available only by prescription.

The Cox-2 inhibitors do have some disadvantages. They may interact with certain drugs, such as beta-blockers, anti-arrhythmic medications, and tricyclic antidepressants. And unlike aspirin, they do not have antiplatelet effects, so they won't help prevent heart attack. Since its chemical structure includes a sulfa molecule, you should not take Celebrex if you are allergic to sulfa. Vioxx does not contain sulfa.

Other Non-Narcotic Pain Relievers

Acetaminophen (Tylenol) is an effective over-the-counter analgesic that relieves both acute and chronic pain. It also reduces fever. Acetaminophen does not, however, reduce inflammation, which is a major disadvantage in treating many ailments. It is the safest of all analgesics. However, large doses can cause liver damage.

Tramadol (Ultram) is used for moderate to moderately severe pain. Available by prescription only, it is approved for low back pain, osteoarthritis, peripheral neuropathy, and postoperative and orthopedic pain. Your body absorbs Tramadol rapidly, so you may feel relief within an hour. Its primary side effects are nausea, vomiting, and dizziness. It should not be used with opioid drugs or if you are pregnant.

Narcotics

Also known as "painkillers," narcotics are an extremely powerful class of drugs. Morphine is the prototype, upon which all others are based. Because of their addictive potential, narcotics are known as "controlled drugs," and are strictly regulated. They are sometimes called opiates or opioid drugs because they are synthetic drugs that behave like opium. Examples of narcotics include: propoxyphene (Darvocet), pentazocine (Talwin), hydrocodone (Lorcet), dihydrocodeine (Panlor), oxycodone (Percocet, Percodan), methadone, hydromorphone (Dilaudid), meperidine (Demerol), and morphine. Longer acting oral narcotics (Oxcontin and MS Contin) are available, as well as long-acting patches (Duragesic patch).

Narcotics are effective for severe acute or chronic pain. Unfortunately, narcotics have many potential side effects. Because they are available by prescription only, you will need to thoroughly discuss these drugs with your physician.

Antidepressants

Depression can amplify pain and limit your ability to deal with discomfort and anxiety. By relieving depression and anxiety, antidepressants can help reduce pain.

There are three major classes of antidepressants. All are prescription-only. Selective serotonin reuptake inhibitors (SSRIs) are the newest. Prozac, Paxil, and Zoloft are among the most well known. Because they have fewer side effects than older drugs — and they still have plenty — most doctors prescribe these SSRIs first.

If SSRIs are ineffective, the next course of action is often a tricyclic antidepressant. These include imipramine (Tofranil), amitriptyline (Elavil), clomipramine (Anafranil), doxepin (Sinequan), or trimipramine (Surmontil).

Phenelzine (Nardil) and other monoamine oxidase (MAO) inhibitors are usually the last choice of treatment for depression, used when other types of antidepressants have been ineffective.

Finally, there are several new antidepressants that don't fit into these three categories. They include Bupropion (Wellbutrin), Venlafaxine (Effexor), Mirtazapine (Remeron), and Trazodone (Desyrel).

MUSCLE RELAXANTS AND TRANQUILIZERS

Muscle spasms can exacerbate your pain. Adequately addressing these spasms can give you significant relief. Muscle relaxants step up to the plate by helping to curb tension and decrease spasms associated with low back and neck pain. Among the most commonly used muscle relaxants are: diazepam (Valium), cyclobenzaprine (Flexeril), methocarbamol (Robaxin), metaxalone (Skelaxin), baclofen (Lioresal), dantrolene (Dantrium), orphenadrine (Norflex), and tizidium (Zanaflex).

ANTICONVULSANT DRUGS

In addition to controlling seizures, these medications are "membrane sta-bilizing agents," which can relieve certain types of pain. Chronic pain syndromes, such as diabetic peripheral neuropathy, neuropathic pain, complex regional pain syndrome (RSD), migraines, and post-herpetic neuralgia, respond best to this treatment. The anticonvulsants most frequently prescribed for pain are: gabapentin (Neurontin), carbamazepine (Tegretol), phenytoin (Dilantin), and mexiletine (Mexitil).

HYPNOTICS

Often, when you're in pain, you get trapped in an endless cycle. You can't sleep because of your pain; then you're so exhausted that everything hurts even more. Hypnotics break this cycle by allowing you to sleep. If your pain is keeping you awake, you may want to consider zolpidem (Ambien) or zaleplon (Sonata).

NERVE AND MUSCLE BLOCKS

Traditional Nerve Blocks

When other pain therapies don't work, it's sometimes necessary to resort to more heavy-duty options. One possibility is a nerve block. Just as its name implies, this intervention blocks the transmission of pain signals through your nerves. A traditional nerve block can relieve pain for several days to weeks and, in some cases, months to years. However, you may experience numbness, tingling, muscle paralysis, or loss of feeling in the area affected by the nerve. You'll also need injections several times a year.

Other Nerve Blocks

Stellate ganglion block
We do this procedure most frequently when we suspect that a patient has Reflex Sympathetic Dystrophy (RSD) (see Chapter 8). It is both diagnostic and therapeutic. The stellate ganglion is a junction point for your sympathetic nerves, which control some of the involuntary functions of your body, such as opening and narrowing blood vessels. When we block this "circuit box," it can suppress pain and other symptoms. However, a stellate ganglion

block is a technically difficult procedure that is fraught with side effects and complications.

SI joint block

It's been estimated that in as many as one in six cases of chronic low back problems, the pain actually comes from the sacroiliac (SI) joint, but it masquerades as back pain. An SI joint block can differentiate between the two problems, and ensure an accurate diagnosis. It is therapeutic as well as diagnostic.

Sarapin blocks

Nerve blocks traditionally use conventional injection chemicals, such as lidocaine, procaine, phenol, and steroids. However, Sarapin, a botanical chemical harvested from the pitcher plant (*Sarraceniaceae*), is also listed in the *Physicians' Desk Reference* as a useful injection medium. I believe that we need more research to prove its effectiveness.

Muscle Blocks

Blocks can also be performed on muscles. These procedures are especially helpful for treating dystonias, which are painful neurological ailments that cause slow, sustained contractions of muscles that commonly cause twisting movements and abnormal posturing. They are frequently painful and can disturb your sleep.

The latest treatment for dystonias is somewhat surprising: botulism toxin, once only known as a horrifying poison. In an FDA-approved preparation called Myobloc, botulism toxin is now extolled for its therapeutic value in cervical (neck) dystonias. Botox, another botulism preparation, is also available.

Unlike nerve blocks, which interrupt pain transmission in your nerves, Myobloc works by interrupting the transmissions between your nerve and the affected muscle, so the treated muscle relaxes. We can decrease the pain, without the risk of sensory complications. And the effects are sustained. There are risks, however, including skin bruising and inadvertent paralysis of muscles.

Trigger Point and Tender Point Injection and Deactivation

The late Dr. Janet Travell, JFK's physician, along with Dr. David Simons, discovered that the hallmark clinical feature of the myofascial pain syndrome (see Chapter 12) is something she named the "trigger point." Dr.

Travell spent many years mapping out the anatomical locations for trigger points throughout the body. She published her work in a now-famous textbook. The term trigger point has long since achieved widespread acceptance. In recent years, Dr. Andrew Fisher has furthered our understanding of trigger points through his novel anatomical observations.

Trigger points are discrete, tender spots located in a muscle. When pressed, they cause a sudden triggering of pain throughout the muscle's zone of reference, which follows the trajectory of the muscle's fibers. Injecting a solution of an anesthetic called lidocaine into these trigger points helps deactivate them.

Dr. Travell also advocated using a vapocoolant ethyl chloride and florimethane spray to help stretch muscles, a technique we call "spray and stretch." The spray, produced by the Gebauer family in Cleveland, relaxes the muscle so it stretches more easily. Another technique pioneered by this impressive woman is ischemic compression, which is somewhat akin to acupressure. By pressing on the trigger point for sixty seconds, we can relieve the pain.

As part of a multidisciplinary pain program, these techniques are important strategies for treating MPS, fibromyalgia, and other painful conditions.

Spinal Interventional Procedures and Surgery

When conservative measures have failed to lessen pain in your spine, it might be time to consider a variety of spinal interventional procedures, or surgery. However, these are beyond the scope of this book.

14

—

Foods That Heal

A diet that includes certain nutrients can speed healing, prevent or slow down the development of painful ailments, and reduce pain and inflammation. Here's a brief summary of important pain-related nutrients and their food sources.

Fat

Cholesterol, saturated, monounsaturated, and polyunsaturated are the four types of dietary fats. It's important to reduce your total fat intake to 30 percent or less of your calories and to limit your saturated fat intake to 10 percent of your diet. But it is *critical* to avoid trans-fatty acids and hydrogenated or partially hydrogenated oils, which are found in margarines, mayonnaise, salad dressings, chocolate bars, and snack foods. Besides raising LDL cholesterol (so-called bad cholesterol) levels, these fats lead to the premature oxidation of cell membranes and to the development of chronic illnesses, such as arthritis, diabetes, cardiovascular disease, and degenerative nerve and muscular diseases.

On the other hand, olive oil, which is the basis of the Mediterranean diet, has been linked to lower risk for heart disease and other chronic illnesses.

Essential Fatty Acids

Omega-3 (linolenic acid) and omega-6 (linoleic acid) fatty acids, which are types of polyunsaturated fats, are called "essential fatty acids (EFAs)" because our bodies can't produce them; we have to get them from food.

EFAs are very important when we think about pain. Omega-3 fats help fight inflammation, while omega-6 fats contribute to inflammatory processes. More than the absolute amount of each of these fatty acids in your diet, what's important is the *ratio* between the two. To reduce pain and inflammation, increase your intake of omega-3s. Dietary sources are:

- Coldwater fish, such as mackerel, salmon, bluefish, flounder, herring, sardines, halibut, striped bass, sable fish (black cod), anchovies, and tuna. Strive to eat fish at least three times a week.
- Wild game, walnuts, wheat germ, and flaxseeds.
- Canola, grapeseed, walnut, hemp, and flaxseed oils. These oils are highly unstable. To prevent them from turning rancid, buy them in dark containers, if possible, and keep them in the refrigerator. Because heating these oils destroys the omega-3s, put them on salads, or add them to foods after cooking. Grapeseed oil is your best choice for frying; its omega-3s are less likely to be destroyed since it has a higher boiling point than the others.

To fight pain, it's equally important to cut back on linoleic acid, gamma-linolenic acid, and arachidonic acid, all members of the omega-6 family. Your body uses them to produce substances called prostaglandins and leukotrienes, which contribute significantly to inflammation and pain. Foods high in linoleic acid are cottonseed, corn, and other types of vegetable oils, except for canola, safflower, soybean, and olive oils. Meat is high in arachidonic acid. Duck and pork are the worst culprits, while beef and lamb contain smaller amounts.

Protein

Proteins, which build and repair body tissue, are made of amino acids. Specific amino acids, and even certain types of protein-rich foods, have an influence on pain. Tryptophan, for example, reduces sensitivity to pain. Your body uses it to produce 5-hydroxytryptophan (5-HTP), which is used in the manufacture of the neurotransmitter serotonin. The important part serotonin plays in pain and inflammation is just now unfolding. For example, people with fibromyalgia often have low serotonin levels in their blood.

Increasing your intake of tryptophan, and therefore your serotonin levels, may help reduce chronic pain. To do this, you must reduce the total amount of protein in your diet *and* focus on carbohydrates and foods that contain high levels of tryptophan, including salmon, tuna, soy flour, bulgur, garbanzo beans, meat, turkey, bananas, pineapple, yogurt, and dairy products.

Phenylalanine, another amino acid, seems to influence certain chemicals in the brain that relate to pain sensation. It has been useful in treating chronic pain conditions, such as osteoarthritis and rheumatoid arthritis. The richest food sources are seaweed, kelp, dairy products, pumpkin, sunflower seeds, poultry, fish, eggs, and collard greens.

In addition, soy may reduce pain. A groundbreaking study at Johns Hopkins University demonstrated that rats on a soy-based diet had decreased pain sensitivity. It's certainly worth a try, especially given soy's many other benefits. Soy may help prevent the development of breast, stomach, and skin tumors. It also may relieve the hot flashes of menopause and prevent osteoporosis. Besides soybeans, you can get soy milk, ice cream, and protein. Other soy products are miso, tofu, and tempeh.

Vitamins

Vitamins are organic nutrients necessary to regulate many of your body's chemical processes. Many vitamins help reduce pain and inflammation.

Vitamin A improves your body's ability to heal. It acts as a major antioxidant, and promotes cell differentiation, which helps maintain cell membranes, tissues, and the skin. This nutrient also promotes good vision and supports your immune system and healthy bones. There are two forms of vitamin A. Retinol is found in cod liver oil, liver, kidneys, eggs, and dairy. Beta-carotene is an orange pigment and a vitamin A precursor, found in plants. Good sources are yellow-orange fruits and vegetables, such as carrots, sweet potatoes, pumpkin, cantaloupe, apricots, and peaches as well as dark leafy greens, including collards, mustard, and spinach.

Vitamin C blocks the effects of inflammatory substances and is involved in wound healing. It is also a powerful antioxidant that protects cells and cell membranes from free radical damage. You use vitamin C to make collagen, which strengthens muscles, blood vessels, bones, teeth, gums, skin, tendons, ligaments, and joints. Food sources of this nutrient are rosehips, black currants, broccoli, cauliflower, oranges, green and red bell peppers, tangerines and other citrus fruits, strawberries, kale, kiwi fruit, papaya, mangoes, brussels sprouts, cabbage, potatoes, and tomatoes.

Foods high in vitamin C tend to contain **bioflavonoids,** such as rutin, hesperidin, quercitin, and genistein. They are not vitamins, but they have anti-inflammatory properties.

Vitamin E is a powerful antioxidant. It protects white and red blood cells, lipids, vitamin A, and other components of cells and their membranes from destruction. Research involving patients with rheumatoid arthritis suggests that vitamin E also reduces pain. Food sources include avocado, fresh wheat germ, and safflower oil, broccoli, leafy greens, peanuts, soybeans, whole grains, nuts, and seeds.

Vitamin B1 (Thiamin) and Vitamin B2 (Riboflavin) are both involved in your cells' energy production, and in nerve function. Food sources include low-fat dairy products, lean meat, leafy green vegetables, sea vegetables, whole grain breads and cereals, legumes, spinach, broccoli, acorn squash, watermelon, and sunflower seeds.

Vitamin B3 (Niacin) is essential for energy metabolism. It also supports normal vision, maintains healthy skin, and is key to a smoothly functioning nervous and digestive system. It's found in milk, eggs, meat, fish, legumes, poultry, spinach, avocado, and sweet potatoes.

Pantothenic acid (Vitamin B5) synthesizes neurotransmitters, steroid hormones, and hemoglobin. It's also involved in metabolizing glucose and fatty acids. Best sources are whole grains, breads, cereals, nuts, and beans.

Pyridoxine (B6) reduces muscle spasms, cramps, and skin inflammation. It also is essential for the production of serotonin. Low levels of this neurotransmitter are linked to pain and inflammation. Vitamin B6 is found in meat, fish, milk, eggs, whole grains, fresh vegetables, dried yeast, bananas, nuts, and potatoes.

Folic acid (B9) is a natural anti-inflammatory. Food sources include leafy greens, wheat germ, whole grains, nuts, eggs, bananas, oranges, legumes, and organ meats.

Vitamin B12 is involved in the breakdown of fatty and amino acids and the synthesis of new cells. It maintains the sheath that surrounds and protects nerve fibers, and it may help prevent muscle weakness and neurological conditions, such as peripheral neuropathies. Best food sources are meat, fish, shellfish, poultry, dairy products, eggs, sea vegetables, and soy products.

Biotin works with the B vitamins to reduce muscle aches and pains. It's found in nuts, fruit, beef liver, egg yolks, milk, kidneys, brewer's yeast, and cauliflower.

Vitamin D is essential for metabolizing calcium. Dietary sources include vitamin D–fortified milk, sardines, fresh mackerel, herring, salmon, and shrimp.

Minerals and Trace Elements

These inorganic chemical substances are also necessary for various body processes.

Calcium is essential for strong, dense bones. Adequate intake and absorption prevents the bone loss associated with osteoporosis. Calcium is also helpful if you have leg cramps. Food sources include low-fat dairy products, leafy greens, salmon, eggs, beans, nuts, tofu, and canned sardines.

Magnesium repairs and maintains your body cells. Good food sources are brown rice, millet, oats, soybeans, leafy greens, nuts, brewer's yeast, whole wheat flour, legumes, and milk.

Zinc is essential for wound healing, and for a healthy immune system. Zinc-rich foods include seafood, turkey, yogurt, lentils, tofu, green peas, green beans, ricotta cheese, lean meat, sunflower seeds, and garbanzo beans.

Copper can help reduce pain and inflammation. It also helps prevent free radical formation. The best source for this trace element is oysters; you can also get it from liver, shellfish, nuts, fruit, kidney, legumes, seeds, cereal, and potatoes.

Selenium works in concert with vitamin E to protect you against free radicals. Brazil nuts are the best source of selenium (one nut gives you all you need for the day); other sources are seafood, meat, and whole grains.

Cobalt promotes a healthy nervous system and maintains the sheath that surrounds your nerves, which can affect how pain is transmitted. Food sources include fresh leafy greens, meat, liver, milk, oysters, and clams.

Chromium acts as a helper to insulin. Considerable research exists on its ability to help diabetes, which is linked to many painful ailments. Food sources of chromium include legumes, soybeans, lima beans, pinto beans, miso, tofu, cooked greens, mushrooms, pumpkin seeds, red meat, and fish.

Silicon, important for bone formation in animals, is found in whole grain breads and cereals and root vegetables.

Bromelain

This enzyme is an all-purpose anti-inflammatory. Promoted extensively throughout Europe for many forms of musculoskeletal injury, arthritis, menstrual cramps, and for use after surgery, it's also listed in the German E Monographs as an agent helpful in reducing post-traumatic swelling.

I suggest taking it in its natural form, rather than in supplements. The best source is pineapple juice. Try drinking one twelve-ounce glass of juice three times daily, or make yourself the delicious Pineapple Smoothie found on page 154. Bromelain may interact with blood-thinning medications, sedatives, and antibiotics.

Fiber

Adequate fiber prevents and controls diabetes, helps lower cholesterol, prevents diverticulosis and hemorrhoids, and helps you maintain a healthy weight. The best sources are whole grains, raw vegetables and fruits, and legumes. You can also drink fresh vegetable juices (without added sugar).

15

Manual Muscle Strategies

Practitioners of manual healing methods rely primarily on their hands to gather information, diagnose, and treat you. Using physical touch, pressure, and movement, they manipulate soft tissues, realign your body, promote endorphin release, and improve circulation. In so doing, they aim to bring localized areas of your body back to optimum health, and restore your body's overall equilibrium and well-being.

Chiropractic

Spinal ailments—low back and neck pain—account for most chiropractic visits. Unfortunately, there isn't sufficient scientific data to prove the safety and effectiveness of chiropractic for *all* types of chronic pain and other ailments. I'm most likely to refer my patients to chiropractors for low back pain; that's the area where the research is strongest.

Currently, a number of major studies supported by the National Center for Complementary and Alternative Medicine of the National Institutes of Health are investigating the use of chiropractic for pain syndromes and other problems, so we should know more in the near future.

Most chiropractic visits involve adjustment or manipulation of your spine. There are (remote) risks associated with chiropractic care. For the most part, they are direct complications of spinal manipulation, such as ruptured discs, increased pain, paralysis, stroke, or other neurological problems. If you have fractures, cancer that has metastasized, or a structural anomaly of your spine, chiropractic is not a good idea.

Osteopathy

Historically, osteopaths differed from conventional doctors because of their reliance on manipulation, nutrition, and lifestyle. Today, though, osteopathy is a separate but equal branch of conventional medicine; a growing number of osteopaths gravitate toward physiatry because of its focus on conservative management of the musculoskeletal system.

Osteopathic manipulation is used primarily for low back, neck, or joint pain, headaches, sports injuries, sciatica, and other musculoskeletal ailments. It can involve anything from gentle manipulation of your joints and spine, to light pressure on your muscles or other soft tissues, to high-velocity thrusts on your joints.

Other than a bit of soreness for a day or two, osteopathic manipulation has no side effects. However, if you have bone or joint disease, including cancer, infection, or osteoporosis, manipulation is probably not a good idea. The same is true if you've had spinal fusion, or have disk problems.

Massage Therapy

Massage doesn't just feel good; it's an effective way to fight pain. When you're hurt, one of your natural defenses is to stiffen your muscles and joints. Massage relaxes tense muscles, so it relieves the pain. It also enhances mobility, improves your range of motion, and increases serotonin and endorphins, your body's natural painkillers. And by helping you relax, therapeutic massage also alleviates the psychological and emotional toll of pain.

Scientific research has shown massage therapy to be effective for back pain, cancer pain, anxiety, PMS, chronic fatigue syndrome, fibromyalgia, and headaches. In addition, massage can be helpful during pregnancy, labor, and childbirth.

Massage is not a good idea when you have a skin infection, fever, open wounds, or burns, or if performed directly over a tumor. If you have a low blood platelet count, massage may cause bruising.

Shiatsu

Shiatsu (Japanese for "finger pressure") is based on the theory that illness is caused by a disturbance in vital energy (*qi* in Chinese and *ki* in Japanese). Shiatsu practitioners use their fingers, thumbs, palms, elbows, knees, and feet to massage and apply pressure to these points to unblock *ki*. Although there is little science to explain shiatsu's effects, one theory is that it may release endorphins, or reduce levels of adrenaline and other stress hormones.

Rolfing

Rolfing is a form of deep tissue manipulation and rigorous massage, used to strengthen and realign your body. It focuses on your fascia, sheets of connective tissue that bind muscle fiber together, attach muscles and bones, shape and support your body, and cover your organs, nerves, and blood vessels, holding everything in place. Injury, emotional trauma, or poor posture can damage your fascia, throw your skeleton out of alignment, and cause pain. Rolfers attempt to stretch the distorted fascias back to normal, realigning your bones and muscles, and allowing your body to return to equilibrium.

16

―

Nature's Remedies

Although they are very different, homeopathy and herbal medicine both rely on remedies derived from natural substances. Both are highly popular methods of self-care for painful conditions.

Herbal Medicine

Herbal medicines are integral to complementary care. A growing number of scientific studies are being conducted to validate the effectiveness of specific herbs and some of the results are very encouraging. Herbs are used by a variety of practitioners; in addition, many people treat themselves. However, I strongly recommend consulting with your doctor before you try any herbal remedy. Many herbs can interact with medications and cause serious side effects. This is especially important if you are pregnant or breast-feeding, taking prescription medication, or undergoing chemotherapy or radiation therapy. And if you are going to have surgery, inform the surgeon and anesthesiologist about *all* medicines—including herbals—that you take.

Herbs aren't used only to treat disease. Many products support your body's ability to withstand disease and some of the stressors that might be precursors to illness.

Still, herbal remedies can be tricky. You can't assume that something is safe just because it's natural. Since passage of the Dietary Supplement Health and Education Act (DSHEA) in 1994, herbal products are not regulated by the Food and Drug Administration (FDA), except as dietary supplements. Therefore, they have not been tested in this country for therapeutic effectiveness or safety. As a result, herbal preparations vary widely in content, purity, and potency.

If you're thinking of giving herbal medicines a try, see your doctor first, so you don't delay receiving a proven treatment. Besides, certain ailments are best treated conventionally. For example, bacterial infections usually clear up rapidly when remedied with antibiotics. And herbal medicines are not meant as solo treatments for serious conditions.

The two most scientifically respected sources of herbal information are: *The Complete German Commission E Monographs: Therapeutic Guide to Herbal Medicines*, edited by Mark Blumenthal, and *PDR for Herbal Medicines*, edited by Georg Gruenwald et al.

Homeopathy

Many homeopathic medicines are derived from herbal extracts, but homeopathy is not a form of herbalism. By the time any substance is a homeopathic remedy, it has been diluted to such a point that it no longer has any resemblance to the plant from which it came. And some homeopathic remedies are based on animal and mineral substances.

Homeopathic medicines, which are regulated by the FDA, aim to stimulate your body's innate ability to heal itself in a safe, gentle way, without using strong medications that have toxic side effects. You can buy many of them over the counter. Those used to treat serious conditions have to be dispensed under the care of a licensed practitioner.

Solid research about the effectiveness of homeopathy is hard to find, and skepticism about its validity is rampant. You can use homeopathy as an adjunct to conventional therapy.

17

Exercise for Relief and Prevention

The healing power of exercise never ceases to amaze me. The general health benefits of exercise are well known. But every day in my practice, I see that exercise also effectively relieves pain. And, by reducing your risk of injuries, exercise can prevent pain from occurring in the first place.

Researchers have done laboratory experiments to show that exercise does indeed reduce pain. More impressive, though, are the clinical studies. A sampling of recent research from credible medical journals shows that patients with chronic pain syndromes, including low back pain, temporomandibular disorders (TMD), complex regional pain syndromes, tension-type headache, and irritable bowel syndrome, all benefited from aerobic exercise. In addition, aerobic exercise relieved the symptoms of fibromyalgia, and rheumatoid and osteoarthritis. And isometric strength training helped reduce neck and shoulder pain among women industrial workers who had work-related pain.

In addition, exercise may break a vicious cycle I often see with my patients: When you live with pain, particularly chronic pain, you're much more likely to suffer from depression. Then, when you're depressed and anxious, you are less able to tolerate pain. That's why your doctor may suggest that you take antidepressant medication for pain.

Instead of popping another pill, however, you may prevent yourself from spiraling into depression and more pain with regular exercise. Researchers have been studying the role of exercise in improving mental well-being for more than twenty years, and there is substantial evidence that exercise reduces depression. That's why exercise is sometimes called "Nature's Prozac."

It's never too late to start exercising. However, it's important to check with your physician before starting a new routine. If you have painful or debilitating ailments, your doctor can help you find a program that matches your level of fitness and physical condition.

I recommend that you develop a varied regimen that includes aerobic exercise, stretching or flexibility training, and strength or resistance training. Each of these major types of exercise provides different, worthwhile benefits. Besides, playing the "fitness field" can help prevent injuries and keep you from getting bored with your routine.

Aerobic exercise strengthens your heart and lungs, and improves your overall fitness by increasing your body's ability to use oxygen. Brisk walking, swimming, aerobic dancing, bicycling, running, dancing, jumping rope, cross-country skiing, and playing tennis are all aerobic exercise.

Stretching improves physical performance, increases the supply of blood and nutrients to your joints, reduces soreness, improves posture and balance, expands your range of motion, and decreases the risk of low back pain, torn ligaments, and muscle strain.

Strength training helps you avert injuries. Stronger muscles are less vulnerable. In addition, they better support weak joints, helping to prevent sore hips, knees, and shoulders. By stressing your muscles, you also stimulate bone growth, which can prevent osteoporosis. And resistance training is the best exercise for controlling or losing weight. Remember, if you're overweight, you're more vulnerable to injury and disease.

Specific Exercises

THE PELVIC TILT
1. Lie flat on your back, with your knees bent and your feet flat on the floor.
2. Tighten your buttock and belly muscles.
3. Push your lower back and pelvis down against the floor, as if you were trying to squash a pea.
4. Hold the position for 3 seconds (count 1-2-3).
5. Begin with 5 repetitions and, as you get stronger, slowly increase the number of reps in intervals of 5.
6. As a variation, raise both arms over your head while you are in the pelvic tilt. Be sure to keep your lower back flat.

HALF SIT-UP
1. Lie on your back, with your knees slightly bent.
2. Cross your arms on your chest.

3. Slowly lift your head and shoulders off the floor, to about 45 degrees. Be sure to keep your lower back firmly on the floor.
4. Hold for a slow count to 6 and then lower.
5. Repeat 10 times.

LEG RAISES

1. Lie on the floor with your right knee bent and the right foot flat.
2. Slowly raise your left leg until it is perpendicular. Point your toes to the ceiling.
3. As you exhale, keep your leg straight and lower it to the floor. Be sure to keep your lower back on the floor.
4. Repeat, 5 times on each side.

SEATED LOW BACK STRETCH

1. Sit in a chair with your knees apart. Your feet should reach the floor.
2. Bend forward toward the floor. Don't bend so far that it hurts, but you should feel a comfortable stretch in your lower back.
3. Hold for 15 to 20 seconds.

KNEE TO CHEST RAISE

1. Lie on your back on the floor, with both knees bent and your feet flat.
2. Grasp your right leg below the knee and pull it toward your right shoulder.
3. Hold for 5 seconds. You should feel the stretch in your lower back or buttock area.
4. Repeat this exercise 3 times with each leg.

LOWER BACK-PIRIFORMIS STRETCH

1. Lie on your back on the floor, with your legs outstretched.
2. Grasp one knee from behind and pull it toward your chest.
3. Using your hands, pull the knee toward the opposite hip.
4. As you move your knee, slowly straighten the leg, pointing your toes toward the floor.
5. Hold for 10 seconds, then relax.
6. Repeat this exercise 3 times with each leg.

SIDE STRETCHES

1. Sit or stand in a comfortable position.
2. Bend your head slowly to one side, bringing the ear close to the shoulder.
3. Relax and hold for 5 to 10 seconds.

4. Return your head to center.
5. Repeat on the other side.

CHIN TUCK
1. Sit or stand comfortably. Pinch your shoulder blades together.
2. Bring your chin in line with your right shoulder and hip.
3. Look straight ahead, not up or down.
4. Relax and hold for 5 to 20 seconds; then, return your head to center.
5. Repeat on the left side.

HAMSTRING STRETCH
1. Stand up, with the heel of your injured leg resting on a stool or chair that is about 15 inches off the ground. Your knee should be straight.
2. Bend forward from your hips until you feel a stretch in the back of your thigh. Do not twist, round your shoulders, or bring your head toward your toe. Your aim is to stretch your hamstrings, not your low back.
3. Hold 30 to 60 seconds.
4. Repeat 3 times.

PATELLAR MOBILITY EXERCISE
Do not attempt this if it's painful to move your kneecap.
1. Sit with your injured leg straight out in front of you. Keep the muscles in your thigh relaxed.
2. With your index finger and thumb, gently press your kneecap down toward your foot.
3. Hold 10 seconds and return to starting position.
4. Pull your kneecap toward your waist.
5. Hold 10 seconds and return to starting position.
6. Try to gently push your kneecap in, toward your other leg.
7. Hold 10 seconds.
8. Repeat these steps 5 times.

QUADRICEPS STRETCH
1. Stand an arm's length away from a wall, with your uninjured side facing the wall. Brace yourself on the wall with your hand.
2. With your other hand, grab the ankle of your injured leg and pull your heel toward your buttocks. Don't arch or twist.
3. Hold 30 seconds.
4. Repeat 3 times.

QUADRICEPS SET

1. Lie on a firm flat surface, with your legs straight out.
2. Tense your left extended knee and push down the kneecap.
3. Maintain this pressure for 10 seconds and then release.
4. Repeat with right leg.
5. Repeat 10 times with each leg. Do it 4 times a day.

LEG LIFTS

1. Sit comfortably in a chair.
2. Straighten your right knee (extension) and raise your leg as high as the seat of your chair.
3. Hold in this position for 10 seconds and then lower your leg.
4. Repeat with left leg.
5. Do 5 times with each leg.

STRAIGHT LEG RAISE

1. Sit on the floor with your injured leg straight out. Keep your other leg bent, with the foot flat on the floor.
2. Flex the toes of your injured leg toward you as far as you can.
3. Raise your leg 6 to 8 inches off the floor.
4. Hold 3 to 5 seconds and slowly lower your leg.
5. Do 3 sets of 10.

HEEL SLIDE

1. Sit on the floor with your legs straight out in front of you.
2. Bend your knee, slowly sliding the heel of your injured leg toward your buttocks.
3. Straighten your leg and repeat 20 times.

PRONE KNEE FLEXION

1. Lie on your stomach with a rolled-up towel under your injured thigh, just above the knee.
2. Slowly, bend your injured knee and try to touch your heel to your buttock.
3. Return your leg to the starting position.
4. Repeat 10 times.
5. As this becomes easier, you can add 3 to 5 pound weights.

WALL SQUAT

1. Stand with your back, shoulders, and head against a wall. Your feet should be one foot away from the wall, about shoulder-width apart. Try to keep your shoulders relaxed.

2. Keep your head against the wall and slowly squat. You should be almost in a sitting position, but your thighs will not be quite parallel to the floor.
3. Hold for 10 seconds.
4. Slide back up.
5. Repeat 10 times.

CALF STRETCH WITH TOWEL
1. Sit on a firm surface, with your injured leg straight out in front of you.
2. Loop a towel around the ball of your foot.
3. Pull the towel toward you.
4. Hold 30 seconds, then relax.
5. Repeat 3 times.

STANDING CALF STRETCH
1. Face the wall, with both hands at about eye level on the wall.
2. With your uninjured leg forward, put the injured leg back about 12 to 18 inches. Keep your leg straight with your heel on the floor.
3. Bend the knee of the forward leg and lean into the wall until you feel a stretch in your calf muscle.
4. Hold 30 to 60 seconds, then relax.
5. Repeat 3 times.

ACTIVE RANGE-OF-MOTION OF THE ANKLE
1. Sit or lie down with your legs straight out.
2. Bend your ankle to move the foot up and down, in and out, and in circles. Do not bend your knee. Push hard in all directions.
3. Repeat 20 times in each direction.

HEEL RAISES
1. Stand with your hands on a counter, table, or chair for balance.
2. Raise yourself up onto your toes, then slowly lower.
3. Do 2 sets of 10.

SITTING TOE RAISES
1. Sit with your feet flat on the floor.
2. Keep your heel on the floor and raise the toes off the floor.
3. Do 3 sets of 10.
4. When you can do this with ease, progress to standing toe raises (see below).

STANDING TOE RAISES
1. Stand with your feet flat on the floor.
2. Rock back onto your heels and lift your toes off the floor.
3. Hold 5 seconds.
4. Do 3 sets of 10.

WRIST RANGE-OF-MOTION
1. Bend your wrist forward and backward as far as you can.
2. Repeat 10 times.
3. Do 3 sets of 10.

FOREARM RANGE-OF-MOTION
1. With your arm at your side, bend your elbow 90 degrees.
2. Face your palm upward and hold 5 seconds.
3. Slowly turn your palm facedown and hold 5 seconds.
4. Do 3 sets of 10.

ELBOW RANGE-OF-MOTION
1. With your arm by your side, palm up, bring your hand up toward your shoulder. In other words, flex your elbow.
2. Straighten out, or extend, your elbow as far as you can.
3. Do 3 sets of 10.

WRIST STRENGTHENING EXERCISES
Start these exercises by holding a soup can or hammer handle. As you get stronger, you can increase the weight.
Wrist flexion:
1. Hold the weight with your palm up.
2. Slowly bend your wrist up.
3. Slowly lower the weight and return to the starting position.
4. Do 3 sets of 10.
Wrist extension:
1. Hold the weight with your palm facing down.
2. Gently bend your wrist up.
3. Slowly lower the weight and return to the starting position.
4. Do 3 sets of 10.
Wrist radial deviation strengthening:
1. Hold the weight with your wrist sideways and your thumb up.
2. Gently bend your wrist up with your thumb reaching toward the ceiling.

3. Slowly lower to the starting position.
4. Do not move your forearm throughout this exercise.
5. Do 3 sets of 10.

Pronation and supination strengthening:
1. Hold the weight with your elbow bent 90 degrees.
2. Slowly rotate your hand, first palm up and then palm down.
3. Do 3 sets of 10.

STAIR STRETCH
1. Stand with the ball of your injured foot on a stair.
2. Slowly lower your heel toward the step below until you feel a good stretch in the arch of your foot.
3. Hold 30 seconds, then relax.
4. Repeat 3 times.

ONE LEG BALANCE
1. Stand with both feet together. Take a couple of deep breaths, in and out.
2. Bending it at the knee, lift your uninjured leg and try to balance on the injured side.
3. Hold for 30 seconds.
4. When you can do that, try closing your eyes and balancing.
5. Repeat 3 times.

HEEL BOUNCE
1. While standing, raise and lower your heels, one at a time.
2. Keep your toes on the ground at all times.
3. Do this 20 times.

FOOT BOUNCE
1. Sit down with your feet flat.
2. Keep your heels on the ground and raise your feet, one at a time.
3. Repeat 20 times.

PLANTAR FASCIA STRETCH
1. Put your hands on a wall and lean on them, with your uninjured foot on the floor in front of you and your injured foot placed behind you so that the heel is not touching the floor.
2. Gently bounce or bob up and down.

GASTROC STRETCH

1. Stand on the edge of a step.
2. Rise up on your toes and lower yourself slowly as far as you can until you feel a stretch in your calf.
3. Hold one or two seconds.
4. Repeat 10 to 20 times.

SOLEUS STRETCH

Same as above, except with knees bent.

BICYCLE STRETCH

1. Lie on your side with your top leg straight.
2. Bend your knee up toward your nose until you feel a stretch in your hamstring (in back of your thigh).
3. With your top leg, start pedaling as if you were on a bicycle.
4. Repeat 10 to 30 times with each leg.

18

Mind-Body Therapies

Your mind and your body are inseparable. Your experience of pain, and the meaning you give to it, depends to a great extent on your emotional state. The therapies in this chapter take that all-important fact as their starting point.

Relaxation and Meditation Techniques

Tense muscles and anxiety make pain worse. With some ailments, such as headaches or low back pain, tension may even be the root of the problem. Relaxation, meditation, and imaging help you reduce pain by altering your mental state, and reducing tension. They are also particularly useful if your pain comes from cancer or another disease that makes you fearful.

Belly Breathing

I recommend that you try this simple exercise once or twice a day for ten or twenty minutes. You'll find that it reduces stress and brings you a sense of inner peace.

1. Find a comfortable position. You can lie on your back with your knees bent, or sit cross-legged with your back straight.
2. Put one hand on your belly, just below your navel, and the other on your chest. As you breathe in through your nose, your belly—and nothing else—should move. Do not push your belly out; this is a small, gentle movement.
3. As you exhale, your belly should contract. Imagine pain and stress leaving your body with each breath.

Relaxation

With Progressive Muscle Relaxation, you systematically focus on reducing muscle tension in all of your major muscle groups by first tensing and then relaxing them.

1. Set up a relaxing environment by putting on soft music, dimming the lights, lighting a candle, or doing anything else you find calming.
2. Lie on a flat surface—the floor, a couch, or a bed. Be sure to wear comfortable clothes and take your shoes off.
3. Starting at your feet and working up, gradually tighten and relax all the muscles in your body. Don't forget your neck, face, and head.
4. Lie, completely relaxed, until you are ready to get up.

Meditation

There are many forms of meditation. In addition to seated forms, there are moving types of meditation, such as tai chi, the walking meditation of Zen Buddhism, and yoga.

Whatever type of meditation you choose, your goal is to quiet the hubbub of your mind, to achieve a state of relaxed but alert awareness. This brings profound psychological and physical benefits. Research-documented effects of relaxation and meditation include reduced pain, anxiety, depression, and use of pain medications in patients with chronic diseases, as well as lower blood pressure and stress relief.

It takes a while to learn this powerful therapy. You'll probably have more success if you make it a habit and do it at the same time every day.

1. Wear comfortable clothing that is not restrictive. (No tight jeans or compressive bra.)
2. Sit somewhere quiet, warm, and well ventilated. Assume an erect sitting position that helps you relax but keeps you awake. Keep your back straight and your shoulders relaxed. Use a pillow for support, if you need it. Rest your hands in your lap or on your knees, whichever is more comfortable.
3. Close your eyes. Breathe deeply, in and out through your nose.
4. Slowly and consciously, begin to relax your body—your shoulders, arms, hands, fingers, toes, feet, legs, neck, and face.
5. Begin to focus on one word or phrase.
6. If other thoughts come into your head, take notice of them and let them go. Don't get upset if you can't stop thinking; no one can. After some practice, repeating your phrase will help keep other thoughts at bay.

7. Continue to meditate for fifteen minutes to one-half hour.

8. When you are ready to stop, take a deep breath in, exhale, gently stretch your limbs, and open your eyes.

Autogenic Training

By directing your mind to physical sensations, this technique promotes release of stress and pain. It's best done three times a day, after each meal.

Get into a relaxed state. Then, in your mind's eye, put yourself in a peaceful environment. Focus on one of the following: easy, natural breathing; warmth in your arms and legs; a sensation of heaviness throughout your body; coolness on your forehead; or the steady beat of your heart.

Imagery

With imagery, often referred to as visualization, you use the power of your imagination to help you change your physical or emotional state. You can do this with audiotapes, music, or meditation. The idea is to encourage your mind to focus on pictures that represent changes you want to occur in your body. What's key is that you come up with images that are personal and meaningful for you.

Imagery has been used successfully for pain control, especially for cancer and other chronic pain, tension and migraine headaches, and neck and back pain. It helps reduce anxiety and depression, and can relieve the side effects of surgery, radiation, and chemotherapy.

Here's a simple way to start doing imagery on your own. First, get into a relaxed, meditative state (see above). Then:

- Turn your pain into an image. For example, if you have burning pain, imagine it as a fire. Then picture yourself fighting the pain. In this example, call in the fire brigade to quench the fire with lots of cold water.
- Picture a place where you feel happy—see it, smell the air, feel the breeze, listen to the sounds around you. Then put yourself into the picture as a pain-free woman.

Biofeedback

This is a method for learning how to become aware of and control what are usually involuntary, or autonomic, body processes. Autonomic pain responses include skin temperature, muscle tension, pulse, blood pressure, and heart rate. It's probably best to start with a course of biofeedback training. However, once you master this technique, you should be able to do it on your own.

Biofeedback is often used for stress-related illnesses or for ailments related to muscle tension. A recent study found that biofeedback was a successful treatment for neuropathic, or nerve-related, pain. Here's an example of a simple "low tech" biofeedback exercise:

1. In a quiet place, stretch out and get into a relaxed state by progressively and consciously working your way through all of your muscles, from your toes to your head. If it helps you relax, you can listen to music as you do this exercise.
2. Be sure you are breathing deeply; in other words, that your belly, not your chest, is moving up and down.
3. Once you are relaxed, focus on bringing the blood to your hands. You'll know you are successful when your hands start to feel warm.

Hypnosis

Hypnosis, once dismissed as the mumbo jumbo of magic shows, can help you harness the power of your mind to reduce pain. By entering a state of deep relaxation and eliminating all distractions, you allow your subconscious mind to take over. Because you are better able to concentrate, and because your subconscious is more receptive to suggestion, you can direct your brain to meet your needs, whether it's coping with pain or reducing anxiety.

In 1995, the National Institutes of Health, in a Technology Assessment Conference Statement, endorsed the use of hypnosis as an adjunct to conventional treatment in alleviating cancer pain. In research published in 1998, approximately one-third of patients with chronic pain syndromes, including low back pain, fibromyalgia syndrome, temporomandibular disorders, complex regional pain syndromes, tension-type headaches, and irritable bowel syndrome, got some benefit from hypnosis. And hypnosis reduces anxiety and depression, which helps you sleep, increases energy, and makes pain more bearable.

Aromatherapy

Fragrances stimulate a part of your brain that affects emotion, blood pressure, heart rate, and breathing. Aromatherapy, which means "treatment using scents," is a branch of herbal medicine that uses concentrated plant oils, called essential oils, to heal. Aromatherapy can relax your mind and body, relieve pain, and restore balance, although it may take several weeks of treatment before you see results.

Music Therapy

Music therapy consists of listening to music, making music, or creating music. Chanting, an integral part of the Hasidic, Tibetan, Buddhist, Native American, and other traditions, is also associated with healing. During my acupuncture treatments, I routinely play traditional Chinese "Five Element Music."

Music can reduce anxiety and fear, which both aggravate pain, and it helps relieve fatigue and depression. In addition to these indirect effects, music decreases pain response. For example, a study of women in labor found that music diverted their attention from their pain. Similarly, music can significantly decrease hospitalized cancer patients' awareness of pain. When music is played in operating rooms, patients have fewer postsurgical complications and less pain. And there's also evidence that the use of music during postoperative care can reduce pain reactions and requests for pain medication.

Humor Therapy

Research shows that laughter has physiological effects. It may reduce pain, lower levels of stress hormones, boost immune function, trigger endorphin release, and decrease blood pressure.

We can't say conclusively that laughing speeds healing. But it can distract you from your pain. Besides, it's free, and it has no side effects!

Yoga

The goal of a yoga practice is to prevent illness by maintaining balance within your mind and body. Like many complementary therapies, there isn't a lot of solid research about yoga and pain, but studies have shown that yoga may lower the incidence and severity of migraine headaches, reduces chronic neck and shoulder pain, and helps relieve symptoms of carpal tunnel syndrome and osteoarthritis. Yoga may also help if you have lower back pain, other nerve disorders, menstrual problems, joint pain, and chronic pain.

If you're interested in yoga, mention it to your doctor, especially if you have high blood pressure, arthritis, or spinal disc injuries. Begin by taking lessons from an experienced teacher. Performing postures incorrectly can cause muscle strain or tears.

Yoga Postures

ALTERNATING LEG LIFTS

1. Lie down on your back.
2. Press the small of your back onto the floor. This activates your abdominal muscles.
3. Take a deep breath in; at the same time, slowly and smoothly raise your left leg.
4. Keep your leg steady.
5. Maintain your back flat on the floor while keeping your body relaxed. Hold the position for a few breaths.
6. Gradually, lower your leg and exhale.
7. Repeat with the right leg.
8. Repeat the exercise 10 times, alternating legs.

BOAT POSE

1. Lie on your stomach, with your arms stretched out in front of you and your forehead on the floor.
2. Breathe in and lift your arms, legs, and head.
3. Hold for 3 seconds, then breathe out and relax.
4. Repeat 1 to 3 times.

As you get stronger, try these two variations:

1. Get into Boat Pose. On an exhale, sweep your arms out sideways. Hold for 3 seconds, then return to Boat Pose. Exhale again and relax.
2. Get into Boat Pose. On an exhale, sweep your arms behind you, clasping your hands. Hold for 3 seconds, then return to Boat Pose. Exhale and relax.

BOW POSE

1. Lie on your stomach with forehead on the floor and your arms at your sides.
2. On an exhalation, bend your knees, bringing your feet up toward your buttocks.

3. Reach back with your arms and take hold of your left ankle with your left hand and your right ankle with the right hand. Flex your feet.

4. Inhale deeply. As you exhale, raise your head, chest and legs. Try to get your thighs off the floor. Your ribs and pelvis should be lifted so your belly bears the full weight of your body. Hold for a few breaths and release.

CAT POSE

1. Get onto your hands and knees, with your hands under your shoulders and your knees under your hips.

2. As you inhale, curl your toes into the floor, lift your head, and drop your belly, gently arching your back.

3. As you exhale, flatten your toes, drop your head, and round your back, pushing it up toward the ceiling.

4. Repeat this sequence 10 times.

CHAIR POSE

1. Stand upright, feet together, hands at sides. Imagine your head stretching up toward the ceiling.

2. As you exhale, bend your knees until your thighs are perpendicular to your shins.

3. Bend your torso forward, as if you were going to sit in a chair.

4. Raise your arms up over your head, keeping them apart with your palms facing.

5. Continue breathing, and hold, working up to 30 seconds.

CHILD'S POSE

1. Sit on your knees, with your buttocks resting on your feet. Your knees should be together and your feet slightly apart.

2. Inhale deeply and lift your head toward the ceiling, elongating your spine.

3. Bend at your hips, moving your torso forward until your forehead rests on the floor. Tuck your chin into your chest to lengthen your neck.

4. Place your hands alongside your torso, palms up.

5. Allow gravity to absorb the weight of your body. Relax and breathe deeply, feeling your back expand with every breath.

COBRA

Stop this pose if you experience any low back pain.

1. Lie on your belly with your forehead touching the floor. Bend your

elbows and place your hands flat on the floor, underneath your shoulders. Keep your elbows tucked into your side.

2. Press your pelvis into the floor and bring your shoulder blades together.

3. Inhale and roll your head back, slowly raising your forehead, nose, and chin. Continuing to inhale, raise your shoulders and upper back off the floor. Roll your neck back and look up. Keep your pelvis and legs pressing into the floor. Use your hands only for balance. Breathe in and out a few times.

4. If you can, on your next inhalation, use your arms to push yourself up higher, but keep your belly button on the floor.

5. On an exhalation, slowly unroll—first your belly, then your upper body, then your chin, nose, and forehead—back to the floor.

DOWNWARD-FACING DOG

1. This traditional pose is excellent for strengthening bones in your upper and lower body. Get onto all fours on the floor, with your hands directly under your shoulders and your knees directly under your hips.

2. Point your fingers forward and spread them apart.

3. Curl your toes under, and gradually straighten your legs, raising your buttocks into the air. Stop before your legs are completely straight.

4. With your knees still slightly bent, push your buttocks toward the wall in back of you. Slowly straighten your legs until your body forms a "V," and your heels approach the floor (they may not reach).

5. Let your head and neck hang loosely. Keep pressing your buttocks toward the ceiling and at the same time, bring your chest between your arms.

6. Hold the pose for 10 to 15 seconds, pressing your hands into the floor.

7. Release on an exhalation, returning to all fours.

8. As you get stronger, hold the pose longer.

GARUDASANA (EAGLE POSTURE)

1. Stand upright with your feet together.

2. Bend your left knee and wrap it around your right calf with your toes curled around your calf.

3. Wrap your left arm around the right arm in a similar fashion.

4. Join the hands together, raise them and point them outward like a beak.

5. Repeat with the opposite side.

GUPTASANA (CONCEALED POSTURE)

1. Sit on the floor, legs outstretched, with your heels and toes touching.
2. Bend your left leg in until you are sitting on your foot.
3. Using your hands to raise yourself up, bring in your right leg and sit on your right foot. So you are now sitting on your feet, in a cross-legged position.
4. Rest with your hands palms up on your knees.
5. Look straight ahead.

HEAD TO KNEE POSE

1. Sit straight with your legs straight in front of you.
2. Inhale, and bring both arms up, shoulders next to your ears. Stretch your head up toward the ceiling.
3. Exhale and lean forward from your hips. Keeping your back and legs straight, reach forward and grab your shins, ankles, or feet, depending on your flexibility. Your goal is to bring your chest as close to your knees as possible.
4. Hold for 30 seconds.
5. Inhale and bring up your head and shoulders, still holding on to your feet.
6. Exhale and go back down. Hold 30 seconds.
7. Inhale and bring your arms back up next to your ears. Slowly come up as you press your buttocks and legs into the floor. If you have back problems, just slide your hands up your legs as you come back to sitting.

KAGASANA (CROW POSTURE)

1. Squat on the ground by bending your legs and resting your rear on your heels.
2. Cup your hands over your knees, keeping your neck straight.
3. Gaze forward and hold.

KNEELING FOOT STRETCH

1. Begin on your hands and knees. Your legs and feet should be together, with the tops of your feet and your ankles on the floor.
2. Exhale and walk your hands back, placing them on your knees.
3. Sit back on your heels.
4. Using your hands if necessary, curl your toes into the floor.
5. Allow the weight of your body to settle onto your toes. Go slowly and stop if you feel any pain.
6. Hold for 1 or 2 breaths.

LOCUST POSE

If you have low back problems, consult your doctor before trying this.

1. Lie flat on your stomach on a mat or blanket on the floor.
2. Make your hands into fists and put them under your body, inside your hips and near your ovaries.
3. Keep your chin and upper body on the floor and, exhaling, raise your legs as high as you can without hurting yourself. Keep your feet together and your legs straight.
4. Breathe deeply through your nose. Hold for as long as you can, working up to 1 to 3 minutes.
5. Then, while exhaling, lower your legs, make a pillow out of your hands, rest your head and relax, breathing deeply. Allow yourself to melt into the floor.

MODIFIED BRIDGE POSE

1. Lie on your back on a mat or blanket on the floor.
2. Bend your knees and put your feet on the floor close to your buttocks, keeping them parallel and about hip width apart.
3. With your arms beside you, palms down, exhale and press your feet firmly into the floor as you slowly raise your hips and back off the floor.
4. Hold, making sure that your knees are pointing forward.
5. Meanwhile, squeeze your pelvic floor muscles tight and hold while you slowly breathe in and out 3 times.
6. When you're ready to release, slowly roll down, one vertebra at a time.

OVERHEAD ARM EXTENSION (URDHVA HASTASANA)

1. Stand straight with your feet parallel and your arms at your sides. This promotes blood flow to the hands.
2. Raise your arms out in front of you with your elbows and fingers straight and your palms facing the floor.
3. Slowly raise your arms above your head, inhaling through your nose.
4. Keep your throat and shoulders relaxed.
5. Hold 15 to 30 seconds. Continue to breathe through your nose.
6. As you exhale, slowly lower your arms to your sides.

PASCHIMOTTANASANA (POSTERIOR-STRETCH POSTURE)

Do not attempt this posture if you have backache, cervical spondylitis, or sciatica.

1. Sit on the floor with your legs together, stretched out in front of you.
2. Raise both arms above your head and take a deep breath.

3. Exhale as you bend over and reach for your ankles. If possible, try for your toes.
4. Continuing to bend forward as far as possible, try to touch your forehead to your knees.

SANKATASANA (CONTRACTED POSTURE)
1. Stand with your feet together and your arms at your sides with palms facing in.
2. Shift your weight to your right foot and twist your left leg over your right one.
3. Raise your arms, interlock your fingers, and twist your hands so that your knuckles face the front and back, rather than the sides, of your body.
4. Hold for 15 to 30 seconds.
5. Repeat with the other side.

SHAVASANA (CORPSE POSTURE)
1. Lie on your back with your legs stretched out, about a foot apart, so your hips are relaxed.
2. Put your arms at your sides, a few inches away from your body. Your palms may be up or down, whichever is more comfortable.
3. Close your eyes and relax.

SIDDHASAN (PERFECT POSTURE)
1. Sit on the floor with your legs stretched out and apart.
2. Bring the heel of your left foot in, toward your groin.
3. Bring in your right foot and wedge the toes of each foot between your thighs and calves.
4. Place your hands on your knees, palms up, and gaze straight ahead.
5. Inhale and exhale deeply and hold as long as you comfortably can.

SPINAL TWIST
1. Sit up tall in a comfortable cross-legged position, with your hands on your knees.
2. Put your left hand in back of you, fingers facing back.
3. Inhale. Then, on the exhale, slowly twist, moving your right hand to your left knee. Turn your entire body to the left, including your head. Gaze back and to the left.
4. With each inhalation, stretch up through your spine. On each exhalation, see if you can extend the twist.

5. Return to the front on an exhale.
6. Repeat on the opposite side.

STANDING FORWARD BEND

1. Stand upright; lift your arms over your head with your palms facing forward and stretch upwards.
2. Take a couple of deep breaths. On an exhalation, bend slowly forward.
3. Rest your fingertips or palms on either side of your feet and inhale. If you have lower back problems, keep your knees slightly bent.
4. Continue to breathe, sinking down a bit further on each exhalation. Hold, allowing gravity to lengthen your spine.
5. On an inhalation, press your feet into the floor and slowly roll back up.

STANDING YOGA MUDRA

1. Stand with your legs apart and your arms at your sides.
2. Inhale and raise your arms in front of you.
3. Exhale and sweep your arms around in back of you, squeezing your shoulder blades. Interlace your fingers and begin to raise your arms up as far as you can.
4. Pushing your chest forward, gradually bend forward from the hips. Push your buttocks back and continue moving down from the hips, extending your torso forward and then down, bringing your head toward the floor. At the same time, you continue to raise your arms away from your buttocks. You can bend your knees to relieve any pressure on your lower back.
5. Hold for 10 to 20 seconds.
6. Pushing your feet into the floor, slowly roll up, bringing your arms down as you do. Allow your head to come up last.
7. Unclasp your hands and slowly return your arms to your sides.

TREE POSE

1. Stand with your feet together and your arms at your sides.
2. Shift your weight to your right foot and, using your hands, place your left foot on your right ankle, calf, or thigh (whichever you can reach).
3. Find a point of focus on the floor or wall in front of you.
4. Place your palms together in front of your heart and raise them overhead, with elbows straight.
5. Balance evenly on the inner and outer edges of your right foot.
6. Slowly push your raised leg more to the side and back, opening your hip.

7. For better balance, tighten your abdominal muscles.
8. Hold for 15 to 30 seconds.
9. Repeat with the other side.

TRUNK EXTENSION (DANDASANA)

1. Sit in a chair.
2. With arms at your sides, press the palms of your hands into your seat. Do not tense your shoulders or neck.
3. Press your shoulders back and down.
4. Hold for 30 seconds.
5. Breathe through your nose.
6. Relax and repeat.

UTKATASANA (SQUATTING POSTURE)

1. Squat on the ground, balanced on your feet, with your elbows resting on your knees.
2. Intertwine your fingers and rest your chin on them.
3. Shift weight completely to your toes.
4. Hold for 30 to 45 seconds.

VAJRASANA (ADAMANTINE POSTURE)

1. Sit on your knees.
2. Keep your back straight and place your hands on your knees.
3. Look straight ahead.
4. Hold 20 to 60 seconds, then release.

VIRASANA (HERO'S POSTURE)

1. Kneel on the floor with your knees together and your feet about 18 inches apart.
2. Rest your buttocks on the floor. If you can't reach the floor, use a small pillow or rolled-up towel under your buttocks. Do not put any weight on your feet. Your feet should be on the sides of your thighs, with the inner side of each calf touching the outer side of its respective thigh.
3. Keep your toes pointing back and touching the floor.
4. Put your hands on your knees palms facing up. With each hand, form a circle with your thumb and index finger and keep your other fingers extended.
5. Hold the position, breathing deeply, as long as you can.

19

Acupuncture and Reflexology

Acupuncture

Since I completed my training in medical acupuncture, I have incorporated this indispensable art into my everyday practice, with fantastic results. I believe it is one of the safest, most effective tools in the pain relief arsenal. Its lack of side effects is another big advantage. Still, like most complementary therapies, I see it as an adjunct to medical care, not a substitute.

A variety of techniques fall under the rubric of acupuncture. What they have in common is that they all stimulate locations on the skin called acupuncture points. These points are the gateways to your meridians, through which your *qi*, or vital energy, flows. There are points connecting to every part of the body and to every organ. The continuous flow of *qi* is vital to your health. Pain is also the result of congested *qi*. By getting the *qi* moving again, acupuncture reduces swelling, relieves pain, and promotes healing.

Of all the complementary medical practices, acupuncture may just be the most thoroughly researched and well documented. When master acupuncturist Dr. Joseph Helms conducted a comprehensive, worldwide literature survey of all human clinical research studies relating to acupuncture, he found that 25 percent of all studies focused on pain-related disorders, with as many as 65 percent of them related to musculoskeletal disease. In short, acupuncture and pain is a well-studied area.

Two highly respected groups—the World Health Organization and a Consensus Panel convened by the National Institutes of Health—have endorsed the use of acupuncture, either alone or in combination with other treatments, for a variety of ailments. It's appropriate for many painful conditions, including sinusitis, neck, myofascial, and low back pain, headaches, tennis elbow, tendinitis, sciatica, osteoarthritis, postoperative dental pain, menstrual cramps, fibromyalgia, and carpal tunnel syndrome.

Using acupuncture also reduces the need for conventional painkilling drugs so it reduces the risk of their side effects, too. By combining painkillers and acupuncture we can bring complete pain relief to some patients. Acupuncture also helps people relax, reduces anxiety, and relieves spasms.

Acupressure

Acupressure, a needle-less form of treatment, is another part of the system of traditional Chinese medicine. Acupressure is also thought to release blocked vital energy, or *qi*, allowing your body to heal itself. However, because it does not involve penetration of the skin, acupressure is not as potent or precise. Still, it has one big advantage: you can do it yourself. Here is what I teach my patients to do:

Use your index finger or fingers, your thumb or your whole hand. Gently explore the specific acupressure point until you find a slight indentation. (Points on your hands and feet are under thicker skin, so you may need to probe a bit more to find them.) Press the point firmly and steadily for about 30 seconds until you feel a dull ache, or a tingling that spreads around the area. Strong pressure that causes pain is not necessary or helpful. You can use direct pressure, a circular massaging motion, or both. Maintain the pressure for another 30 to 60 seconds; you may feel the tension under your fingers relax. Then, release. The dull ache may continue for a few minutes. Meanwhile, move on to the other points you wish to massage.

If a point feels extremely sensitive, don't work on it for very long. It may take several sessions for it to release. For chronic ailments, try five minutes twice a day. For acute problems, such as migraines, you can work for a minute or two on each point; then stop. If necessary, you can go back to those points after a few minutes.

Avoid acupressure points on your legs, belly, and in the web between your thumb and first finger during pregnancy. You should also avoid working points on your legs if you have varicose veins or phlebitis.

Reflexology

Although there are similarities, reflexology is not the same as acupressure. This form of regional massage focuses on specific points only on your ears, hands, and feet. Still, the locations of reflex points and acupuncture points overlap considerably. And both techniques share the idea that applying pressure to these points will ease pain or promote healing in other areas of your body.

The jury is still out when it comes to solid scientific evidence for the effectiveness of reflexology in treating specific disorders. But because pain is so intimately interwoven with tension and anxiety, I recommend reflexology to my patients as a nonpharmaceutical, noninvasive means of reducing pain through relaxation.

Reflexology is a complementary therapy; it's not a substitute for medical treatment. If you're in pain, see your medical doctor first to be sure you don't have a condition that needs conventional treatment. And although reflexology is quite safe, discuss it with your doctor if you have a foot injury, clots, phlebitis, or other vascular problems in your legs.

The technique I prefer for applying pressure to reflex points was imparted to me by an experienced reflexology master, Beryl Crane:

- The Rotating Knuckle, Finger, Thumb Pressure Technique:
    1. Explore the area to find the indentation where the point lies.
    2. Take the pad of your thumb, finger, or knuckle and gently apply it to the reflex point. Avoid any fingernail contact with point.
    3. Maintaining constant pressure, firmly press the point. You may feel a dull ache.
    4. Simultaneously rotate around the point in a clockwise direction.
    5. Continue pressure for another 30 to 60 seconds, then release.
    6. Move on to the next point.

Other techniques you can use include:

- Rubbing or friction — Use your thumb and forefinger to pincer the point (i.e., put the thumb on one side and the forefinger on the other) and rub. If you're working the edges of your foot, use your palms.
- Kneading — This technique works well for your heels, or other thick-skinned areas. Make a fist and use your knuckles in a circular motion on the point. Or knead the area like dough.
- Walking — When you want to apply gentle pressure to a large area, such as the top of your hand or foot, put your thumb on one side of your hand or foot and two or three fingers on the other. Start at the toes or fingers and "finger-walk" along your hand or foot, ending at your ankle or wrist.

The Future of Pain Management for Women

In writing this book, I seek to validate what you probably already know—that there are pain issues unique to you, as a woman. I also hope that the book will serve as an inspiration to my esteemed colleagues in medicine to keep an open mind, to continue to recognize the importance of mind *and* body in pain management, and to recognize the diversity of human experience. Men and women are fundamentally different, and they require a customized, individualized approach to pain management.

Medical care has changed enormously over the last few decades. Scientists have made astounding leaps in comprehending the basic mechanisms of illness and pain. And treatments such as organ transplants and genetic therapy—once only possible in the realm of science fiction—are now an everyday reality.

To a great extent, though, pain is still a black box. Still, the newborn field of gender-based research has begun to bear fruit. Perhaps nowhere else in contemporary medical science are the results so likely to alleviate human suffering. If we put our hearts and minds into advancing gender medicine, the future will be bold, exciting, and rewarding. I believe that we must press forward on many fronts.

Gender is a basic human variable that we have to take into account when designing and analyzing the results of all pharmaceutical, biomedical, and health research. No longer should men be considered "the norm." We need basic research to study the fundamental anatomical, physiological, and genetic differences between men and women. We must also develop a more nuanced understanding of the neurobiology of pain. Do our pain responses vary during childhood or adolescence? When do our differences begin to manifest themselves and how do they affect aging? And how do genetic differences, hormones, and/or past experiences shape our reactions to pain?

Clinical research also requires a healthy infusion of gender awareness, even if it's expensive or complicated to do so. There are many questions to answer: Why do some illnesses disproportionately affect men or women? And why, even when they have the same disease, do men and women have different symptoms?

We must also consider gender when it comes to treatment. Already, we know that certain types of pain receptors, known as Kappa receptors, are more closely linked to analgesia in women than in men. Now we need to apply that knowledge as we develop better pain medications. As a pain researcher and doctor, I believe that failure to take advantage of gender differences to improve palliative care is tantamount to a cardinal sin.

I'm also excited by advances we are making in understanding and quantifying pain. Pain assessment has always been bedeviled by the lack of objectivity. To a great extent, pain is "in the eye of the beholder." But better means for measuring pain are slowly emerging. For example, functional MRIs and other imaging studies help us see what's actually going on in the brain when someone is in pain.

Advances in molecular biology are allowing us to study pain at the level of the gene. Pain researchers are working to define which of our genes are involved in transmitting and controlling pain messages and whether specific mutations are associated with pain conditions. We are also learning about the mechanisms of pain, both our "pain wiring" and the chemical pain mediators, such as serotonin, substance P, and nerve growth factor, that affect how we feel, transmit, and respond to pain. This work is crucially important because it will help us develop innovative therapies, such as "designer drugs," tailored to our individual needs.

Meanwhile, our conventional arsenal for pain relief is growing rapidly. The new Cox-2 inhibitor medications relieve pain without the side effects of older non-steroidal anti-inflammatory drugs (NSAIDS). We are just beginning to see that these drugs may also decrease the risk of colorectal cancer. More powerful Cox-2 drugs are in the pipeline. And we've also learned how to use other drugs, such as antidepressants and anticonvulsants, to treat severe chronic pain.

But the new, exciting paradigm of pain management that is on the horizon encompasses far more than state-of-the-art pharmaceuticals and biomedical technology. It also pays homage to the richness and bounty of ancient healing traditions and respects the profound benefits we can reap from complementary medicine.

Spearheaded by the National Center for Complementary and Alternative Medicine, we will learn how complementary therapies work. Are central and peripheral nervous system receptors activated during acupuncture and acupressure? Is magnet therapy a useful treatment or is it bogus? What role does prayer and spirituality play in pain treatment? Through basic science, we will begin to unlock the tangled relationship between mind and body. Just what happens during hypnosis and biofeedback, or when you breathe in the essential oil of, say, lavender? Perhaps we will learn to harness the power of one of the great medical mysteries—the placebo effect.

Even without understanding their mechanisms, we are amassing a substantial body of literature about when, and for what ailments, complementary therapies work. Already, growing numbers of academic medical centers and hospitals have embraced some complementary treatments. I am confident that in the near future, nutrition will also be recognized as a critical component of pain modulation. Throughout this book, I've tried to include some of the latest thinking on how vitamins, minerals, and other nutrients influence pain and inflammation.

I also believe that major pharmaceutical houses will, more and more, look toward botanicals to find treatments for pain. This will be driven not only by public demand and a burgeoning interest in going back to the basics, but because these natural compounds work. At the same time, the manufacture of herbal medicines will change from a cottage industry to a more advanced quasi-pharmaceutical enterprise. My hope is that an increasing level of scrutiny from federal authorities and improved industry standards of purity and composition will bring herbal remedies into the legitimate limelight in this country, as they are in much of Europe.

But why not get the best of both worlds? When we combine new medical technologies with complementary approaches, such as mind-body research, we can develop therapies that positively leap into the future. For example, psychologists are exploring clinical applications for virtual reality (VR), or interactive artificial worlds created by computers. This astounding treatment is already being used to treat agonizing pain, phobias, posttraumatic stress disorder, and eating disorders.

As we begin the twenty-first century, I am enormously excited and optimistic about the revolution in pain management. Ironically, though, to take full advantage of these new frontiers, we have to pay much more attention to something that goes back to the beginning of time—the difference between men and women.

REFERENCES

(A complete list of references, by chapter, can be found on Womenandpain.com)

Armitage, K. J., Schneiderman, L. J., Bass, R. A. 1979. *JAMA* 241(20), May 18: 2186–2187.

Bendelow, Gillian. 2000. *Pain and Gender*. Prentice Hall Publishers.

Bendich, A., and Deckelbaum, R. J. 2000. *Nutrition: Primary and Secondary Prevention*. Humana Press.

Berkley, Karen J. 1997. "Sex Differences in Pain." *Behavioral and Brain Sciences* 20(3): 371–380.

Berman, B. M., and Swyers, J. P. 1997. "Establishing a Research Agenda for Investigating Alternative Medical Interventions for Chronic Pain." *Primary Care* 24: 4, 743–758.

Blumenthal, M., et al. 1998. *The Complete German Commission E Monographs: Therapeutic Guide to Herbal Medicines*. Integrative Medicine Communications.

Braddom, R. L. 2000. *Physical Medicine and Rehabilitation*, 2nd ed. W. B. Saunders Company.

Calderone, Karen L. 1990. "The Influence of Gender on the Frequency of Pain and Sedative Medication Administered to Postoperative Patients." *Sex Roles* 23: 11–12.

Campbell, J. N. 2001. "Women and Treatment of Pain." *Journal of Women's Health & Gender-Based Medicine* 10, No. 4, May.

Cleeland, C. S., Gonin, R., Hatfield, A. K., Edmondson, J. H., Blum, R. H., et al. 1994. "Pain and Its Treatment in Outpatients with Metastatic Cancer." *New England Journal of Medicine* 330: 592–596.

DeLisa, J. A., Gans, B. A., and Bockenek, W. *Rehabilitation Medicine: Principles and Practice*. Lippincott, Williams & Wilkins.

Eisenberg, D. M., et al. 1998. "Trends in Alternative Medicine Use in the USA." *JAMA* 280(18), November 11: 1569–1575.

"Exploring the Biological Contributions to Human Health: Does Sex Matter?" Institute of Medicine Report, 2001.

"FDA Approval Process Still Not Catching Risks of Prescription Drugs to Women." 2001. Reuters Health, February 8.

Feine, Jocelyne S., et al. 1991. "Sex Differences in the Perception of Noxious Heat Stimuli." *Pain* 44: 255–262.

Fillingim, Roger B. *Sex, Gender, and Pain: Progress in Pain Research and Management*, Volume 17. International Association for the Study of Pain (IASP Press).

Fishbain, David A., et al. 1986. "Male and Female Chronic Pain Patients Categorized by DSM-III Psychiatric Diagnostic Criteria." *Pain* 26: 181–197.

Gear, R. W., Miaskowski, C., Gordon, N. C., et al. 1996. "Kappa-opioids Produce Significantly Greater Analgesia in Woman Than Men." *Nature Medicine* 2: 1248–1250.

———. 1999. "The Kappa-opioid Nalbuphine Produces Gender and Dose Dependent Analgesia and Antianalgesia in Patients with Postoperative Pain." *Pain* 83(2): 339–345.

Giamberardino, M. A., and Berkley, K. J. 1997. "Pain Threshold Variations." *Pain* 71: 187–197.

Gnatz, S. M., and Childers, M. 2000. "Acute Pain." In *Physical Medicine & Rehabilitation* by Grabois M., Garrison, et al. Blackwell Science, pp. 1001–1015.

Greeberger, P. 2001. "Women, Men, and Pain." *Journal of Women's Health & Gender-Based Medicine* 10, May 4.

Gruenwald, J., Brendler, T., and Jaenicke, C. 2001. *PDR for Herbal Medicines* 2001. Medical Economics Company.

Haythornthwaite, J. A., Menefee, I. A., Heinberg, I. J., and Clark, M. R. 1998. "Pain Coping Strategies Predict Perceived Control Over Pain." *Pain* 771(1): 33–39.

Helms, J. M. 1997. *Acupuncture Energetics: A Clinical Approach for Physicians*. Medical Acupuncture Publishers.

Hohmann, A. A. 1989. "Gender Bias in Psychotropic Drug Prescribing in Primary Care." *Med Care* 27(5), May: 478–490.

Komisaruk, B. R., and Whipple, B. 1995. "The Suppression of Pain by Genital Stimulation in Females." *Annals of Review of Sexual Research* 6: 151–186.

Lamberg, Lynne. 1998. "Venus Orbits Closer to Pain Than Mars, Rx for One Sex May Not Benefit the Other." [Medical News & Perspectives] *JAMA* 280(2), July 8: 120–124.

LaResche, L. 1995. "Gender Differences in Pain: Epidemiological Perspectives." *Pain Forum* 4: 228–230.

Legato, M. J. 2000. "Is There a Role for Gender Specific Medicine in Today's Health Care System?" *Journal of Gender-Specific Medicine* 3, Issue 3, April: 12–21.

Loeser, ed. *Bonica's Management of Pain*, 3rd ed. 2001. Lippincott, Williams, & Wilkins.

McDonald, D. 1994. "Gender and Ethnic Stereotyping and Narcotic Analgesic Administration." *Research in Nursing & Health* 17: 45–49.

McDonald, D., and Bridge, R. G. 1991. "Gender Stereotyping and Nursing Care." *Research in Nursing & Health* 14: 373–378.

Melzack, R., and Wall, P. D. 1965. "Pain Mechanisms: A New Theory." *Science* 150(699), November 19: 971–979.

Merkatz, R. B., Temple, R., Subel, S., Fieden, K., Kessler, D. A. 1993. "Women in Clinical Trials of New Drugs: The Working Group of Women in Trials." *New England Journal of Medicine* 329: 292–296.

Miaskowski, C. 1997. "Women and Pain." *Critical Care Nursing Clinics of North America* 9(4): 453–458.

Miaskowski, C., Levine, J. D. 1999. "Does Opioid Analgesia Show a Gender Preference for Females?" *Pain Forum* 8(1): 34–44.

Mogil, J. S., Yu, L., Basbaum, A. J. 2000. "Pain Genes?: Natural Variations and Transgenic Mutants." *Annu Rev Neurosci* 23: 777–811.

Myles, P. S., McLeod, A. D., Hunt, J. O., Fletcher, H. 2001. "Sex Differences in Speed of Emergence and Quality of Recovery after Anaesthesia: Cohort Study." *BMJ* 322(7288), March 24: 710–711.

National Institute of Health Conference/NIH Pain Research Consortium. 1998. "Gender and Pain: A Focus on How Pain Impacts Women Differently Than Men." Bethesda, Maryland, April 7–8.

"Nociceptors and Pain." 1995. *Brain Briefings*. Society for Neuroscience, Winter.

O'Young, B. J., Young, M. A., Stiens, S. A. 1995. *PM&R Secrets*, 1st ed. Hanley & Belfus Publishers.

Pardue, M. I., and Magasanik, B. 2001. "Exploring the Biological Contributions to Human Health: Does Sex Matter?" Institute of Medicine Report Preface.

Pasternak, G. W. 1993. "Pharmacological Mechanisms of Opioid Analgesics." *Clinical Neuropharmacology* 16: 1–18.

Patil, J., Guarino, A., and Staats, P. 2001. "Chronic Pain." In *PM&R Secrets*, 2nd ed., ed. O'Young, B. J., Young, M. A., Stiens, S. A. Hanley & Belfus Publishers.

Pear, Robert. 2000. "Research Neglects Women, Studies Find; Reports Say Health Trials Often Disregard Differences in the Sexes." *New York Times*, April 29.

———. 2001. "Sex Differences Called Key in Medical Studies." *New York Times*, April 25.

Peyron, J. G., Altman, R. D. 1992. "The Epidemiology of Osteoarthritis." In Moskowitz, R. W., Howell, D. S., et al., eds. *Osteoarthritis, Diagnosis and Medical/Surgical Management*, 2nd ed. W. B. Saunders, Inc., pp. 15–37.

Reisine, T., Pasternak, G. 1996. "Opioid Analgesics and Antagonists." In Hardman, J. G., Limbard, L. E., eds., Goodman and Gilman's *The Pharmacological Basis of Therapeutics*, 9th ed. McGraw-Hill, pp. 521–555.

Rubin, Rita. 2001. "Researchers Urged to Consider Gender." *USA Today*, April 25.

Ruda, M. A. 1993. "Gender and Pain." *Pain* 53: 1–2.

Sarton, E., Olofsen, E., Romberg, R., den Hartigh, J., Kest, B., Nieuwenhuijs, D., Burm, A., Teppema, L., Dahan, A. 2000. "Sex Differences in Morphine Analgesia: An Experimental Study in Healthy Volunteers." *Anesthesiology* 93(5), November: 1245–1254.

Sheiner, E. K., Sheiner, E., Shoham-Vardi, J., Mazor, M., Katz, M. 1999. "Ethnic Differences Influence Care Giver's Estimates of Pain During Labour." *Pain* 81(3), June: 299–305.

Simoni-Wastila, L. 1998. "Gender and Psychotropic Drug Use." *Med Care* 36(1), January: 88–94.

Stretcher, R. M. 1975. "Heberden's Nodes: A Clinical Description of Osteoarthritis of the Finger Joint." *Annals of Rheumatic Disease* 34: 379–387.

Turk, D. C., and Okifuzi, A. 1998. "Does Sex Make a Difference in Chronic Pain?" *Pain* 82: 127–138.

Unruh, A. M. 1996. "Gender Variations in Clinical Pain Experience." *Pain* 65: 123–167.

Walker, J. S., and Carmody, J. J. 1998. "Experimental Pain in Healthy Human Subjects: Gender Differences in Nociception and in Response to Ibuprofen." *Anesth Analg* 86(6), June: 1257–1262.

Wesselman, U. 1998. "Gender Differences in Chronic Pain Syndromes of the Reproductive Organs." National Institute of Health Gender and Pain Conference, April.

Young, M. A. 2001. "Acupuncture in Headache: A Critical Review." *The Integrative Medicine Consult*, April.

Young, M. A., and Lavin, R. 1995a. *Conservative Care and Spinal Rehabilitation*. Hanley and Belfus Publishers.

——. 1995b. *Spinal Rehabilitation: State of the Art Review*. Hanley and Belfus Publishers.

Zborowski, M. 1969. *People in Pain*. Jossey-Bass.

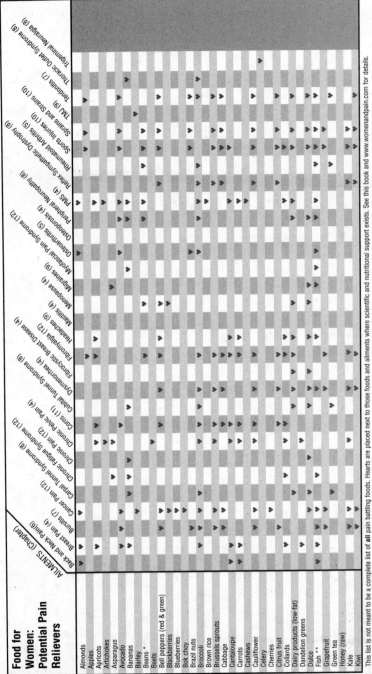

Food for Women: Potential Pain Relievers

This list is not meant to be a complete list of **all** pain battling foods. Hearts are placed next to those foods and ailments where scientific and nutritional support exists. See this book and www.womenandpain.com for details.

* Navy beans, pinto beans, garbanzo, green beans, chickpeas ** Salmon, mackerel, black cod, tuna, trout, sardines, carp, herring

Food for Women: Potential Pain Relievers (cont'd)

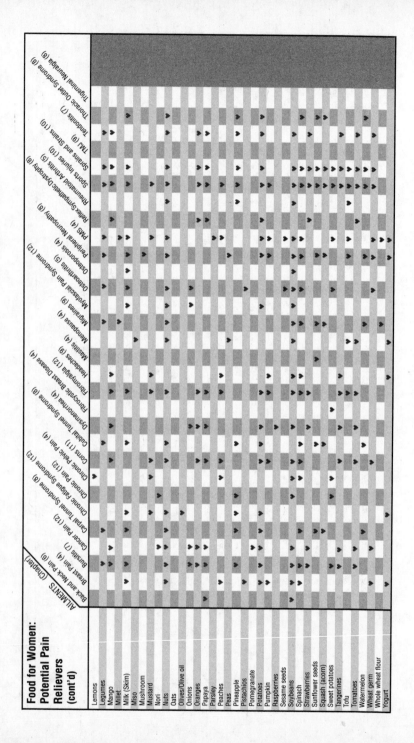

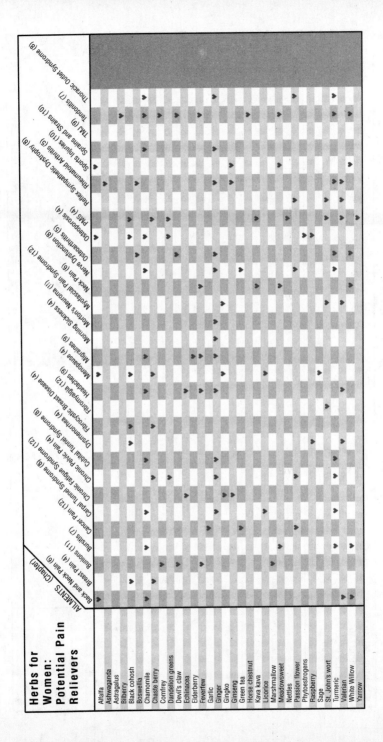

Herbs for Women: Potential Pain Relievers

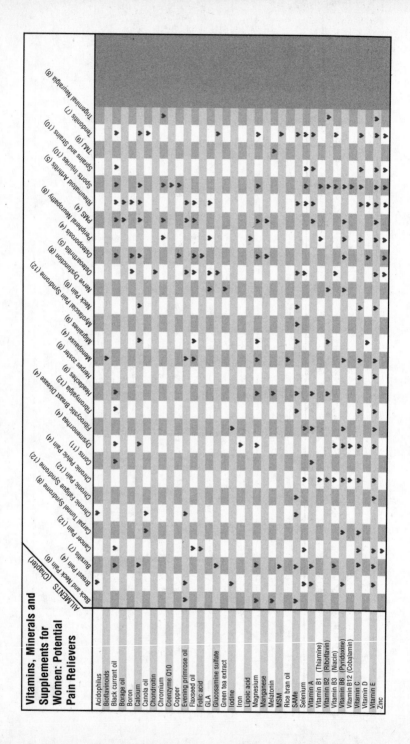

Vitamins, Minerals and Supplements for Women: Potential Pain Relievers